Acute Myocardial Infarction

Acute Myocardial Infarction

Editor: Megan Smith

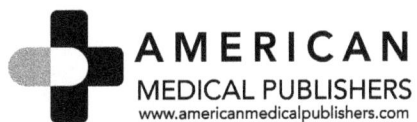

AMERICAN
MEDICAL PUBLISHERS
www.americanmedicalpublishers.com

AMERICAN
MEDICAL PUBLISHERS
www.americanmedicalpublishers.com

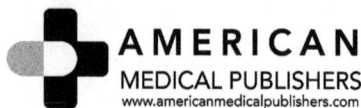

Cataloging-in-Publication Data

Acute myocardial infarction / edited by Megan Smith.
   p. cm.
Includes bibliographical references and index.
ISBN 978-1-63927-012-5
1. Myocardial infarction. 2. Coronary heart disease. 3. Infarction. 4. Heart--Diseases. I. Smith, Megan.
RC685.I6 A28 2022
616.123 7--dc23

American Medical Publishers,
41 Flatbush Avenue,
1st Floor, New York,
NY 11217, USA

ISBN 978-1-63927-012-5 (Hardback)

Contents

Preface

This book has been a concerted effort by a group of academicians, researchers and scientists, who have contributed their research works for the realization of the book. This book has materialized in the wake of emerging advancements and innovations in this field. Therefore, the need of the hour was to compile all the required researches and disseminate the knowledge to a broad spectrum of people comprising of students, researchers and specialists of the field.

Acute myocardial infarction (AMI) occurs when the blood flow to a part of the heart decreases or stops, resulting in damage to the heart muscle. This happens when an atherosclerotic plaque ruptures and blocks the coronary artery. It can also be caused due to coronary artery spasms triggered by cocaine use, emotional stress or extreme cold. The chief symptom is chest discomfort or pain. Faintness, shortness of breath, nausea, exhaustion and cold sweats are also observed. Acute myocardial infarction may cause an irregular heartbeat and result in cardiogenic shock, heart failure or cardiac arrest. Most AMIs occur due to coronary artery disease. ECGs, coronary angiography and blood tests aid in the diagnosis of AMI. Quick management of myocardial infarction is important. Aspirin, nitroglycerin or opioids may be prescribed for its management. Supplemental oxygen may be given to those experiencing shortness of breath. This book explores the emerging aspects of acute myocardial infarction in present day medicine. It provides significant information of this condition to help develop a good understanding of its diagnosis and management. This book includes contributions of experts and scientists which will provide innovative insights into this cardiac condition.

At the end of the preface, I would like to thank the authors for their brilliant chapters and the publisher for guiding us all-through the making of the book till its final stage. Also, I would like to thank my family for providing the support and encouragement throughout my academic career and research projects.

Editor

Association of body mass index with risk of acute myocardial infarction and mortality in Norwegian male and female patients with suspected stable angina pectoris

Heidi Borgeraas[1,2,3*], Jens Kristoffer Hertel[1], Gard Frodahl Tveitevåg Svingen[3], Reinhard Seifert[4], Eva Kristine Ringdal Pedersen[3], Hall Schartum-Hansen[4], Jøran Hjelmesæth[1,2†] and Ottar Nygård[3,4†]

Abstract

Background: A number of previous studies have suggested that overweight or obese patients with coronary artery disease (CAD) may have lower morbidity and mortality than their leaner counterparts. Few studies have addressed possible gender differences, and the results are conflicting. We examined the association between body mass index (BMI) and risk of acute myocardial infarction (AMI), cardiovascular (CV) death and all-cause mortality in men and women with suspected stable angina pectoris.

Method: The cohort included 4164 patients with suspected stable angina undergoing elective coronary angiography between 2000 and 2004. Events were registered until the end of 2006. Hazard ratios (HR) (95% confidence intervals) were estimated using Cox regression by comparing normal weight (18.5-24.9 kg/m^2) with overweight (25–29.9 kg/m^2) and obese (≥30 kg/m^2) patients. Underweight (<18.5 kg/m^2) patients were excluded from the study.

Results: Of 4131 patients with complete data, 72% were males and 75% were diagnosed with significant CAD. The mean (standard deviation (SD)) age in the total population was 62 (10) years. Mean (SD) BMI was 26.8 (3.9) kg/m^2, 34% was normal weight, 48% overweight and 19% obese. During follow up, a total of 337 (8.2%) experienced an AMI and 302 (7.3%) patients died, of whom 165 (4.0%) died from cardiovascular causes. We observed a significant interaction between BMI groups and gender with regards to risk of AMI (p = 0.011) and CV death (p = 0.031), but not to risk of all-cause mortality; obese men had a multivariate adjusted increased risk of AMI (HR 1.80 (1.28, 2.52)) and CV death (HR 1.60 (1.00, 2.55)) compared to normal weight men. By contrast, overweight women had a decreased risk of AMI (HR 0.56 (0.33, 0.98)) compared to normal weight women. The risk of all-cause mortality did not differ between BMI categories.

Conclusion: Compared with normal weight subjects, obese men had an increased risk of AMI and CV death, while overweight women had a decreased risk of AMI. These findings may potentially explain some of the result variation in previous studies reporting on the obesity paradox.

Keywords: Acute myocardial infarction, Body mass index, Cardiovascular disease, Obesity paradox

* Correspondence: heibor@siv.no
†Equal contributors
[1]Morbid Obesity Center, Vestfold Hospital Trust, Tønsberg, Norway
[2]Institute of Clinical Medicine, University of Oslo, Oslo, Norway
Full list of author information is available at the end of the article

Background

Cardiovascular disease (CVD) is the leading cause of death globally: the majority dying from ischemic heart disease [1]. Overweight and obesity, most commonly defined according to body mass index (BMI), has been characterized as a major modifiable risk factor for cardiovascular (CV) morbidity and mortality by the American Heart Association and the American College of Cardiology [2].

As recently reviewed, some studies of patients with coronary artery disease (CAD) suggest that being overweight or obese has beneficial effects in terms of reduced risk of CV events and/or mortality; a phenomenon known as the obesity paradox. However, there is no broad consensus regarding the obesity paradox, as several studies are unsupportive of this conclusion [3].

Moreover, despite the fact that both body fat percentage and distribution vary by gender [4], only a limited number of studies among patients with CAD or suspected CAD have examined the association between BMI and risk of coronary events and mortality in men and women separately, and the reported results are conflicting [5-9]. There is, however, a tendency towards a non-disadvantageous [5,6,9] or even a beneficial [7] effect of overweight and obesity among women, while obesity appears to increase the risk of coronary events in men [5,6].

In the present study we examined the association between BMI and risk of incident acute myocardial infarction (AMI), CV death and all-cause mortality in a large population of men and women with suspected CAD. We hypothesized that overweight and/or obesity, as compared to normal weight, was associated with an increased risk of AMI, CV death and all-cause mortality among men, but not among women.

Methods

Study design and patient population

The patients recruited for the present investigation are described in detail elsewhere [10]. In brief, 4164 patients undergoing elective coronary angiography for suspected stable angina pectoris were recruited from two university hospitals in Western Norway from January 2000 to April 2004. Of these patients, 2573 (62.0%) were enrolled in the Western Norway B Vitamin Intervention Trial (WENBIT) which studied the prognostic impact of B-vitamin supplementation upon incident CV events and mortality (clinicaltrials.gov Identifier: NCT00354081) [11]. Patients for whom there was no BMI data (n = 3) were excluded from the study, as were underweight patients (BMI < 18.5 kg/m^2) (n = 30). This left a total of 4131 subjects eligible for the analyses.

The study protocol met the mandate of the Helsinki Declaration, and was approved by the Western Norway Regional Committee for Medical and Health Research Ethics and the Norwegian Data Inspectorate. Written informed consent was obtained from all participants.

Baseline data and biochemical analyses

Height, weight and blood pressure were measured at baseline by trained study personnel. BMI was calculated by dividing weight by height squared (kg/m^2). Each patient provided information about medical history, risk factors and medications through a self-administered questionnaire, and all information was subsequently validated against medical records. Diabetes mellitus included type 1 and 2. Current smokers included those with self-reported current smoking, those who had quit smoking within <1 month and those with plasma cotinine >85 ng/mL [12]. Patients, who reported to have quit smoking > 1 month prior to inclusion and had plasma cotinine levels ≤85 ng/mL, were categorized as ex-smokers. Pulmonary disease included chronic obstructive lung disease, other chronic lung diseases and pulmonal hypertension. Cancer included active cancer with or without metastases. Family history of early coronary heart disease (CHD) encompassed those reporting to have at least one 1st degree relative suffering from CHD before the age of 55 for men and 65 for women. Left ventricular ejection fraction (LVEF) was determined by ventriculography or echocardiography. The extent of CAD at angiography was scored as 0–3 as has previously been described [11]. Baseline coronary revascularisation procedures, after baseline angiography, included percutaneous coronary intervention (PCI) and coronary artery bypass graft surgery (CABG).

Blood samples were collected by study personnel prior to angiography and stored at –80˚C until analysis. Serum apolipoprotein A-1 (ApoA1), apolipoprotein B (ApoB) and lipoprotein (a) (Lp(a)) were analysed on the Hitachi 917 system (Roche Diagnostics, GmbH, Mannheim, Germany). Serum C-reactive protein (CRP) was measured using a latex, high sensitive assay (Behring Diagnostics, Marburg, Germany). Plasma cotinine was measured by liquid chromatography/tandem mass spectrometry [13]. Low density lipoprotein (LDL) cholesterol was calculated using the Friedewald formula [14] and estimated glomerular filtration rate (eGFR) was estimated using the Chronic Kidney Disease Epidemiology Collaboration formula [15].

Follow-up and end points

The study participants were followed from angiography until they experienced one of the primary endpoints; AMI (fatal or non-fatal), death or till December 31st 2006.

Information on clinical events was collected from The Western Norway Cardiovascular Registry and from the Cause of Death Registry at Statistics Norway as previously described [11]. An event was classified as fatal if death occurred within 28 days after onset. AMI was classified according to the diagnostic criteria of the revised AMI definition published in 2000 [16], and fatal strokes were classified according to diagnostic criteria published in 2001 [17]. Procedure-related non-fatal AMI occurring within 24 h of coronary angiography, PCI or CABG were not included in the end-point. CV death included causes of death coded I00-I99 or R96, according to the International Statistical Evaluation of Disease, Tenth Revision system. An endpoints committee adjudicated all events.

Statistical analysis

Continuous variables are presented as means (standard deviation (SD)). Categorical variables are reported as counts (percentage). Non-normally distributed variables (diastolic blood pressure, serum creatinine, CRP, plasma glucose, serum triglycerides and Lp(a)) were log transformed. BMI groups were created using established BMI cut-offs; Normal weight (BMI 18.5-24.9 kg/m^2), overweight (BMI 25–29.9 kg/m^2) and obesity (BMI ≥30 kg/m^2). Underweight patients (n = 30) were eliminated due to the possibility of reverse causation. Between group differences were tested by one-way analysis of variance (ANOVA) or independent samples t-test for continuous variables, and by chi square test for categorical variables. Post hoc tests were applied for multiple comparisons where appropriate.

The relationships between baseline BMI and subsequent risk of AMI, CV death and all-cause mortality were evaluated across BMI groups. Hazard ratios (HR) and 95% confidence intervals (CI) of endpoints associated with BMI categories were estimated with Cox proportional hazard models using the BMI normal weight category as reference. The time, in days, from angiography until endpoint (AMI, CV death and all-cause mortality) or end of study (December 31st 2006) was used as time scale. Proportionality assumptions were tested by visual examination of log minus log plots and calculating Schoenfeld residuals. Covariates in the multivariate adjusted models were selected based on clinical relevance and the change-in-estimate method [18], with a limit for inclusion of 10% change in the risk ratio. The final multivariate model included gender, age (continuous), LVEF (%), current smoking (yes/no), angiotensin converting enzyme (ACE) -inhibitors (yes/no), loop diuretics (yes/no) and pulmonary disease (yes/no). Further adjustment of the multivariate Cox model did not alter the results in the total population or in gender stratified analyses; systolic and diastolic blood pressure (mmHg), diabetes mellitus (yes/no), previous AMI (yes/no), extent of significant CAD (0–3), serum creatinine levels (μmol/L), CRP (mg/L), total cholesterol (mmol/L), vitamin B6 (yes/no) or folate/B12 (yes/no) intervention status (data not shown).

Effect modifications by gender were investigated by including the product of gender and BMI categories as an interaction term in the multivariate adjusted Cox model.

All tests were 2-sided, and a p-value <0.05 was considered significant. Statistical analyses were performed with SPSS 17 (SPSS Inc, Chicago, IL) and R 2.14.2 (The R-Foundation for Statistical Computing, Vienna, Austria).

Results

Baseline characteristics

The cohort consisted of 4131 patients (72% males), and the mean (SD) age in the total population was 62 (10) years. Baseline characteristics across BMI groups are presented in Table 1. The mean (SD) BMI was 26.8 (3.9) kg/m^2, and 34% of the patients had a BMI within the normal weight range, 48% were overweight and 19% were obese.

Compared to the overweight and obese groups, the normal weight group was characterised by older age and a higher proportion of current smokers and subjects with a history of peripheral arterial disease. Mean blood pressure was lower in this group, as was the prevalence of diabetes. The extent of CAD at baseline did, however, not differ between the BMI categories. Compared to normal weight patients, overweight and obese patients were more often discharged with aspirin, statins and beta-blockers, while ACE inhibitors and loop diuretics were more often prescribed to obese patients.

The levels of eGFR, serum CRP, plasma glucose, HbA1c, Hb, serum ApoB, triglyceride and Lp(a) increased across incremental BMI groups, while serum ApoA1 and HDL cholesterol levels declined.

Baseline characteristics according to gender

Among men, 32% were normal weight, 51% overweight and 17% obese, whereas the respective proportions were 38%, 40% and 22% among women. Mean (SD) BMI was 26.8 (3.7) kg/m^2 among men and 26.8 (4.7) kg/m^2 among women.

Baseline characteristics according to gender and BMI groups are presented in Table 2. Compared to women, men were generally younger, and there was an inverse relationship between age and BMI among men. Men had worse CV risk profile and more severe CAD, at baseline, than women. Correspondingly, men, compared to women, did more often undergo revascularisation procedures following baseline angiography and were more often discharged with medication.

Follow-up and end-points

During the follow-up period (mean (SD) 4.8 (1.4) years), 337 (8.2%) patients experienced an AMI, of which 101 (30%) were fatal. A total of 302 (7.3%) patients died, of whom 165 (55%) died from cardiovascular causes.

There were statistically significant multivariate adjusted interactions between gender and BMI categories with regards to risk of incident AMI (p-int = 0.011) and

Table 1 Baseline characteristics and laboratory findings according to BMI groups[a]

	Total n = 4131	Normal weight n = 1395	Overweight n = 1970	Obese n = 766	p-value[b]
Demographic characteristics					
Male sex, n (%)	2989 (72.4)	959 (68.7)	1517 (77.0)	513 (67.0)	<0.001
Age (years)[c]	62 (10)	63 (11)	61 (10)	60 (10)	<0.001
Clinical parameters					
Systolic blood pressure (mmHg)	141 (20.7)	139 (21.0)	142 (20.6)	143 (20.3)	<0.001
Diastolic blood pressure (mmHg)	81.3 (10.4)	79.3 (10.3)	82.0 (10.1)	83.3 (10.7)	<0.001
Left ventricular ejection fraction (%)	64.0 (11.3)	63.7 (11.9)	64.4 (10.7)	63.6 (11.8)	0.08
Cardiovascular risk factors, n (%)					
Diabetes[d]	496 (12.0)	123 (8.8)	209 (10.6)	164 (21.4)	<0.001
Current smoker[e]	1061 (25.7)	417 (29.9)	469 (23.9)	175 (22.9)	<0.001
Ex smoker[f]	1933 (46.9)	571 (40.6)	975 (49.6)	387 (50.7)	<0.001
Family history of coronary heart disease[g]	1253 (31.1)	417 (30.8)	573 (29.7)	263 (35.1)	0.02
Cardiovascular history, n (%)					
Previous acute myocardial infarction	1670 (40.4)	564 (40.4)	784 (39.8)	322 (42.0)	0.56
Previous cerebrovascular disease	286 (6.9)	100 (7.2)	128 (6.5)	58 (7.6)	0.55
Previous peripheral vascular arterial disease	371 (9.0)	153 (11.0)	148 (7.5)	70 (9.1)	<0.01
Previous percutaneous coronary intervention	794 (19.2)	250 (17.9)	396 (20.1)	148 (19.3)	0.29
Previous coronary artery bypass graft surgery	477 (11.5)	150 (10.8)	238 (12.1)	89 (11.6)	0.49
Extent of coronary artery disease at baseline as assessed by coronary angiography, n (%)					
No significant coronary artery disease	1030 (24.9)	367 (26.3)	467 (23.7)	196 (25.6)	0.21
1-vessel disease	958 (23.2)	306 (21.9)	482 (24.5)	170 (22.2)	0.18
2-vessel disease	923 (22.3)	308 (22.1)	440 (22.3)	175 (22.8)	0.92
3-vesseldisease	1220 (29.5)	414 (29.7)	581 (29.5)	225 (29.4)	0.99
Comorbidity at baseline, n (%)					
Pulmonary disease	367 (8.9)	139 (10.0)	140 (7.1)	88 (11.5)	<0.001
Cancer	4 (0.1)	2 (0.1)	1 (0.1)	1 (0.1)	0.66
Medication following baseline coronary angiography, n (%)					
Acetylsalisylic acid	3376 (81.7)	1114 (79.9)	1638 (83.1)	624 (81.5)	0.05
Statins	3310 (80.1)	1064 (76.3)	1626 (82.5)	620 (80.9)	<0.001
β-blockers	2994 (72.5)	970 (69.5)	1456 (73.9)	568 (74.2)	0.01
ACE inhibitors	858 (20.8)	243 (17.4)	403 (20.5)	212 (27.7)	<0.001
Loop diuretics	447 (10.8)	127 (9.1)	182 (9.2)	138 (18.0)	<0.001
Coronary revascularization following baseline coronary angiography, n (%)					
Percutaneous coronary intervention	1348 (32.6)	432 (31.0)	663 (33.7)	253 (33.0)	0.26
Coronary artery bypass graft surgery	892 (21.6)	302 (21.6)	438 (22.2)	152 (19.8)	0.39
Biochemical markers					
Creatinine (μmol/L)	92.6 (31.1)	92.5 (33.4)	93.0 (32.0)	91.8 (23.4)	0.34
eGFR (mL/min)	87.8 (17.3)	86.2 (17.7)	88.5 (16.6)	88.9 (17.8)	<0.001
CRP (mg/L)	3.69 (7.17)	3.34 (7.93)	3.59 (6.67)	4.60 (6.85)	<0.001
Glucose (mmol/L)	6.35 (2.40)	5.93 (2.24)	6.32 (2.28)	7.20 (2.79)	<0.001
HbA1c (mmol/L)	6.22 (1.38)	6.12 (1.28)	6.18 (1.41)	6.51 (1.45)	<0.001
Hemoglobin (g/dL)	14.2 (1.24)	13.9 (1.24)	14.4 (1.18)	14.4 (1.29)	<0.001
ApoA1 (g/L)	1.32 (0.27)	1.37 (0.29)	1.30 (0.25)	1.27 (0.26)	<0.001
ApoB (g/L)	0.90 (0.25)	0.87 (0.24)	0.91 (0.24)	0.93 (0.26)	<0.001

Table 1 Baseline characteristics and laboratory findings according to BMI groups[a] *(Continued)*

Total cholesterol (mmol/L)	5.07 (1.17)	5.02 (1.14)	5.08 (1.18)	5.10 (1.19)	0.13
LDL cholesterol (mmol/L)	3.09 (1.03)	3.05 (1.02)	3.12 (1.00)	3.11 (1.10)	0.11
HDL cholesterol (mmol/L)	1.29 (0.38)	1.42 (0.43)	1.25 (0.34)	1.17 (0.32)	<0.001
Triglycerides (mmol/L)	1.78 (1.22)	1.43 (0.90)	1.86 (1.28)	2.22 (1.39)	<0.001
Lp(a) (mmol/L)	0.42 (0.39)	0.41 (0.39)	0.43 (0.39)	0.42 (0.39)	0.03
WENBIT intervention trial, n (%)	2560 (62.0)	797 (57.1)	1283 (65.1)	480 (62.7)	<0.001
B6, n (% of WENBIT participants)	1275 (49.8)	394 (49.4)	657 (51.2)	224 (46.7)	<0.01
Folate/B12, n (% of WENBIT participants)	1282 (50.1)	409 (51.3)	649 (50.6)	224 (46.7)	0.04

ACE, angiotensin converting enzyme; ApoA1, apolipoprotein A1; ApoB, apolipoprotein B; BMI, body mass index; CRP, c-reactive protein; eGFR, esitimated glomerular filtration rate; HDL, high density lipoprotein; LDL, low density lipoprotein; Lp(a), lipoprotein (a).
[a]Normal weight (BMI 18.5-24.9 kg/m^2), overweight (BMI 25–29.9 kg/m^2) and obese (BMI $\geq$ 30 kg/m^2).
[b]Based on between group differences calculated by one-way analysis of variance (ANOVA) for continuous variables and Chi squared test for categorical variables.
[c]Mean (SD).
[d]Includes DM type 1 and 2.
[e]Smokers included self-reported current smoking, those who quit smoking within <1 month and patients with plasma cotinine >85 ng/mL.
[f]Patients reported to have quit smoking > 1 month prior to inclusion.
[g]Included those reporting to have at least one 1st degree relative suffering from CAD before the age of 55 for men and 65 for women.

CV-death (p-int = 0.031), but not to all-cause mortality (p-int = 0.427).

A total of 115 (8.2%) normal weight patients, 127 (6.4%) overweight patients and 60 (7.8%) obese patients died. The risk of all-cause mortality did not differ significantly between BMI categories in any analyses; compared to the normal weight group, the multivariate adjusted HR (95% CI) was 0.95 (0.74, 1.23) in the overweight group and 1.16 (0.84, 1.60) in the obese group.

Analyses were repeated in subgroups of patients with significant CAD or without diabetes only, and the results were not significantly different from those reported (data not shown).

Gender stratified analyses
A total of 267 (8.9%) men and 70 (6.1%) women suffered an AMI. Further, 241 (8.1%) men and 61 (5.3%) women died, whereof 132 (55%) male deaths and 33 (54%) female deaths were characterised as CV deaths.

Obese men had a significantly higher multivariate adjusted risk of both incident AMI; HR 1.80 (1.28, 2.52), and CV death; HR 1.60 (1.00, 2.55), compared to normal weight men (Table 3).

Overweight women had a significantly lower multivariate adjusted risk of AMI; HR 0.56 (0.33, 0.98), compared to normal weight women (Table 4). By contrast, the multivariate adjusted HR for AMI between normal weight women and obese women did not differ significantly.

Discussion
Principal findings
In this large longitudinal prospective cohort study of more than 4000 patients with suspected stable angina pectoris, we demonstrate that obese male patients had a 1.8 fold and 1.6 fold increased risk of incident AMI and CV death compared to normal weight men. By contrast,

compared to normal weight women, obese women had similar risk of AMI and CV death, while overweight women had nearly half the risk of incident AMI. The risk of all-cause mortality associated with BMI was similar among men and women, and did not differ significantly across BMI categories.

BMI and risk of AMI, CV death and all-cause mortality in men and women
Strong associations between overweight/obesity and risk of CVD and death have been demonstrated in the general population [19,20]. By contrast, several studies of patients with CAD have demonstrated that overweight and/or obese patients may have a better morbidity and mortality prognosis than their leaner counterparts; although as one recent review points out, this observation is not supported by all [3].

Only a few studies of patients with CAD have examined the association between BMI and risk of CV events and mortality in men and women separately. Our finding of an increased risk of cardiovascular events among obese men are in accordance with the results from a previous US study of patients with stable CVD, whereof 85% had CHD, as well as with a multi-ethnic sample study of patients with established CAD [5,6]. However, while these studies did not observe any significant associations between BMI and risk of major adverse coronary events in women, we report a nearly halved adjusted risk of AMI among overweight women as compared to their normal weight counterparts.

In the present study, there was no interaction between BMI and gender with regards to all-cause mortality. Moreover, the risk of death did not differ between BMI groups. These findings are in accordance with a previous study conducted among European patients with CAD [21]. To the best of our knowledge only two studies,

Table 2 Baseline characteristics and laboratory findings according to gender and BMI groups[a]

	Men					Women					
	Total	Normal weight	Overweight	Obese	p-value[b]	Total	Normal weight	Overweight	Obese	p-value[c]	p-value[d]
	n = 2989	n = 959	n = 1517	n = 513		n = 1142	n = 436	n = 453	n = 253		
Demographic characteristics											
Age (years)[e]	61 (10)	63 (11)	61 (10)	59 (10)	<0.001	63 (10)	63 (19)	64 (11)	63 (10)	0.52	<0.001
Clinical parameters											
Systolic blood pressure (mmHg)	141 (20.4)	140 (20.5)	141 (20.3)	143 (20.4)	0.03	141 (21.6)	138 (22.1)	143 (21.6)	144 (20.2)	<0.01	0.94
Diastolic blood pressure (mmHg)	81.8 (10.4)	79.6 (10.1)	82.2 (10.0)	84.3 (11.1)	<0.001	80.0 (10.3)	78.4 (10.8)	80.9 (10.1)	81.0 (9.60)	<0.001	<0.001
Left ventricular ejection fraction (%)	63.1 (11.8)	62.6 (12.4)	63.7 (11.1)	62.1 (12.4)	<0.01	66.5 (9.81)	65.9 (10.3)	66.9 (9.21)	66.8 (9.93)	0.30	<0.001
Cardiovascular risk factors, n (%)											
Diabetes[f]	361 (12.1)	97 (10.1)	158 (10.4)	106 (20.7)	<0.001	135 (11.8)	26 (6.0)	51 (11.3)	58 (22.9)	<0.001	0.82
Current smoker[g]	803 (26.9)	305 (31.8)	375 (24.8)	123 (24.0)	<0.001	258 (22.7)	112 (25.7)	94 (20.8)	52 (22.7)	0.16	<0.01
Ex smoker[h]	1595 (53.4)	448 (46.7)	842 (55.6)	305 (59.6)	<0.001	338 (29.7)	123 (28.2)	133 (29.5)	82 (32.7)	0.47	<0.001
Family history of coronary heart disease[i]	844 (29.0)	258 (27.8)	417 (28.1)	169 (33.9)	0.03	409 (36.4)	159 (37.3)	156 (34.9)	94 (37.6)	0.69	<0.001
Cardiovascular history, n (%)											
Previous acute myocardial infarction	1346 (45.9)	429 (44.7)	668 (44.0)	249 (48.5)	0.20	324 (28.4)	135 (31.0)	116 (25.6)	73 (28.9)	0.21	<0.001
Previous cerebrovascular disease	203 (6.9)	69 (7.2)	101 (6.7)	33 (6.4)	0.82	83 (7.3)	31 (7.1)	27 (6.0)	25 (9.9)	0.16	0.59
Previous peripheral vascular arterial disease	276 (9.2)	114 (11.9)	115 (7.6)	47 (9.2)	<0.01	95 (8.3)	39 (8.9)	33 (7.3)	23 (9.1)	0.59	0.36
Previous percutaneous coronary intervention	641 (21.4)	193 (20.1)	340 (22.4)	108 (21.1)	0.39	153 (13.4)	57 (13.1)	56 (12.4)	40 (15.8)	0.42	<0.001
Previous coronary artery bypass graft surgery	394 (13.2)	116 (12.1)	205 (13.5)	73 (14.2)	0.44	83 (7.3)	34 (7.8)	33 (7.3)	16 (6.3)	0.77	<0.01
Extent of coronary artery disease at baseline as assessed by coronary angiography, n (%)											
No significant coronary artery disease	538 (18.0)	179 (17.7)	280 (18.5)	88 (17.2)	0.77	492 (43.1)	197 (45.2)	187 (41.3)	108 (42.7)	0.21	<0.001
1-vessel disease	704 (23.6)	218 (22.7)	373 (24.6)	113 (22.0)	0.38	254 (22.2)	88 (20.2)	109 (24.1)	57 (22.5)	0.16	0.37
2-vessel disease	731 (24.5)	236 (24.6)	360 (23.7)	135 (26.3)	0.50	192 (16.8)	72 (16.5)	80 (17.7)	40 (15.8)	0.59	<0.001
3-vessel disease	1016 (34.0)	335 (34.9)	504 (33.2)	177 (34.5)	0.66	204 (17.9)	79 (18.1)	77 (17.0)	48 (19.0)	0.42	<0.001
Comorbidity at baseline, n (%)											
Pulmonary disease	276 (9.2)	96 (10.0)	115 (7.6)	65 (12.7)	0.04	91 (8.0)	43 (9.9)	25 (5.5)	23 (9.1)	0.50	0.20
Cancer	4 (0.1)	2 (0.20)	1 (0.10)	1 (0.20)	0.59	0 (0.0)	0	0	0	-	0.22
Medication following baseline coronary angiography, n (%)											
Acetylsalisylic acid	2546 (85.2)	810 (84.5)	1306 (86.1)	430 (83.8)	0.13	830 (72.7)	304 (69.7)	332 (73.3)	194 (76.7)	0.34	<0.001
Statins	2492 (83.4)	759 (79.1)	1296 (85.4)	437 (85.2)	<0.001	818 (71.6)	305 (70.0)	330 (72.8)	183 (72.3)	0.61	<0.001
β-blockers	2229 (74.6)	684 (71.3)	1155 (76.1)	390 (76.0)	0.02	765 (67.0)	286 (65.6)	301 (66.4)	178 (70.4)	0.42	<0.001
ACE inhibitors	644 (21.5)	171 (17.8)	320 (21.1)	153 (29.8)	<0.001	214 (18.7)	72 (16.2)	83 (18.3)	59 (23.3)	0.08	0.05
Loop diuretics	297 (9.9)	90 (9.4)	128 (8.4)	79 (15.4)	<0.001	150 (13.1)	37 (8.5)	54 (11.9)	59 (23.3)	<0.001	<0.01

Table 2 Baseline characteristics and laboratory findings according to gender and BMI groups[a] (Continued)

Coronary revascularization following baseline coronary angiography, n (%)

	Men All	Men Normal weight	Men Overweight	Men Obese	p[b]	Women All	Women Normal weight	Women Overweight	Women Obese	p[c]	p[d]
Percutaneous coronary intervention	1065 (35.6)	545 (35.9)	327 (34.1)	193 (37.6)	0.38	283 (24.8)	105 (24.1)	118 (26.0)	60 (23.7)	0.72	<0.001
Coronary artery bypass graft surgery	731 (24.5)	363 (23.9)	248 (25.9)	120 (23.4)	0.46	161 (14.1)	54 (12.4)	75 (16.6)	32 (12.6)	0.15	<0.001
Biochemical markers											
Creatinine (μmol/L)	96.4 (31.7)	96.6 (30.5)	95.9 (23.3)		0.93	82.8 (26.5)	83.9 (36.7)	81.4 (14.5)	83.4 (21.5)	0.35	<0.001
eGFR (mL/min)	89.3 (17.0)	87.5 (16.6)	91.2 (16.9)		<0.001	84.1 (17.3)	83.4 (17.6)	84.6 (16.1)	84.2 (18.7)	0.58	<0.001
CRP (mg/L)	3.66 (7.59)	3.55 (8.91)	4.07 (6.49)		0.39	3.79 (5.93)	2.88 (5.17)	3.62 (5.43)	5.66 (7.42)	<0.001	0.59
Glucose (mmol/L)	6.41 (2.38)	6.08 (2.42)	7.26 (2.77)		<0.001	6.20 (2.46)	5.60 (1.75)	6.30 (2.68)	7.06 (2.82)	<0.001	0.01
HbA1c (mmol/L)	6.17 (1.39)	6.16 (1.11)	6.62 (1.49)		<0.001	6.36 (1.38)	6.10 (1.36)	6.11 (1.37)	6.46 (1.43)	<0.001	<0.001
Hemoglobin (g/dL)	14.6 (1.16)	14.2 (1.21)	14.8 (1.16)		<0.001	13.4 (1.05)	13.3 (1.04)	13.5 (1.04)	13.5 (1.05)	<0.01	<0.001
ApoA1 (g/L)	1.26 (0.25)	1.31 (0.27)	1.20 (0.23)		<0.001	1.46 (0.27)	1.49 (0.28)	1.45 (0.26)	1.42 (0.27)	<0.01	<0.001
ApoB (g/L)	0.90 (0.25)	0.86 (0.24)	0.93 (0.27)		<0.001	0.92 (0.25)	0.88 (0.24)	0.94 (0.26)	0.94 (0.25)	<0.01	<0.01
Total cholesterol (mmol/L)	4.98 (1.17)	5.18 (1.12)	5.25 (1.16)		0.30	5.28 (1.14)	5.18 (1.12)	5.39 (1.14)	5.25 (1.16)	0.02	<0.001
LDL cholesterol (mmol/L)	3.05 (1.02)	3.03 (1.01)	3.07 (1.13)		0.64	3.19 (1.03)	3.08 (1.02)	3.30 (1.03)	3.18 (1.04)	<0.01	<0.001
HDL cholesterol (mmol/L)	1.22 (0.33)	1.33 (0.38)	1.09 (0.26)		<0.001	1.47 (0.42)	1.57 (0.44)	1.45 (0.39)	1.34 (0.37)	<0.001	<0.001
Triglycerides (mmol/L)	1.85 (1.28)	1.48 (0.97)	2.32 (1.52)		<0.001	1.62 (1.03)	1.34 (0.72)	1.67 (1.18)	2.00 (1.07)	<0.001	<0.001
Lp(a) (mmol/L)	0.41 (0.37)	0.43 (0.41)	0.47 (0.40)		0.79	0.46 (0.42)	0.43 (0.41)	0.48 (0.45)	0.47 (0.40)	0.11	<0.01
WENBIT intervention trial, n (%)	2047 (68.5)	1072 (70.7)	614 (64.0)	361 (70.4)	<0.01	513 (44.9)	183 (42.0)	211 (46.6)	119 (47.0)	0.29	<0.001
B6, n (% of WENBIT participants)	1043 (34.9)	553 (51.9)	320 (52.1)	170 (47.1)	0.19	239 (20.9)	89 (48.6)	96 (45.5)	54 (45.4)	0.94	<0.001
Folate/B12, n (% of WENBIT participants)	1031 (34.5)	555 (51.8)	301 (49.0)	175 (48.5)	0.03	244 (21.4)	93 (50.8)	102 (48.3)	49 (41.2)	0.92	<0.001

ACE, angiotensin converting enzyme; ApoA1, apolipoprotein A1; ApoB, apolipoprotein B; BMI, body mass index; CRP, c-reactive protein; eGFR, esitimated glomerular filtration rate; HDL, high density lipoprotein; LDL, low density lipoprotein; Lp(a), lipoprotein (a).

[a]Normal weight (BMI 18.5-24.9 kg/m^2), overweight (BMI 25-29.9 kg/m^2), and obese (BMI $\geq$ 30 kg/m^2).

[b]Based on differences between BMI groups among men, and was calculated by ANCVA for continuous variables and Chi squared test for categorical variables for differences between men and women.

[c]Based on differences between BMI groups among women, and was calculated by ANOVA for continuous variables and Chi squared test for categorical variables for differences between men and women.

[d]Based on between group differences in men vs. women, and was calculated by independent samples t-test for continuous variables and Chi squared test for categorical variables.

[e]Mean (SD).

[f]Includes DM type 1 and 2.

[g]Smokers included self-reported current smoking, those who quit smoking within <1 month and patients with plasma cotinine >85 ng/mL.

[h]Patients reported to have quit smoking > 1 month prior to inclusion.

[i]Included those reporting to have at least one 1st degree relative suffering from CAD before the age of 55 for men and 65 for women.

Table 3 BMI groups[a] and risk of acute myocardial infarction and cardiovascular death in men

Model	Acute myocardial infarction				Cardiovascular death			
	Events, n (%)	HR	95% CI	p-value	Events, n (%)	HR	95% CI	p-value
Univariate								
Normal weight	84 (8.8)	1.00			51 (5.3)	1.00		
Overweight	117 (7.7)	0.88	0.66, 1.16	0.37	49 (3.2)	0.61	0.41, 0.90	0.01
Obese	66 (12.9)	1.51	1.09, 2.08	0.01	32 (6.2)	1.19	0.76, 1.85	0.45
Multivariate adjusted[b]								
Normal weight		1.00				1.00		
Overweight		1.11	0.84, 1.48	0.47		0.85	0.57, 1.28	0.44
Obese		1.80	1.28, 2.52	<0.01		1.60	1.00, 2.55	0.05

BMI, body mass index; CI, confidence interval; HR, hazard ratio.
[a]Normal weight (BMI 18.5-24.9 kg/m^2), overweight (BMI 25–29.9 kg/m^2) and obese (BMI ≥ 30 kg/m^2).
[b]Age (continuous), current smoking (yes/no), left ventricular ejection fraction (%), pulmonary disease (yes/no), angiotensin converting enzyme-inhibitors (yes/no) and loop diuretics (yes/no).

of patients with CAD, have examined the association between BMI and all-cause mortality in men and women separately [7,8]. First, a study of Danish patients with AMI showed that normal weight, overweight and obese men had similar risk of death, whereas overweight women had a slightly decreased risk (HR (95% CI); 0.78 (0.68, 0.90)) of death, as compared to their normal weight counterparts. Furthermore, in a follow up study of the CADILLAC trial, they observed significantly lower in-hospital mortality (0.9% vs. 2.7%), 30 days (1.1% vs. 3.8%) and 1- year (1.8% vs. 7.5%) mortality in obese patients with AMI undergoing PCI when compared to normal weight patients. Statistical significance was, however, only reached in males.

Possible explanations

BMI is often used to quantify overweight and obesity owing to a high fat percentage correlation, but does not account for fat distribution. Men have a tendency to store excessive fat in visceral fat deposits, whereas women usually store fat in peripheral subcutaneous distributions [4]. Excessive visceral fat is associated with an increased risk of developing metabolic syndrome, putting men at a greater risk of developing CVD, while subcutaneous fat in the femoral-gluteal region may be associated with a more favourable CV risk profile [22]. Furthermore, overweight and obese postmenopausal women may benefit from the increase in circulating levels of estrogen produced by the adipose tissue [23,24].

Moreover, at baseline, men were more often affected by CV risk factors and had more severe CAD. Inclusion of these potential confounding variables in stratified multivariate analyses did not alter our results. Differing health status at baseline is thus unlikely to be the cause of the observed gender interaction.

Strengths and limitations of the study

The main strength of the present study is its, well defined population with complete follow up of clinical endpoints.

Table 4 BMI groups[a] and risk of acute myocardial infarction and cardiovascular death in women

Model	Acute myocardial infarction				Cardiovascular death			
	Events, n (%)	HR	95% CI	p-value	Events, n (%)	HR	95% CI	p-value
Univariate								
Normal weight	33 (7.6)	1.00			16 (3.7)	1.00		
Overweight	21 (4.6)	0.61	0.35, 1.05	0.08	13 (2.9)	0.78	0.38, 1.63	0.51
Obese	16 (6.3)	0.84	0.46, 1.53	0.57	4 (1.6)	0.43	0.14, 1.28	0.13
Multivariate adjusted[b]								
Normal weight		1.00				1.00		
Overweight		0.56	0.33, 0.98	0.04		0.71	0.34, 1.50	0.37
Obese		0.80	0.43, 1.47	0.46		0.38	0.21, 1.16	0.09

BMI, body mass index; CI, confidence interval; HR, hazard ratio.
[a] Normal weight (BMI 18.5-24.9 kg/m^2), overweight (BMI 25–29.9 kg/m^2) and obese (BMI ≥ 30 kg/m^2).
[b] Age (continuous), current smoking (yes/no), left ventricular ejection fraction (%), pulmonary disease (yes/no), angiotensin converting enzyme-inhibitors (yes/no) and loop diuretics (yes/no).

Limitations include the single baseline measurements of BMI and other time dependent cofactors such as medication. We did not have sufficient data on possible confounders such as physical activity, socioeconomic status or cardio- respiratory fitness and intentional vs. unintentional weight loss, and thus we cannot exclude the possibility that residual confounding from unmeasured causal factors unevenly distributed between BMI groups may have influenced our results. Unfortunately, we did not have data on recent weight loss prior to inclusion, but as underweight patients (BMI <18.5 kg/m^2) were excluded, and adjustment for possible confounders such as cancer, pulmonary disease, extent of significant CAD and LVEF did not significantly alter our results, reverse causation is unlikely. BMI was positively associated with common obesity related characteristics such as higher blood pressure, diabetes, an unfavourable lipid profile, higher eGFR and CRP. Adjustment for these variables did not have a significant effect on our results, but we would in any case not include these variables in a final multivariate adjusted survival model because of the possibility of over-adjustment bias. We did, however, adjust for use of ACE inhibitors and loop diuretics as a proxy of heart failure, and there is the possibility that these variables may have mediated some of the effect of BMI.

It has previously been suggested that BMI is an inadequate marker of overweight and obesity in patients with CAD [25], with waist circumference or waist to hip ratio suggested as better predictors of cardiovascular events, especially in women [6,26]. Studies supporting an obesity paradox have almost exclusively used BMI as an index of obesity [3]. We thus suspect that the diverging findings among such studies may be the result of BMI's inadequacy as a quantifier of true body fatness and fat distribution.

Given that there were relatively few females in the study population and the event rate was low, we thus had a low statistical power to by which to detect the possible effects of BMI on risk of events among women. Further, we cannot rule out that the relatively lower incidence rate of AMI among women is a result of detection bias; women, compared to men, are more likely to experience atypical symptoms of AMI and may consequently delay seeking medical care for symptoms or be misdiagnosed by healthcare providers [27]. Finally, the inclusion of predominantly white subjects limits the ability to generalise our findings to non-white populations.

Conclusion

Among 4131 men and women with suspected stable angina pectoris, obese men carried an 80% and 60% higher risk of AMI and CV death, respectively, compared to normal weight men, whereas being overweight, compared to normal weight, was associated with a 50% lower risk

of AMI among women. These findings may potentially explain some of the result variation in studies reporting on the obesity paradox, with further investigation of the interaction between gender and BMI in terms of risk of CV events and mortality therefore warranted.

Competing interests

The authors declare that they have no competing interests.

Authors' contributions

ON conceived of the study and contributed to the study design; GFTS, EKRP, HSH and ON conducted research; HB, RS analyzed data or performed statistical analysis; HB, JKH, GFTS, JH and ON wrote the paper; HB had primary responsibility for final content; HB, JKH, JH and ON interpreted data; HB, JKH, GFTS, EKRP, HSH, JH and ON critically revised the manuscript. All listed authors take responsibility for all aspects of the reliability and freedom from bias of the data presented and their discussed interpretation. All authors read and approved the final manuscript.

Acknowledgements

We thank all WENBIT coworkers at Haukeland and Stavanger University Hospitals, Norway, as well as the Endpoints Committee: Marta Ebbing (HUS), Leik Woie (SUS), Eva Ringdal Pedersen (UiB), Hall Schartum-Hansen (UiB), Per Lund Johansen (UiB) (Chair). We would also like to thank all those who participated in the study for their time and effort. Thanks are also due to Matthew McGee for proofreading the manuscript.

Author details

^{1}Morbid Obesity Center, Vestfold Hospital Trust, Tønsberg, Norway. ^{2}Institute of Clinical Medicine, University of Oslo, Oslo, Norway. ^{3}Department of Clinical Science, University of Bergen, Bergen, Norway. ^{4}Department of Heart Disease, Haukeland University Hospital, Bergen, Norway.

References

1. The top 10 causes of death. http://www.who.int/mediacentre/factsheets/fs310/en/.
2. Goff DC Jr, Lloyd-Jones DM, Bennett G, Coady S, D'Agostino RB Sr, Gibbons R, Greenland P, Lackland DT, Levy D, O'Donnell CJ, Robinson J, Schwartz JS, Shero ST, Smith SC Jr, Sorlie P, Stone NJ, Wilson PWF: 2013 ACC/AHA guideline on the assessment of cardiovascular risk: a report of the American College of Cardiology/American Heart Association Task Force on Practice Guidelines. Circulation 2013,
3. Chrysant SG, Chrysant GS: New insights into the true nature of the obesity paradox and the lower cardiovascular risk. J Am Soc Hypertens 2013, 7(1):85–94.
4. Lemieux S, Prud'homme D, Bouchard C, Tremblay A, Despres JP: Sex differences in the relation of visceral adipose tissue accumulation to total body fatness. Am J Clin Nutr 1993, 58(4):463–467.
5. Domanski MJ, Jablonski KA, Rice MM, Fowler SE, Braunwald E, Investigators P: Obesity and cardiovascular events in patients with established coronary disease. Eur Heart J 2006, 27(12):1416–1422.
6. Dagenais GR, Yi Q, Mann JF, Bosch J, Pogue J, Yusuf S: Prognostic impact of body weight and abdominal obesity in women and men with cardiovascular disease. Am Heart J 2005, 149(1):54–60.
7. Kragelund C, Hassager C, Hildebrandt P, Torp-Pedersen C, Kober L: Impact of obesity on long-term prognosis following acute myocardial infarction. Int J Cardiol 2005, 98(1):123–131.
8. Nikolsky E, Stone GW, Grines CL, Cox DA, Garcia E, Tcheng JE, Griffin JJ, Guagliumi G, Stuckey T, Turco M, Negoita M, Lansky AJ, Mehran R: Impact of body mass index on outcomes after primary angioplasty in acute myocardial infarction. Am Heart J 2006, 151(1):168–175.
9. Wessel TR, Arant CB, Olson MB, Johnson BD, Reis SE, Sharaf BL, Shaw LJ, Handberg E, Sopko G, Kelsey SF, Pepine CJ, Merz NB: Relationship of physical fitness vs body mass index with coronary artery disease and cardiovascular events in women. JAMA 2004, 292(10):1179–1187.
10. Svingen GF, Ueland PM, Pedersen EK, Schartum-Hansen H, Seifert R, Ebbing M, Loland KH, Tell GS, Nygard O: Plasma dimethylglycine and risk of incident acute myocardial infarction in patients with stable angina pectoris. Arterioscler Thromb Vasc Biol 2013.

11. Ebbing M, Bleie O, Ueland PM, Nordrehaug JE, Nilsen DW, Vollset SE, Refsum H, Pedersen EK, Nygard O: **Mortality and cardiovascular events in patients treated with homocysteine-lowering B vitamins after coronary angiography: a randomized controlled trial.** *JAMA* 2008, **300**(7):795–804.

12. Benowitz NL, Jacob P III, Ahijevych K, Jarvis MJ, Hall S, LeHouezec J, Hansson A, Henningfield J, Tsoh J, Hurt RD, Velicer W for the The SRNT Subcommittee on Biochemical Verification: **Biochemical verification of tobacco use and cessation.** *Nicotine Tob Res* 2002, **4**(2):149–159.

13. Midttun O, Hustad S, Ueland PM: **Quantitative profiling of biomarkers related to B-vitamin status, tryptophan metabolism and inflammation in human plasma by liquid chromatography/tandem mass spectrometry.** *Rapid Commun Mass Spectrom* 2009, **23**(9):1371–1379.

14. Friedewald WT, Levy RI, Fredrickson DS: **Estimation of the concentration of low-density lipoprotein cholesterol in plasma, without use of the preparative ultracentrifuge.** *Clin Chem* 1972, **18**(6):499–502.

15. Levey AS, Stevens LA, Schmid CH, Zhang YL, Castro AF 3rd, Feldman HI, Kusek JW, Eggers P, Van Lente F, Greene T, Coresh J: **A new equation to estimate glomerular filtration rate.** *Ann Intern Med* 2009, **150**(9):604–612.

16. Alpert JS, Antman E, Apple F, Beller G, Breithardt G, Armstrong PW, Bassand JP, Baye's de Luna A, Chaitman BR, Clemmensen P, Falk E, Fishbein MC, Galvani M, Garson A Jr, Grines C, Hamm C, Hoppe U, Jaffe A, Katus H, Kjekshus J, Klein W, Klootwijk P, Lenfant C, Levy D, Levy RI, Luepker R, Marcus F, Näslund U, Ohman M, Pahlm O, *et al*: **Myocardial infarction redefined–a consensus document of The Joint European Society of Cardiology/American College of Cardiology Committee for the redefinition of myocardial infarction.** *Eur Heart J* 2000, **21**(18):1502–1513.

17. Cannon CP, Battler A, Brindis RG, Cox JL, Ellis SG, Every NR, Flaherty JT, Harrington RA, Krumholz HM, Simoons ML, Van De Werf FJJ, Weintraub WS, Mitchell KR, Morrisson SL, Anderson HV, Cannom DS, Chitwood WR, Cigarroa JE, Collins-Nakai RL, Gibbons RJ, Grover FL, Heidenreich PA, Khandheria BK, Knoebel SB, Krumholz HL, Malenka DJ, Mark DB, Mckay CR, Passamani ER, Radford MJ, *et al*: **American College of Cardiology key data elements and definitions for measuring the clinical management and outcomes of patients with acute coronary syndromes. A report of the American College of Cardiology Task Force on Clinical Data Standards (Acute Coronary Syndromes Writing Committee).** *J Am Coll Cardiol* 2001, **38**(7):2114–2130.

18. Greenland S: **Modeling and variable selection in epidemiologic analysis.** *Am J Public Health* 1989, **79**(3):340–349.

19. Grundy SM, Pasternak R, Greenland P, Smith S Jr, Fuster V: **Assessment of cardiovascular risk by use of multiple-risk-factor assessment equations: a statement for healthcare professionals from the American Heart Association and the American College of Cardiology.** *Circulation* 1999, **100**(13):1481–1492.

20. Eckel RH: **Obesity and heart disease: a statement for healthcare professionals from the Nutrition Committee.** *Am Heart Assoc Circul* 1997, **96**(9):3248–3250.

21. De Bacquer D, De Backer G, Ostor E, Simon J, Pyorala K, Group EIS: **Predictive value of classical risk factors and their control in coronary patients: a follow-up of the EUROASPIRE I cohort.** *Eur J Cardiovasc Prev Rehabil* 2003, **10**(4):289–295.

22. Snijder MB, van Dam RM, Visser M, Seidell JC: **What aspects of body fat are particularly hazardous and how do we measure them?** *Int J Epidemiol* 2006, **35**(1):83–92.

23. Silva TC, Barrett-Connor E, Ramires JA, Mansur AP: **Obesity, estrone, and coronary artery disease in postmenopausal women.** *Maturitas* 2008, **59**(3):242–248.

24. Castracane VD, Kraemer GR, Ogden BW, Kraemer RR: **Interrelationships of serum estradiol, estrone, and estrone sulfate, adiposity, biochemical bone markers, and leptin in post-menopausal women.** *Maturitas* 2006, **53**(2):217–225.

25. Romero-Corral A, Somers VK, Sierra-Johnson J, Jensen MD, Thomas RJ, Squires RW, Allison TG, Korinek J, Lopez-Jimenez F: **Diagnostic performance of body mass index to detect obesity in patients with coronary artery disease.** *Eur Heart J* 2007, **28**(17):2087–2093.

26. Rexrode KM, Carey VJ, Hennekens CH, Walters EE, Colditz GA, Stampfer MJ, Willett WC, Manson JE: **Abdominal adiposity and coronary heart disease in women.** *JAMA* 1998, **280**(21):1843–1848.

27. Maas AH, van der Schouw YT, Regitz-Zagrosek V, Swahn E, Appelman YE, Pasterkamp G, Ten Cate H, Nilsson PM, Huisman MV, Stam HC, Eizema K, Stramba-Badiale M: **Red alert for women's heart: the urgent need for more research and knowledge on cardiovascular disease in women: proceedings of the workshop held in Brussels on gender differences in cardiovascular disease, 29 September 2010.** *Eur Heart J* 2011, **32**(11):1362–1368.

2

Predictors of non-invasive therapy and 28-day-case fatality in elderly compared to younger patients with acute myocardial infarction: an observational study from the MONICA/KORA Myocardial Infarction Registry

Ute Amann[1,2*], Inge Kirchberger[1,2], Margit Heier[1,2], Christian Thilo[3], Bernhard Kuch[3,4], Annette Peters[2] and Christa Meisinger[1,2]

Abstract

Background: A substantial proportion of patients with acute myocardial infarction (AMI) did not receive invasive therapy, defined as percutaneous coronary intervention and/or coronary artery bypass grafting. Aims of this study were to evaluate predictors of non-invasive therapy in elderly compared to younger AMI patients and to assess the association between invasive therapy and 28-day-case fatality.

Methods: From the German population-based registry, 3475 persons, consecutively hospitalized with an AMI between 2009 and 2012 were included. Data were collected by standardized interviews and chart review. All-cause mortality was assessed on a regular basis. Multivariable logistic regression analyses were conducted.

Results: The sample consisted of 1329 patients aged 28–65 years (age category [AC] 1), 1083 aged 65–74 years (AC 2), and 1063 aged 75–84 years (AC 3). The proportion of patients receiving non-invasive therapy was 10.7, 17.7, and 35.8 % in AC 1, 2, and 3, respectively. Predictors of non-invasive therapy in all ACs were non-ST segment elevation MI, bundle branch block, reduced left ventricular ejection fraction, prior stroke, absence of hyperlipidemia, and low creatine kinase. Elderly women (≥65 years) were less likely to receive invasive therapy. Stratifying the models by type of AMI revealed fewer predictors in patients with ST segment elevation MI. Regarding 28-day-case fatality, strong inverse relations with invasive therapy were seen in all AC: odds ratio of 0.35 (95 % confidence interval [CI] 0.15–0.84), 0.45 (95 % CI 0.22–0.92), and 0.39 (95 % CI 0.24–0.63) in AC 1, 2 and 3, respectively.

Conclusion: In today's real-life patient care we found that predictors of non-invasive therapy were predominantly the same in all age groups, but differed particularly by type of AMI. Further research is necessary to investigate the real reasons for non-invasive therapy, especially among elderly women. Moreover, we confirmed that receiving invasive therapy was inversely associated with 28-day-case fatality independent of age.

Keywords: Myocardial infarction, Mortality, Invasive therapy, Predictors

* Correspondence: ute.amann@helmholtz-muenchen.de
[1]MONICA/KORA Myocardial Infarction Registry, Central Hospital of Augsburg, Stenglinstr. 2, 86156 Augsburg, Germany
[2]Institute of Epidemiology II, Helmholtz Zentrum München, German Research Center for Environmental Health (GmbH), Neuherberg, Germany
Full list of author information is available at the end of the article

Background

Percutaneous coronary intervention (PCI) and coronary artery bypass grafting (CABG) are today's standard invasive treatment options for patients with acute coronary syndrome (ACS) independent of patient's chronological age [1–5]. Over the last years, an increasing trend in use of these invasive procedures in patients with an acute myocardial infarction (AMI) was reported in several registry studies [6–9]. Nevertheless, there is still a substantial proportion of AMI patients who neither receive PCI nor CABG, even though being eligible for invasive therapy. Earlier studies have determined reasons for the underuse of reperfusion therapy in ST-segment elevation myocardial infarction (STEMI) patients and found that several factors such as older age, female sex, delayed presentation, comorbidities, prior stroke, prior MI, contraindications to the use of fibrinolytic agents and/or mechanical reperfusion (e.g., bleeding risk) are related with no reperfusion therapy in the acute setting [7, 9–13]. To our knowledge, previous studies have not investigated predictive factors of invasive treatment in patients with non-ST segment elevation myocardial infarction (NSTEMI) and did not distinct between younger and elderly persons beneath consideration of short-term survival. The aim of this study was firstly to evaluate predictive factors for non-invasive treatment in elderly and younger AMI patients including the type of AMI (e.g., STEMI, NSTEMI). Secondly, to assess the association between invasive compared to non-invasive therapy and 28-day-case fatality by age group in real-life patient care.

Methods

Study design and data source

The present study is based on data from the population-based MI registry in Augsburg, Germany, which was established in 1984 as part of the World Health Organization MONICA Project (MONItoring Trends and Determinants in CArdiovascular disease). After the termination of MONICA in 1995, the MI registry became part of the framework of KORA (Cooperative Health Research in the Region of Augsburg). Since 1984, coronary deaths and non-fatal (at least 24 h surviving) AMI cases of the 25- to 74-year old inhabitants of the city of Augsburg and 2 adjacent counties (about 600,000 inhabitants) have been continuously registered. About 80 % of all AMI cases of the study region are treated in the region's major hospital, Klinikum Augsburg, a tertiary care center offering 24/7 interventional cardiovascular procedures, as well as heart surgery facilities. From 2009 onwards, the registry was extended for the elderly up to 84 years. The methods of case identification, diagnostic classification of events, and data quality control have been described in detail elsewhere [14, 15]. Since 2001, diagnostic criteria according to the European Society of Cardiology and American College of Cardiology criteria were used for case identification, including assessment of troponin levels especially for identification of NSTEMI [16].

Data collection

Patients were interviewed during hospital stay by trained nurses using a standardized questionnaire to collect sociodemographic characteristics, cardiovascular risk factors, medical history of previous MI, stroke and comorbidities, and information on the acute event. Further information on type of AMI, treatment procedures and complications during hospital stay, vital signs, medical history, and medication use during hospitalization were collected by review of medical chart. Information provided by the patient concerning the medical history had to be confirmed by chart review. Information on renal dysfunction was collected by review of medical chart. Data collection of the MONICA/KORA MI registry has been approved by the ethics committee of the Bavarian Medical Association (Bayerische Landesärztekammer) and all study participants gave written informed consent.

Study population

The present study included all consecutive patients aged 25–84 years, who were hospitalized with a non-fatal AMI between January 1, 2009, and December, 31, 2012 and survived longer than 24 h. From 3669 persons, we excluded 194 (5.3 %) individuals with missing information on any of the relevant covariables. Thus, the final study population covered 3475 cases (2397 males and 1078 females) with AMI. Excluded patients due to missing covariable information were older (median age 72 vs. 69 years, p <0.0001), had more frequently a NSTEMI (67.5 vs. 53.3 %) or bundle branch block (BBB) (12.4 vs. 9.5 %, p <0.0001), were less likely to receive an invasive therapy (52.1 vs. 79.5 %, p <0.0001) and coronary angiography (61.9 vs. 89.2 %, p <0.0001), and showed a higher rate of 28-day-case fatality (23.7 vs. 7.4 %, p <0.0001) compared to patients included in the study population.

Definitions and outcome

The following 3 age categories (AC) were analyzed: AC 1) patients aged 25–64 years, AC 2) patients aged 65–74 years, and AC 3) patients aged 75–84 years. Patients were grouped regarding their in-hospital treatment strategy: invasive therapy was defined as PCI with stent implantation or balloon dilatation or/and CABG; non-invasive (conservative) therapy included patients treated with thrombolysis and/or receiving coronary angiography but without a treatment procedure. The type of AMI was defined as STEMI, NSTEMI, or BBB. The BBB group contains newly developed left BBB, right BBB, and pre-known BBB. Because we do not exactly know whether all patients with a BBB had a newly developed left BBB, which is considered as STEMI equivalent, we displayed the BBB group as separate category.

The outcome of this study was 28-day-case fatality after AMI. Mortality was assessed by checking the vital status of all registered persons of the MONICA/KORA MI registry on a regular basis. Death certificates were obtained from local health departments.

Data analysis

Categorical variables were expressed as absolute numbers and percentages (%), continuous variables as median with interquartile range (25th and 75th percentiles). For descriptive purpose, the 3 ACs were compared using Chi^2-test or Fisher's exact test for categorical variables and the Kruskal-Wallis test (Wilcoxon Analysis) for continuous variables.

To identify predictors that determined the selection of in-hospital treatment strategy (invasive or conservative therapy), multivariable logistic regression analyses were performed for each AC and further stratified by type of AMI. Variables analyzed as potential predictive factors were sex (male/female), smoking (current smoker/ex-smoker/never-smoker/missing), living alone (yes/no/missing), body mass index ≥ 30 kg/m^2 (yes/no), prior MI, prior stroke, medical history of diabetes, hyperlipidemia, hypertension, angina pectoris, and chronic obstructive pulmonary disease (yes/no), renal dysfunction reported in medical chart (yes/no), pre-hospital time (symptom onset to arrival) [min] (continuous), left ventricular ejection fraction (LVEF) (> 30 %/$\leq$ 30 %/not assessed or missing), type of AMI (STEMI/NSTEMI/BBB), and peak serum creatine phosphokinase (CPK) level (U/l) during hospitalization (continuous). As criterion for entry in the models, the explanatory variables must meet the 0.05 significance level in at least 1 AC in the bivariate analysis with the in-hospital treatment strategy. The models of the sub-samples by type of AMI included only factors which significantly ($p < 0.05$) contributed to the model using forward selection technique.

To investigate the associations between in-hospital treatment strategy and 28-day-case fatality, further multivariable logistic regression models for each AC were performed. In addition to the above mentioned variables, the following potential confounding factors were considered: in-hospital cardiac arrest (yes/no), any other in-hospital complication (cardiogenic shock or ventricular fibrillation or ventricular tachycardia or recurrent infarction or pulmonary edema or bradycardia [heart rate <50/min] or stroke or any major bleeding complication [intracranial or retroperitoneal or any other major spontaneous bleeding]) (yes/no), married (yes/no/missing),

and use of the following evidence-based medication regarded as cornerstone of long-term medical therapy in ACS patients [1–5]: dual antiplatelet therapy, beta-blockers, angiotensin-converting-enzyme inhibitors or angiotensin receptor blockers (ACEIs/ARBs), and statins. We considered a model for each AC adjusted for sex and a full model with additional adjustment for all bivariately significant ($p < 0.05$) variables. A forward stepwise selection technique was used. Variables with more than 2 characteristic (e.g., yes/no/missing) were 'dummy'-coded.

All analyses were performed using SAS version 9.2 (SAS Institute Inc., Cary, North Carolina).

Results

The study population consisted of 3475 patients (69.0 % men) with a median age of 69.0 years (interquartile range 58–76 years). There were 1329 (38.2 %) patients in AC 1, 1083 (31.2 %) in AC 2, and 1063 (30.6 %) in AC 3. Baseline characteristics, in-hospital procedures and in-hospital medications according to ACs are shown in Tables 1 and 2. The 3 ACs significantly differed from each other in terms of the analyzed variables except for pre-hospital time and the use of at least 1 antiplatelet agent. The proportion of patients not receiving an invasive therapy was 10.7, 17.7, and 35.8 % in AC 1, 2, and 3; in the sub-group of STEMI patients it was 3.4, 7.6, and 16.4 %, respectively. In general, patients with NSTEMI or BBB were less likely to receive coronary angiography, invasive therapy and the evidence-based medication (except for beta-blockers) compared with STEMI patients (Table 2). The highest proportion of patients treated conservatively was observed in AC 3 in patients with BBB (47.6 %) and with NSTEMI (41.9 %); both subgroups showed the lowest rate of angiography of 71.7 and 74.0 %, respectively (Table 2).

Factors associated with in-hospital treatment strategy

The multivariable logistic regression models revealed that type of AMI (NSTEMI vs. STEMI and BBB vs. STEMI), LVEF (LVEF $\leq$30 vs. LVEF >30 % and LVEF not assessed or missing vs. LVEF >30 %), prior stroke, no hyperlipidemia, and low peak CPK level were strong predictors of non-invasive therapy in all ACs (Table 3). Being a woman was a significant predictor in AC 2 (odds ratio [OR] 1.80; 95 % confidence interval [CI] 1.24–2.61) and AC 3 (OR 1.38; 95 % CI 1.03–1.85); whereas renal dysfunction and prior MI was significantly associated with non-invasive therapy in AC 1 and 2. Stratifying the models by type of AMI showed more differentiated results. For example, in patients with STEMI 3 factors were associated with non-invasive therapy: prior stroke in AC 1 (OR 11.2; 95 % CI 2.58–48.7), female sex in AC 2 (OR 2.35; 95 % CI 1.06–5.21), and LVEF (reduced

Table 1 Baseline characteristics of the study population by age category ($n = 3475$)

Variable	Age category			
	25–64 years $n = 1329$ (38.2)	65–74 years $n = 1083$ (31.2)	75–84 years $n = 1063$ (30.6)	p Value
Sociodemographics				
Age (years)[a]	55 (49–60)	70 (68–72)	79 (77–81)	<0.0001
Female sex	251 (18.9)	327 (30.2)	500 (47.0)	<0.0001
Married[b]	885 (69.6)	777 (75.6)	607 (61.9)	<0.0001
Living alone[b]	255 (20.1)	189 (18.4)	278 (28.4)	<0.0001
Body mass index ≥30 kg/m^2	413 (31.1)	255 (23.6)	183 (17.2)	<0.0001
Smoker				<0.0001
Current smoker	714 (53.7)	201 (18.6)	74 (7.0)	
Ex-smoker	337 (25.4)	403 (37.2)	308 (29.0)	
Never-smoker	234 (17.6)	391 (36.1)	476 (44.8)	
missing/not known	44 (3.3)	88 (8.1)	205 (19.3)	
Medical history[c]				
Prior MI	181 (13.6)	228 (21.1)	244 (23.0)	<0.0001
Prior stroke	51 (3.8)	117 (10.8)	171 (16.1)	<0.0001
Diabetes	353 (26.6)	439 (40.5)	439 (41.3)	<0.0001
Hypertension	910 (68.5)	885 (81.7)	943 (88.7)	<0.0001
Hyperlipidemia	631 (47.5)	538 (49.7)	453 (42.6)	0.004
Angina pectoris	135 (10.2)	187 (17.3)	210 (19.8)	<0.0001
Chronic obstructive pulmonary disease	50 (3.8)	92 (8.5)	92 (8.7)	<0.0001
Clinical characteristics				
Type of AMI				<0.0001
STEMI	625 (47.0)	369 (34.1)	298 (28.0)	
NSTEM	651 (49.0)	603 (55.7)	599 (56.4)	
Bundle branch block	53 (4.0)	111 (10.2)	166 (15.6)	
Peak serum CPK level (U/l)[a,b]	744 (265–1915)	530 (212–1292)	395 (173–991)	<0.0001
LVEF				<0.0001
> 30 %	1141 (85.8)	841 (77.7)	711 (67.0)	
≤ 30 %	73 (5.5)	87 (8.0)	123 (11.5)	
not assessed/missing	115 (8.7)	155 (14.3)	229 (21.5)	
Renal dysfunction[d]	54 (4.1)	159 (14.7)	306 (28.8)	<0.0001
Pre-hospital time/symptom onset to arrival (min)[a]	159 (79–585)	175 (77–613)	188 (75–565)	0.95

Data are presented as number (percentage) unless otherwise indicated. P values were calculated for comparison of the age categories

AMI acute myocardial infarction, STEMI ST-elevation myocardial infarction, NSTEMI non-ST-elevation myocardial infarction, CPK creatine phosphokinase, LVEF left ventricular ejection fraction

[a] Presented as median values (25th, 75th percentiles)

[b] Values were calculated without patients with missing data regarding married ($n = 195$), living alone status ($n = 195$), and peak serum CPK level ($n = 23$)

[c] Patient-reported medical history of known comorbidities before the acute event, which was collected with a standardized interview during hospital stay and further data were gathered in a concluding chart review. If the information on comorbidities from patient-report and medical chart differed, the chart information was used

[d] Information on renal dysfunction was collected by review of medical chart

LVEF and/or LVEF not assessed/missing) in all ACs. In patients with NSTEMI, LVEF was seen as predictor in all ACs, whereas patients with renal dysfunction, prior MI and history of chronic obstructive pulmonary disease demonstrated higher odds of receiving conservative therapy in AC 1 and 2. Prior stroke was observed as strong predictor in AC 3 with NSTEMI (Table 3).

Association between invasive therapy and 28-day-case fatality

In addition to baseline characteristics previously reported, Table 4 shows that the 3 ACs significantly differed from each other in terms of the analyzed outcome and several complications during hospitalization except for ventricular fibrillation, bradycardia, stroke, and any

Table 2 In-hospital procedures and treatment strategy by age category and stratified by type of AMI (n = 3475)

Variable	Age category									p Value
	25–64 years n = 1329 (38.2)			65–74 years n = 1083 (31.2)			75–84 years n = 1063 (30.6)			
Type of AMI	STEMI n = 625 (47.0)	NSTEMI n = 651 (49.0)	BBB n = 53 (4.0)	STEMI n = 369 (34.1)	NSTEMI n = 603 (55.7)	BBB n = 111 (10.2)	STEMI n = 298 (28.0)	NSTEMI n = 599 (56.4)	BBB n = 166 (15.6)	<0.0001
Diagnostic procedure										
Coronary angiography	622 (99.5)	606 (93.1)	48 (90.6)	361 (97.8)	534 (88.6)	94 (84.7)	272 (91.3)	443 (74.0)	119 (71.7)	0.003
Treatment strategy										<0.0001
PCI	554 (88.6)	460 (70.7)	31 (58.4)	295 (79.9)	346 (57.4)	69 (62.2)	215 (72.2)	272 (45.4)	72 (43.4)	
CABG	49 (7.8)	84 (12.9)	9 (17.0)	46 (12.5)	118 (19.6)	17 (15.3)	33 (11.1)	76 (12.7)	15 (9.0)	
No invasive therapy[a]	21 (3.4)	106 (16.3)	13 (24.5)	28 (7.6)	138 (22.9)	24 (21.6)	49 (16.4)	251 (41.9)	79 (47.6)	
Thrombolysis	1 (0.2)	1 (0.2)	0	0	1 (0.2)	1 (0.9)	1 (0.3)	0	0	
Evidence-based medication										
Antiplatelet agents	623 (99.7)	643 (98.8)	52 (98.1)	367 (99.5)	600 (99.5)	109 (98.2)	295 (99.0)	590 (98.5)	164 (98.8)	0.24
DAPT	587 (93.9)	543 (83.4)	44 (83.0)	329 (89.2)	459 (76.1)	82 (73.9)	253 (84.9)	404 (67.5)	117 (70.5)	<0.0001
Beta-blockers	601 (96.2)	635 (97.5)	50 (94.3)	351 (95.1)	581 (96.4)	105 (94.6)	274 (92.0)	565 (94.3)	155 (93.4)	0.0006
Statins	596 (95.4)	612 (94.0)	48 (90.6)	346 (93.8)	562 (93.2)	94 (84.7)	270 (90.6)	521 (87.0)	147 (88.6)	<0.0001
ACEIs/ARBs	587 (93.9)	584 (89.7)	48 (90.6)	337 (91.3)	544 (90.2)	96 (86.5)	255 (85.6)	507 (84.6)	139 (83.7)	<0.0001

Data are presented as number (percentage). *P* values were calculated for comparison of the age categories. Data of the total sample of each age category are not presented in this table, but used for comparison tests

AMI acute myocardial infarction, *STEMI* ST-elevation myocardial infarction, *NSTEMI* non-ST-elevation myocardial infarction, *BBB* bundle branch block, *PCI* percutaneous coronary intervention, *CABG* coronary artery bypass graft, *DAPT* dual antiplatelet therapy, *ACEIs/ARBs* angiotensin-converting enzyme inhibitors or angiotensin-receptor blockers

[a] Invasive therapy was defined as PCI with stent implantation or balloon dilatation or/and CABG

major bleeding complication. The highest 28-day-case fatality of 19.5 % (n = 74) was observed in AC 3 receiving conservative therapy and the lowest (2.4 %; n = 28) in patients aged 28–65 years treated invasively. In general, 28-day-case fatality was lower in the invasively than non-invasively treated patients in all ACs.

In the multivariable logistic regression analyses, invasive therapy showed a strongly inverse relation with 28-day-case fatality compared with the conservative therapy in all ACs. After adjustment for potential confounding variables the full model (model 2) revealed an OR of 0.35 (95 % CI 0.15–0.84), 0.45 (95 % CI 0.22–0.92), and 0.39 (95 % CI 0.24–0.63) in the AC 1, 2 and 3, respectively (Table 5).

Discussion

In the present registry-based study including 3475 consecutively enrolled patients with AMI occurring between 2009 and 2012, we found that several factors such as type of AMI, reduced LVEF, prior stroke, history of no hyperlipidemia, and a low CPK level were strong predictors of a non-invasive therapy independent of age. The sub-group analysis by type of AMI revealed more independent predictors in patients with NSTEMI compared to STEMI. In addition, besides various differences observed between the 3 age groups, we found that an invasive therapy was inversely associated with 28-day-case

fatality with almost similar mortality risk reductions in all age groups.

Our findings that NSTEMI and prior stroke were strong predictive factors are in concordance with an earlier study conducted in 1001 elderly STEMI and NSTEMI patients in Germany, which additionally found age, prior MI, renal failure, pre existing coronary artery disease, Killip Class >II, and supraventricular tachycardia as factors predicting treatment type in patients above 75 years [17]. Our analysis by age groups and type of AMI adds that renal dysfunction and prior MI were significantly associated only in patients presenting with NSTEMI below 75 years. In contrast to our study, where female sex was associated with non-invasive therapy in the total sample above 64 years, Rittger et al. [17] reported that sex had no significant influence on treatment strategy in patients above 75 years. After stratifying the study population by type of AMI, we found that women demonstrated 2-fold higher odds of receiving conservative therapy only in patients aged 65–74 years diagnosed with either STEMI or NSTEMI. Even if other factors such as frailty or severe multimorbidity could have biased sex differences found in observational studies, especially in STEMI patients (see below), one should consider the recently updated clinical practice guideline of the American College of Cardiology and the American Heart Association which highlights that both genders

Table 3 Factors associated with non-invasive therapy by age category for the total sample and stratified by type of AMI

	Age category					
	25–64 years		65–74 years		75–84 years	
	OR [95 % CI]	p Value	OR [95 % CI]	p Value	OR [95 % CI]	p Value
Total sample (n = 3452)[a]	(n = 1324)		(n = 1077)		(n = 1051)	
Sex (women vs. men)	1.28 [0.80–2.06]	0.30	1.80 [1.24–2.61]	0.002	1.38 [1.03–1.85]	0.03
Type of AMI (NSTEMI vs. STEMI)	3.07 [1.81–5.20]	<0.0001	2.54 [1.59–4.05]	<0.0001	2.36 [1.59–3.51]	<0.0001
Type of AMI (BBB vs. STEMI)	4.22 [1.76–10.1]	0.001	2.01 [1.05–3.84]	0.03	2.60 [1.58–4.26]	0.001
Prior stroke (yes vs. no)	2.97 [1.40–6.30]	0.005	1.91 [1.17–3.13]	0.01	1.87 [1.27–2.75]	0.002
Renal dysfunction (yes vs. no)	2.27 [1.06–4.90]	0.04	1.59 [1.03–2.45]	0.04	1.35 [0.97–1.87]	0.07
Prior MI (yes vs. no)	2.08 [1.27–3.41]	0.004	2.00 [1.35–2.95]	0.001	1.27 [0.89–1.81]	0.18
LVEF (LVEF ≤ 30 % vs. LVEF > 30 %)	3.28 [1.60–6.71]	0.001	1.85 [1.02–3.35]	0.04	2.02 [1.30–3.14]	0.002
LVEF (LVEF n/m[b] vs. LVEF > 30 %)	6.58 [4.05–10.7]	<0.0001	5.03 [3.32–7.63]	<0.0001	6.10 [4.27–8.73]	<0.0001
History of hyperlipidemia (yes vs. no)	0.52 [0.34–0.80]	0.003	0.63 [0.44–0.90]	0.01	0.67 [0.49–0.91]	0.01
History of COPD (yes vs. no)	1.89 [0.87–4.13]	0.11	2.26 [1.34–3.81]	0.002	0.83 [0.50–1.39]	0.48
Peak serum CPK level (U/l) (continuous)	1.00 [1.00–1.00]	0.003	1.00 [1.00–1.00]	0.04	1.00 [1.00–1.00]	<0.0001
STEMI (n = 1292)	(n = 625)		(n = 369)		(n = 298)	
Sex (women vs. men)	n/a[c]		2.35 [1.06–5.21]	0.04	n/a[c]	
Prior stroke (yes vs. no)	11.2 [2.58–48.7]	0.001	n/a[c]		n/a[c]	
LVEF (LVEF ≤ 30 % vs. LVEF > 30 %)	3.71 [1.01–13.6]	0.05	2.36 [0.74–7.54]	0.15	1.53 [0.58–4.03]	0.39
LVEF (LVEF n/m[b] vs. LVEF > 30 %)	4.13 [1.22–14.0]	0.02	3.90 [1.30–11.7]	0.02	13.0 [5.72–29.3]	<0.0001
NSTEMI (n = 1838)	(n = 647)		(n = 603)		(n = 588)	
Sex (women vs. men)	n/a[c]		1.63 [1.04–2.53]	0.03	n/a[c]	
Prior stroke (yes vs. no)	n/a[c]		n/a[c]		2.15 [1.34–3.46]	0.002
Renal dysfunction (yes vs. no)	2.76 [1.18–6.45]	0.02	1.80 [1.09–2.99]	0.02	n/a[c]	
Prior MI (yes vs. no)	1.81 [1.03–3.18]	0.04	2.04 [1.30–3.21]	0.002	n/a[c]	
LVEF (LVEF ≤ 30 % vs. LVEF > 30 %)	3.08 [1.15–8.22]	0.03	1.88 [0.86–4.13]	0.12	3.19 [1.75–5.80]	0.001
LVEF (LVEF n/m[b] vs. LVEF > 30 %)	6.24 [3.56–10.9]	<0.0001	5.04 [3.12–8.16]	<0.0001	5.49 [3.54–8.50]	<0.0001
History of hyperlipidemia (yes vs. no)	0.52 [0.32–0.85]	0.01	n/a[c]		0.51 [0.35–0.74]	0.001
History of COPD (yes vs. no)	2.57 [1.05–6.32]	0.04	2.11 [1.16–3.85]	0.01	n/a[c]	
Peak serum CPK level (U/l) (continuous)	1.00 [1.00–1.00]	0.001	n/a[c]		1.00 [1.00–1.00]	0.005
BBB (n = 330)	(n = 53)		(n = 111)		(n = 165)	
Prior MI (yes vs. no)	9.18 [1.62–51.9]	0.01[d]	3.17 [1.10–9.12]	0.03	n/a[c]	
Renal dysfunction (yes vs. no)	18.8 [1.04–340.0]	0.05[d]	n/a[c]		n/a[c]	
History of hypertension (yes vs. no)	0.11 [0.02–0.68]	0.02[d]	n/a[c]		n/a[c]	
LVEF (LVEF ≤ 30 % vs. LVEF > 30 %)	N/A[e]		2.41 [0.65–8.99]	0.19	1.14 [0.46–2.83]	0.79
LVEF (LVEF n/m[b] vs. LVEF > 30 %)	N/A[e]		10.5 [3.27–33.7]	<0.0001	9.44 [3.89–22.9]	<0.0001
Peak serum CPK level (U/l) (continuous	n/a[c]		n/a[c]		1.00 [1.00–1.00]	0.01

The multivariable analysis included as explanatory variables sex, type of AMI ('dummy'-coded), LVEF ('dummy'-coded), renal dysfunction, prior stroke, prior MI, history of diabetes, hypertension, hyperlipidemia, angina pectoris and COPD, pre-hospital time, and peak serum CPK level. In the total sample, variables which meet the 0.05 significance level in at least one age category were included and presented. For the sub-samples by type of AMI only the significant factors in that sub-sample model (forward stepwise selection technique) were included and presented

OR odds ratio, *CI* confidence interval, *AMI* acute myocardial infarction, *STEMI* ST-elevation myocardial infarction, *NSTEMI* non-ST-elevation myocardial infarction, *BBB* bundle branch block, *LVEF* left ventricular ejection fraction, *COPD* chronic obstructive pulmonary disease, *CPK* creatine phosphokinase

[a] As 23 patients had no data on peak serum CPK level, the total sample size was 3452 instead of 3475

[b] n/m, LVEF were not assessed or missing

[c] n/a, OR and p value were not applicable because the analyzed variable did not meet the 0.05 significance level for entry into the model of the sub-sample

[d] P value and OR were assessed in a separate model without the variables regarding LVEF

[e] N/A, not applicable due to quasi-complete separation of data points detected when 'LVEF' was included

Table 4 Clinical complications and outcome by age category and stratified by treatment strategy (n = 3475)

Variable	Age category									p Value
	25–64 years			65–74 years			75–84 years			<0.0001
Treatment strategy	All n = 1329 (100)	IT n = 1187 (89.3)	CT n = 142 (10.7)	All n = 1083 (100)	IT n = 891 (82.3)	CT n = 192 (17.7)	All n = 1063 (100)	IT n = 683 (64.2)	CT n = 380 (35.8)	
Complications during hospital stay										
Cardiac arrest	76 (5.7)	58 (4.9)	18 (12.7)	110 (10.2)	79 (8.9)	31 (16.2)	176 (16.6)	102 (14.9)	74 (19.5)	<0.0001
Cardiogenic shock	54 (4.1)	48 (4.0)	6 (4.2)	77 (7.1)	66 (7.4)	11 (5.7)	101 (9.5)	75 (11.0)	26 (6.8)	<0.0001
Ventricular fibrillation	32 (2.4)	29 (2.4)	3 (2.1)	32 (3.0)	27 (3.0)	5 (2.6)	31 (2.9)	25 (3.7)	6 (1.6)	0.65
Ventricular tachycardia	109 (8.2)	105 (8.9)	4 (2.8)	66 (6.1)	60 (6.7)	6 (3.1)	54 (5.1)	41 (6.0)	13 (3.4)	0.007
Bradycardia	76 (5.7)	72 (6.1)	4 (2.8)	71 (6.6)	67 (7.5)	4 (2.1)	63 (5.9)	51 (7.5)	12 (3.2)	0.68
Re-infarction	10 (0.8)	10 (0.8)	0	18 (1.7)	13 (1.5)	5 (2.6)	26 (2.5)	20 (2.9)	6 (1.6)	0.04
Stroke	5 (0.4)	5 (0.4)	0	9 (0.8)	7 (0.8)	2 (1.0)	8 (0.8)	5 (0.7)	3 (0.8)	0.32
Pulmonary edema	30 (2.3)	25 (2.1)	5 (3.5)	43 (4.0)	33 (3.7)	10 (5.2)	57 (5.4)	41 (6.0)	16 (4.2)	0.0003
Any major bleeding complication[a]	13 (1.0)	11 (0.9)	2 (1.4)	19 (1.8)	14 (1.6)	5 (2.6)	22 (2.1)	16 (2.3)	6 (1.6)	0.08
Any in-hospital complication (without cardiac arrest)	254 (19.1)	236 (19.9)	18 (12.7)	243 (22.4)	208 (23.3)	35 (18.2)	249 (23.4)	185 (27.1)	64 (16.8)	0.02
Outcome										
28-day-case fatality	44 (3.3)	28 (2.4)	16 (11.3)	74 (6.8)	44 (4.9)	30 (15.6)	138 (13.0)	64 (9.4)	74 (19.5)	<0.0001
Death during hospital stay	43 (3.2)	28 (2.4)	15 (10.6)	74 (6.9)	45 (5.1)	30 (15.6)	146 (13.7)	72 (10.5)	74 (19.5)	<0.0001

Data are presented as number (percentage). P values were calculated for comparison of the age categories
IT invasive therapy, CT conservative therapy
[a] Major bleeding complication: intracranial or retroperitoneal or any other major spontaneous bleeding

should be treated in the same way [18]. It is known from earlier studies that prevalence of frailty and multiple co-morbidities influence the likeliness of receiving invasive therapy and also the outcome of elderly ACS patients [5, 19–21], and were found to be more common in women [21–24]. Therefore, for clinical decision-making and evaluation of the prognosis of elderly ACS patients an assessment tool for end-of-life status, which showed comparable usefulness with clinical risk scores such as the Global Registry of Acute Coronary Events (GRACE) score, might be considered to predict the 1-year all-cause mortality and to select the approximately 8 % of patients with an end-stage illness [22].

In the sub-group of STEMI patients we observed that only a small number did not receive invasive therapy, but this proportion increased by age from 3.4 % in AC 1 to 16.4 % in AC 3. Our multivariable analyses revealed only 3 predictive factors for non-invasive therapy in STEMI patients: LVEF in all ACs, prior stroke in patients below 65 years and female sex in patients aged 65–74 years. ORs of 11 (prior stroke) and 4–13 (LVEF) indicate a strong impact of these factors in STEMI patients. Prior stroke was also reported as predictor of non-invasive therapy in earlier studies regarding STEMI patients [11, 13]. Our study adds that reduced LVEF or heart failure and cardiac enzyme levels such as CPK or troponin might be more important than other factors previously reported. Regarding female sex, a discrepancy between previous reported results exists. Gharacholou et al. [11] reported that female sex was identified as strong factor associated with no reperfusion among the reperfusion-eligible STEMI population analyzed from

Table 5 Association between invasive therapy and 28-day-case fatality by age category

	Age category					
	25–64 years		65–74 years		75–84 years	
	OR [95 % CI]	p Value	OR [95 % CI]	p Value	OR [95 % CI]	p Value
Model 1[a]	0.19 [0.10–0.36]	<0.0001	0.28 [0.17–0.46]	<0.0001	0.43 [0.30–0.62]	<0.0001
Model 2[b]	0.35 [0.15–0.84]	0.02	0.45 [0.22–0.92]	0.03	0.39 [0.24–0.63]	<0.0001

[a] Model 1 adjusted for sex for the total sample (n = 3475)
[b] Model 2 adjusted for sex, body mass index ≥30 kg/m², type of AMI, renal dysfunction, prior stroke, prior MI, history of diabetes, hypertension, hyperlipidemia, angina pectoris and chronic obstructive pulmonary disease, any in-hospital complication (without cardiac arrest), pre-hospital time, left ventricular ejection fraction, peak serum creatine phosphokinase (CPK) level, and in-hospital medication: dual antiplatelet therapy, beta-blockers, statins, and angiotensin-converting-enzyme inhibitors or angiotensin receptor blockers. As 23 patients had no data on peak serum CPK level, the total sample size was 3452

226 US hospitals participating in the CRUSADE quality improvement initiative. Another study also reported an association between female sex and not attempting reperfusion in STEMI patients [7]. In contrast, some earlier studies [23, 24] found that being a woman was not an independent predictor in patients presenting with STEMI. As we analyzed factors by age, our study adds the information that female sex might be an independent predictor in patients who were between 65 and 74 years old. However, as mentioned above, missing adjustment for unobserved confounders related with female sex such as frailty, multiple comorbidities or high risk of death could have biased our and previously reported studies. This theory is supported by a recent study in 1104 STEMI patients based on two clinical network registries in Germany which reported that standard of care including performance of primary PCI and procedural success rate were not gender specific, and the adjusted 12-months mortality did not differ between men and women despite significant differences in clinical baseline parameters [25]. However, gender differences in clinical decision-making regarding reperfusion rates and secondary drug treatment prophylaxis were still reported in several countries [26–29]. In contrast to earlier studies in STEMI patients, we did not find diabetes [7, 9, 12], prior MI [9] and delayed presentation (prehospital time) [13, 23, 24] as being predictive factors in this sub-group. The comparison across studies is, however, difficult, since we were not able to adjust our analyses for other potential reasons such as patient preference, dementia [13], or contraindications to the use of reperfusion, prior CABG, spontaneous reperfusion [10] or Killip class risk score [10, 17]. In general, we observed that previous reported results vary considerably depending mainly on study design, time period, analyzed factors, proportion of patients not receiving invasive therapy, and country of origin.

Regarding 28-day-case fatality, we observed a clear short-term survival benefit associated with invasive therapy in all 3 age groups after adjustment for various confounding factors including type of AMI, evidence-based medication and in-hospital complications. In contrast to earlier trials [1, 5, 30], we did not observe greater risk reduction from the invasive therapy in patients above 64 years. The ORs found in our study were almost similar, but showed a narrower CI in the eldest group, which strengthens the benefit of an invasive therapy for reperfusion-eligible patients above 74 years. In addition, the occurrence of major bleeding complications was not significantly different between the ACs in our study, but showed a higher rate in the invasively treated patients only in the oldest age group. However, as we did not know the time point of complications' appearance during hospitalization, we cannot exclude that bleeding complications might have been present before invasive therapy. In summary, our results regarding short-term survival confirmed the previously reported benefit of invasive therapy in AMI patients up to 84 years [5, 31–35]. However, we cannot exclude that the benefit of invasive therapy coexists with a higher risk of major bleeding in patients above 74 years of age as reported previously [1, 5].

Strength and limitations

Major strength of our study is the setting in a population-based registry with patients consecutively hospitalized with all types of AMI and data collection performed soon after the AMI during the hospital stay. Furthermore, our research covers recent data up to 2012. Despite adjustment for a number of variables, residual confounding cannot be entirely excluded due to further unknown comorbidities or complications such as frailty, cancer and cognitive and physical function, which could have influenced decision to perform an invasive therapy and also short-term mortality. As we do not have information on Killip class, GRACE risk score and comorbid anemia for patients included in this study, we were not able to analyze these potential predictors of clinical decision-making in today's real-life patient care. In addition, we were not able to address the issue of contraindications or eligibility to the use of invasive procedures, and documented reasons for non-invasive therapy were not assessed in our registry. Finally, our results are limited to AMI- patients who survived at least 24 h after hospitalization and were between 26 and 84 years old.

Conclusion

In today's real-life patient care we found that NSTEMI, BBB, prior stroke, reduced LVEF, absence of hyperlipidemia, and low CPK level were the strongest predictors for non-invasive therapy in all age groups. Stratifying the analysis by type of AMI revealed more independent predictors in patients with NSTEMI compared to STEMI. Further research is necessary to investigate the real reasons for non-invasive therapy, especially among elderly women. Moreover, we confirmed that invasive therapy was independently associated with short-term survival benefit regardless of patient's age.

Abbreviations

AC, Age category; ACEIs/ARBs, Angiotensin-converting-enzyme inhibitors and/or angiotensin receptor blockers; ACS, Acute coronary syndrome; AMI, Acute myocardial infarction; BBB, Bundle branch block; CABG, Coronary artery bypass grafting; CI, Confidence interval; CPK, Creatine phosphokinase; KORA, Cooperative health research in the region of Augsburg; LVEF, Left ventricular ejection fraction; MI, Myocardial infarction; MONICA, Monitoring trends and determinants in cardiovascular disease; NSTEMI, Non-ST segment elevation myocardial infarction; OR, Odds ratio; PCI, Percutaneous coronary intervention; STEMI, ST-segment elevation myocardial infarction.

Acknowledgements

The KORA research platform and the MONICA Augsburg studies were initiated and financed by the Helmholtz Zentrum München, German Research Center for Environmental Health, which is funded by the German Federal Ministry of Education, Science, Research and Technology and by the State of Bavaria. Since the year 2000, the collection of MI data has been co-financed by the German Federal Ministry of Health to provide population-based MI morbidity data for the official German Health Report (see www.gbe-bund.de). Steering partners of the MONICA/KORA Infarction Registry, Augsburg, include the KORA research platform, Helmholtz Zentrum München and the Department of Internal Medicine I, Cardiology, Central Hospital of Augsburg.

We thank all members of the Helmholtz Zentrum München, Institute of Epidemiology II and the field staff in Augsburg who were involved in the planning and conduct of the study. We wish to thank the local health departments, the office-based physicians and the clinicians of the hospitals within the study area for their support. Finally, we express our appreciation to all study participants.

Funding

None.

Authors' contributions

UA and CM conceived the study. UA performed the statistical analyses and drafted the manuscript. CM, MH, CT, BK and AP contributed to data acquisition. IK, CM, CT, BK, AP and MH critically revised the manuscript. All authors read and approved the final manuscript.

Competing interests

The authors declare that they have no competing interests.

Author details

[1]MONICA/KORA Myocardial Infarction Registry, Central Hospital of Augsburg, Stenglinstr. 2, 86156 Augsburg, Germany. [2]Institute of Epidemiology II, Helmholtz Zentrum München, German Research Center for Environmental Health (GmbH), Neuherberg, Germany. [3]Department of Internal Medicine I - Cardiology, Central Hospital of Augsburg, Augsburg, Germany. [4]Department of Internal Medicine/Cardiology, Hospital of Nördlingen, Nördlingen, Germany.

References

1. Hamm CW, Bassand JP, Agewall S, Bax J, Boersma E, Bueno H, et al. ESC guidelines for the management of acute coronary syndromes in patients presenting without persistent ST-segment elevation: the task force for the management of acute coronary syndromes (ACS) in patients presenting without persistent ST-segment elevation of the European Society of Cardiology (ESC). Eur Heart J. 2011;32:2999–3054.

2. Task Force on the management of ST-segment elevation acute myocardial infarction of the European Society of Cardiology (ESC), Steg PG, James SK, Atar D, Badano LP, Blömstrom-Lundqvist C, et al. ESC Guidelines for the management of acute myocardial infarction in patients presenting with ST-segment elevation. Eur Heart J. 2012;33:2569–619.

3. O'Gara PT, Kushner FG, Ascheim DD, Casey Jr DE, Chung MK, de Lemos JA, et al. 2013 ACCF/AHA guideline for the management of ST-elevation myocardial infarction: a report of the American College of Cardiology Foundation/American Heart Association Task Force on Practice Guidelines. Circulation. 2013;127:e362–425.

4. Jneid H, Anderson JL, Wright RS, Adams CD, Bridges CR, Casey Jr DE, et al. 2012 ACCF/AHA focused update of the guideline for the management of patients with unstable angina/Non-ST-elevation myocardial infarction (updating the 2007 guideline and replacing the 2011 focused update): a report of the American College of Cardiology Foundation/American Heart Association Task Force on practice guidelines. Circulation. 2012;126:875–910.

5. Alexander KP, Newby LK, Cannon CP, Armstrong PW, Gibler WB, Rich MW, et al. Acute coronary care in the elderly, part I: Non-ST-segment-elevation acute coronary syndromes: a scientific statement for healthcare professionals from the American Heart Association Council on Clinical Cardiology: in collaboration with the Society of Geriatric Cardiology. Circulation. 2007;115:2549–69.

6. Jernberg T, Johanson P, Held C, Svennblad B, Lindbäck J, Wallentin L, SWEDEHEART/RIKS-HIA. Association between adoption of evidence-based treatment and survival for patients with ST-elevation myocardial infarction. JAMA. 2011;305:1677–84.

7. Eagle KA, Nallamothu BK, Mehta RH, Granger CB, Steg PG, Van de Werf F, et al. Trends in acute reperfusion therapy for ST-segment elevation myocardial infarction from 1999 to 2006: we are getting better but we have got a long way to go. Eur Heart J. 2008;29:609–17.

8. McNamara RL, Chung SC, Jernberg T, Holmes D, Roe M, Timmis A, et al. International comparisons of the management of patients with non-ST segment elevation acute myocardial infarction in the United Kingdom, Sweden, and the United States: The MINAP/NICOR, SWEDEHEART/RIKS-HIA, and ACTION Registry-GWTG/NCDR registries. Int J Cardiol. 2014;175:240–7.

9. Hall M, Laut K, Dondo TB, Alabas OA, Brogan RA, Gutacker N, et al. Patient and hospital determinants of primary percutaneous coronary intervention in England, 2003–2013. Heart. 2016. doi:10.1136/heartjnl-2015-308616 [Epub ahead of print].

10. Cohen M, Boiangiu C, Abidi M. Therapy for ST-segment elevation myocardial infarction patients who present late or are ineligible for reperfusion therapy. J Am Coll Cardiol. 2010;55:1895–906.

11. Gharacholou SM, Alexander KP, Chen AY, Wang TY, Melloni C, Gibler WB, et al. Implications and reasons for the lack of use of reperfusion therapy in patients with ST-segment elevation myocardial infarction: findings from the CRUSADE initiative. Am Heart J. 2010;159:757–63.

12. Eagle KA, Goodman SG, Avezum A, Budaj A, Sullivan CM, López-Sendón J, GRACE Investigators. Practice variation and missed opportunities for reperfusion in ST-segment-elevation myocardial infarction: findings from the Global Registry of Acute Coronary Events (GRACE). Lancet. 2002;359:373–7.

13. Wood FO, Leonowicz NA, Vanhecke TE, Dixon SR, Grines CL. Mortality in patients with ST-segment elevation myocardial infarction who do not undergo reperfusion. Am J Cardiol. 2012;110:509–14.

14. Meisinger C, Hormann A, Heier M, Kuch B, Löwel H. Admission blood glucose and adverse outcomes in non-diabetic patients with myocardial infarction in the reperfusion era. Int J Cardiol. 2006;113:229–35.

15. Kuch B, Heier M, von Scheidt W, Kling B, Hoermann A, Meisinger C. 20-year trends in clinical characteristics, therapy and short-term prognosis in acute myocardial infarction according to presenting electrocardiogram: the MONICA/KORA AMI Registry (1985–2004). J Intern Med. 2008;264:254–64.

16. Alpert JS, Thygesen K, Antman E, Bassand JP. Myocardial infarction redefined—a consensus document of the Joint European Society of Cardiology/American College of Cardiology Committee for the Redefinition of Myocardial Infarction. J Am Coll Cardiol. 2000;36:959–69.

17. Rittger H, Schnupp S, Sinha AM, Breithardt OA, Schmidt M, Zimmermann S, et al. Predictors of treatment in acute coronary syndromes in the elderly: impact on decision making and clinical outcome after interventional versus conservative treatment. Catheter Cardiovasc Interv. 2012;80:735–43.

18. Amsterdam EA, Wenger NK, Brindis RG, Casey Jr DE, Ganiats TG, Holmes Jr DR, et al. 2014 AHA/ACC guideline for the management of patients with non-ST-elevation acute coronary syndromes: executive summary: a report of the American College of Cardiology/American Heart Association Task Force on Practice Guidelines. Circulation. 2014;130: 2354–94.

19. Mandeep S, Ralph S, Harvey W. Importance of frailty in patients with. Importance of frailty in patients with cardiovascular disease. Eur Heart J. 2014;35:1726–1731.

20. Radovanovic D, Seifert B, Urban P, Eberli FR, Rickli H, Bertel O, et al. Validity of Charlson Comorbidity Index in patients hospitalised with acute coronary syndrome. Insights from the nationwide AMIS Plus registry 2002–2012. Heart. 2014;100:288–94.

21. Murali-Krishnan R, Iqbal J, Rowe R, Hatem E, Parviz Y, Richardson J, et al. Impact of frailty on outcomes after percutaneous coronary intervention: a prospective cohort study. Open Heart. 2015;2, e000294. doi:10.1136/openhrt-2015-000294.

22. Moretti C, Iqbal J, Murray S, Bertaina M, Parviz Y, Fenning S, et al. Prospective assessment of a palliative care tool to predict one-year mortality in patients with acute coronary syndrome. Eur Heart J Acute Cardiovasc Care. 2016; [Epub ahead of print]

23. Cohen M, Gensini GF, Maritz F, Gurfinkel EP, Huber K, Timerman A, et al. Prospective evaluation of clinical outcomes after acute ST-elevation myocardial infarction in patients who are ineligible for reperfusion therapy: preliminary results from the TETAMI registry and randomized trial. Circulation. 2003;108 Suppl 1:III14–21.

24. Cohen M, Gensini GF, Maritz F, Gurfinkel EP, Huber K, Timerman A, et al. The role of gender and other factors as predictors of not receiving reperfusion therapy and of outcome in ST-segment elevation myocardial infarction. J Thromb Thrombolysis. 2005;19:155–61.

25. Birkemeyer R, Schneider H, Rillig A, Ebeling J, Akin I, Kische S, et al. Do gender differences in primary PCI mortality represent a different adherence to guideline recommended therapy? a multicenter observation. BMC Cardiovasc Disord. 2014;14:71. doi:10.1186/1471-2261-14-71.

26. Jneid H, Fonarow GC, Cannon CP, Hernandez AF, Palacios IF, Maree AO, et al. Sex differences in medical care and early death after acute myocardial infarction. Circulation. 2008;118:2803–10.

27. Leurent G, Garlantézec R, Auffret V, Hacot JP, Coudert I, Filippi E. Gender differences in presentation, management and inhospital outcome in patients with ST-segment elevation myocardial infarction: data from 5000 patients included in the ORBI prospective French regional registry. Arch Cardiovasc Dis. 2014;107:291–8.

28. Pilgrim T, Heg D, Tal K, Erne P, Radovanovic D, Windecker S, et al. Age- and Gender-related Disparities in Primary Percutaneous Coronary Interventions for Acute ST-segment elevation Myocardial Infarction. PLoS One. 2015;10, e0137047. doi:10.1371/journal.pone.0137047.

29. Lawesson SS, Alfredsson J, Fredrikson M, Swahn E. A gender perspective on short- and long term mortality in ST-elevation myocardial infarction–a report from the SWEDEHEART register. Int J Cardiol. 2013;168:1041–7.

30. Shanmugasundaram M, Alpert JS. Acute coronary syndrome in the elderly. Clin Cardiol. 2009;32:608–13.

31. Carro A, Kaski JC. Myocardial infarction in the elderly. Aging Dis. 2011;2:116–37.

32. Schiele F, Meneveau N, Seronde MF, Descotes-Genon V, Oettinger J, Ecarnot F, et al. Changes in management of elderly patients with myocardial infarction. Eur Heart J. 2009;30:987–94.

33. Tjia J, Allison J, Saczynski JS, Tisminetzky M, Givens JL, Lapane K, et al. Encouraging trends in acute myocardial infarction survival in the oldest old. Am J Med. 2013;126:798–804.

34. Di Bari M, Balzi D, Fracchia S, Barchielli A, Orso F, Sori A, et al. Decreased usage and increased effectiveness of percutaneous coronary intervention in complex older patients with acute coronary syndromes. Heart. 2014;100: 1537–42.

35. Amann U, Kirchberger I, Heier M, von Scheidt W, Kuch B, Peters A, et al. Acute myocardial infarction in the elderly: treatment strategies and 28-day-case fatality from the MONICA/KORA Myocardial Infarction Registry. Catheter Cardiovasc Interv. 2015. doi:10.1002/ccd.26159.

3

The impact of social deprivation on mortality following acute myocardial infarction, stroke or subarachnoid haemorrhage: A record linkage study

Kymberley Thorne[*], John G. Williams, Ashley Akbari and Stephen E. Roberts

Abstract

Background: The impact of social deprivation on mortality following acute myocardial infarction (AMI), stroke and subarachnoid haemorrhage (SAH) is unclear. Our objectives were, firstly, to determine, for each condition, whether there was higher mortality following admission according to social deprivation and secondly, to determine how any higher mortality for deprived groups may be correlated with factors including patient demographics, timing of admission and hospital size.

Methods: Routinely collected, linked hospital inpatient, mortality and primary care data were analysed for patients admitted as an emergency to hospitals in Wales between 2004 and 2011 with AMI ($n = 30{,}663$), stroke (37,888) and SAH (1753). Logistic regression with Bonferroni correction was used to examine, firstly, any significant increases in mortality with social deprivation quintile and, secondly, the influence of patient demographics, timing of admission and hospital characteristics on any higher mortality among the most socially deprived groups.

Results: Mortality was 14.3 % at 30 days for AMI, 21.4 % for stroke and 35.6 % for SAH. Social deprivation was significantly associated with higher mortality for AMI (25 %; 95 % CI = 12 %, 40 %) higher for quintile V compared with I), stroke (24 %; 14 %, 34 %), and non-significantly for SAH (32 %; −7 %, 87 %).
The higher mortality at 30 days with increased social deprivation varied significantly according to patient age for AMI patients and time period for SAH. It was also highest for both AMI and stroke patients, although not significantly for female patients, for admissions on weekdays and during autumn months.

Conclusions: We have demonstrated a positive association between social deprivation and higher mortality following emergency admissions for both AMI and stroke. The study findings also suggest that the influence of patient demographics, timing of admission and hospital size on social inequalities in mortality are quite similar for AMI and stroke.

Keywords: Mortality, Social deprivation, Risk factors, Acute myocardial infarction, Stroke, Subarachnoid haemorrhage

Background

Acute myocardial infarction (AMI), stroke and subarachnoid haemorrhage (SAH) are all associated with high mortality following hospitalisation [1]. Some research suggests that mortality rates are significantly higher for more deprived than more affluent patients following admission for cardiovascular disease [2–6], stroke [3, 7–13] and SAH [8, 14]. Possible reasons include patient comorbidities, poor diet, obesity and other lifestyle risk factors, as well as differences in health seeking behaviours and inequalities in access to and compliance with treatment and care. However, other studies have reported either no significant association with mortality for cardiovascular diseases [15–17] and stroke [18–20], or that mortality was lower with increased social deprivation for cardiovascular conditions [21, 22] and stroke [23].

There is a lack of evidence for the reasons why social deprivation inequalities in mortality following admission for AMI, stroke or SAH may be affected by factors including patient demographics, timing of admission and the size of the hospital. It is possible that day of the week, year of admission and hospital size could act as

* Correspondence: k.thorne@swansea.ac.uk
College of Medicine, Swansea University, Singleton Park, Swansea SA2 8PP, UK

possible mediators of the relationship between social deprivation and 30 day mortality for AMI, stroke and SAH. If so, we hypothesise that deprived cases would have a worse prognosis if admitted on weekdays and public holidays as any social inequalities in access to urgent investigative and therapeutic services and surgery may be widened by reduced operational levels of services at weekends. Additionally, it has been reported that affluent patients get to hospital sooner following a stroke [9] which may be linked to the admitting hospital's location and size.

In order to explore these possibilities, we investigated associations between social deprivation and mortality following AMI, stroke and SAH in a large population in the UK. The first objective of this study was to determine, for each condition, whether there was higher mortality at 30 days following admission according to social deprivation. Secondly, we determined how any higher mortality for deprived groups may be correlated with factors such as patient demographics, timing of admission and hospital size.

Methods
Study design
To address these study objectives, we used systematic record linkage of national inpatient, mortality and primary care data across Wales (population 3 million). All records were held within the Secure Anonymised Information Linkage (SAIL) Databank, which includes the Patient Episode Database for Wales (PEDW) and the Welsh Administrative Register (AR). All records were linked using a unique anonymised linking field (ALF) for each patient based primarily on the patient's National Health Service (NHS) number and secondly, on other anonymised patient identifiers such as date of birth, gender, postcode and first name and surname by applying a probabilistic matching algorithm MACRAL (Matching Algorithm for Consistent Results in Anonymised Linkage). More details on the SAIL databank and the MACRAL methodology can be found in articles by Lyons et al. and Ford et al. to confirm the accuracy of linkage using this method [24, 25].

To identify all deaths that occurred following discharge from hospital as well as in hospital, the inpatient data were systematically linked to death certificate data from the Office for National Statistics (ONS) and the Welsh AR. Linkage was possible for 100 % of patients in our dataset.

To obtain information on comorbidities recorded from primary care consultations as well as inpatient admissions over the previous 5 years, the inpatient data were also linked to SAIL national primary care data. The SAIL databank has access to 40 % of GP practice data in Wales (approximately 1 million records). We also adjusted for whether each patient had a previous GP or inpatient visit been to eliminate any bias during logistic regression modelling.

Ethics statement
Ethical approval and patient consent for the study data was not required as we were using pseudo-anonymised data. Study approval was obtained instead from the Information Governance Review Panel, which is represented by the National Research Ethics Service, the British Medical Association Ethics Advisor, the Caldicott Guardians and NHS Wales Informatics Service. The linked study data sources we used are publicly available to other researchers.

Inclusion and exclusion criteria
We selected all emergency admissions to Welsh hospitals where AMI, stroke or SAH were recorded as the principal diagnosis on the discharge record. The International Classification of Diseases tenth revision (ICD-10) codes used for the three conditions were I21, I61–64 and I60 respectively. We included patients aged 18 years or over, admitted between January 1st 2004 and December 31st 2011 and followed them up for 12 months. Admissions were excluded if they were not emergencies (e.g. elective) or if they occurred within 365 days of a previous admission's discharge date.

Mortality
Mortality rates at 30 days following the admission were used as the primary outcome measure and at 7 days and 365 days as secondary outcome measures. Thirty day mortality is a common outcome measure in the literature. Mortality was based on all causes of death. We included deaths occurring during the inpatient stay and those occurring following discharge.

Social deprivation
Social deprivation for the Welsh population was measured using the Welsh Index of Multiple Deprivation (WIMD) 2008 [26], produced by the Welsh Assembly Government. It is an area-based measure consisting of seven separate domains of deprivation: 'income' (23.5 % contribution), 'employment' (23.5 %), 'health' (14 %), 'education' (14 %), 'access to services' (10 %), 'housing' (5 %), 'physical environment' (5 %) and 'community safety' (5 %). It is based on 1896 Lower Super Output Areas (average population = ~1500 each) and provides a deprivation score which was ranked and assigned to one of five deprivation quintiles (I = least deprived and V = most deprived quintile).

Risk factors

We assessed the following key risk factors to determine whether they significantly mediated the relationship between social deprivation and mortality at 30 days following admission, comparing the least and most deprived cases, using the least deprived quintile as the reference group.

Patient demographics

The patient's age on admission was collected for each case. Age was grouped into "<65 years", "65 to 74 years", "75 to 84 years" and "85+ years" The patient's gender was also recorded.

Timing of admission

We investigated any impact of the day of admission on mortality by assigning weekdays (Monday 00:00 to Friday 23:59), weekends (Saturday 00:00 to Sunday 23:59) and public holiday (8 per year) with public holidays prioritised over weekdays and weekends in this classification. We also investigated the season of admission (winter = Dec to Feb; spring = Mar to May; summer = Jun to Aug; autumn = Sept to Nov) and grouped year of admission ("2004–2005", "2006–2008" and "2009–2011").

Hospital size

Hospital size at the time of admission was included with the following categories: "Small District General Hospital (DGH) (100–399 beds)", "medium DGH (400–599 beds)", "large DGH (600+ beds)" and "community hospital (less than 100 beds)".

Patient comorbidities

When investigating mortality, we also adjusted for age group, gender and comorbidities. Specifically, we adjusted for any impact of the following 11 major patient comorbidities recorded in any diagnostic position during the admission, or within the previous 5 years from primary and inpatient care records where available: ischaemic heart disease (I20–I25) or other cardiovascular diseases (I00–I15, I26–I52), cerebrovascular disease (I60–I69), other circulatory diseases (I70–I99), malignancies (C00–C97), chronic obstructive pulmonary disease (J40–J44), asthma (J45–J46), diabetes (E10–E14), dementia (F00–F03, F05.1, G30), liver disease (K70–K77) and renal failure (N17–N19) [27].

Sample size calculations

Detecting a 30 % increased risk in adjusted mortality for quintile V compared to quintile I based on mortality rates of 35, 15 and 20 % for AMI, stroke and SAH respectively and using 80 % power and 5 % significance, would require 1150 AMI cases, 805 stroke cases and 360 SAH cases in each quintile.

Methods of analysis

The main study outcome measures were percentage mortality rates and odds of mortality for quintile V versus quintile I at 30 days following admission for each condition. Secondary outcome measures were mortality rates and odds of mortality at 7 and 365 days.

Logistic regression was undertaken to establish, firstly, any increased odds of mortality associated with social deprivation at 7 and 30 days after admission. Secondly, it was used to establish how any higher mortality for deprived groups may be related to key risk factors including patient demographics, timing of admission and hospital size. To do this, we compared mortality in the least and most deprived quintiles, using the least deprived quintile as the reference category, for each individual strata in the risk factors; patient age group, sex, week day, season and time period of admission and hospital size. Thirdly, logistic regression was used to test for any interaction effects on mortality between social deprivation and, respectively, each of the study risk factors.

All logistic regression analyses adjusted for age, gender and the eleven patient comorbidities. To eliminate possible biases in the determination of patient co-morbidities from primary and secondary care diagnoses over the preceding 5 years, we also adjusted for patients with no previous inpatient admissions or primary care consultations. The logistic regression mortality odds ratios were presented with 95 % confidence intervals. Significance was measured at the conventional 5 % level.

There were no missing data for any factor other than patient gender and social deprivation (WIMD). For gender, one case admitted with AMI was missing. For WIMD, data was not available for the patients who were not normally resident in Wales. This equated to 3.2 % of AMI cases, 2.4 % of stroke cases and 3.1 % of SAH cases.

A Bonferroni correction was applied to account for multiple statistical tests for each condition. Results were displayed in tables to indicate whether they were significant before and after the correction was applied, although the text only refers to results significant after the correction was applied.

Results

There were 30,663 cases of AMI, 37,888 cases of stroke and 1753 cases of SAH admitted as emergencies between January 2004 and December 2011. The mean age at admission was 70.9 years ± 13.8 for AMI, 75.7 years ± 12.7 for stroke and 60.7 years ± 16.0 for SAH. Males accounted for 60.2 %, 47.3 % and 36.5 % of cases respectively.

Mortality and social deprivation

Mortality at 30 days was 14.3 % following admission for AMI, 21.4 % for stroke and 35.6 % for SAH (see Table 1). Corresponding mortality at 7 days for AMI, stroke and

Table 1 Admission numbers, mortality rates and adjusted odds ratios at 7, 30 and 365 days following hospitalisation, 2004–2012

Condition	Risk factor	Admissions (n)	7 days mortality rate	7 days OR (95 % CI)[b]	30 days mortality rate	30 days OR (95 % CI)[b]	365 days mortality rate	365 days OR (95 % CI)[b]
AMI	**All cases**	30,663	9.2 %	-	14.3 %	-	24.6 %	-
	Age							
	<65y	9827	2.8 %	-	4.0 %	-	6.2 %	-
	65–74y	7088	7.4 %	-	10.6 %	-	17.2 %	-
	75–84y	8382	12.7 %	-	19.6 %	-	34.3 %	-
	85y+	5366	17.7 %	-	29.5 %	-	52.8 %	-
	Gender							
	Male	18,456	7.7 %	Ref	11.9 %	Ref	20.5 %	Ref
	Female	12,206	11.4 %	**1.09 (1.00, 1.18)**	17.8 %	1.07 (0.99, 1.15)	30.8 %	**1.10 (1.03, 1.17)**
	Social deprivation							
	I (Least deprived)	4776	8.9 %	Ref	14.5 %	Ref	25.3 %	Ref
	II	5527	8.7 %	1.04 (0.90, 1.19)	13.4 %	0.97 (0.86, 1.09)	23.6 %	0.98 (0.89, 1.09)
	III	6579	9.1 %	1.11 (0.97, 1.27)	14.3 %	1.07 (0.96, 1.20)	25.4 %	1.12 (1.01, 1.23)
	IV	6460	9.6 %	**1.23 (1.07, 1.40)**	15.0 %	**1.17 (1.05, 1.31)**	25.3 %	**1.13 (1.02, 1.24)**
	V (Most deprived)	6342	9.9 %	**1.34[a] (1.17, 1.53)**	15.0 %	**1.25[a] (1.12, 1.40)**	25.3 %	**1.20[a] (1.08, 1.32)**
Stroke	**All cases**	37,888	11.6 %	-	21.4 %	-	37.7 %	-
	Age							
	<65y	6779	7.9 %	-	10.9 %	-	5.9 %	-
	65–74y	7989	9.4 %	-	14.9 %	-	25.1 %	-
	75–84y	13,171	11.7 %	-	21.6 %	-	39.6 %	-
	85y+	9949	15.7 %	-	33.4 %	-	60.4 %	-
	Gender							
	Male	17,936	9.8 %	Ref	17.6 %	Ref	32.1 %	Ref
	Female	19,952	13.1 %	**1.25[a] (1.16, 1.33)**	24.7 %	**1.21[a] (1.15, 1.3)**	42.8 %	**1.23[a] (1.17, 1.29)**
	Social deprivation							
	I (Least deprived)	6390	11.3 %	Ref	20.9 %	Ref	37.2 %	Ref
	II	6803	11.3 %	1.01 (0.91, 1.13)	21.7 %	**1.09 (1.00, 1.19)**	39.1 %	**1.13[a] (1.05, 1.22)**
	III	8078	12.2 %	**1.12 (1.01, 1.24)**	22.2 %	**1.12 (1.04, 1.22)**	38.7 %	**1.12 (1.04, 1.21)**
	IV	7817	11.3 %	1.05 (0.95, 1.17)	20.5 %	1.06 (0.97, 1.15)	37.5 %	**1.12 (1.04, 1.20)**
	V (Most deprived)	7886	11.9 %	**1.17 (1.05, 1.30)**	22.0 %	**1.24[a] (1.14, 1.34)**	37.9 %	**1.23[a] (1.15, 1.33)**

Table 1 Admission numbers, mortality rates and adjusted odds ratios at 7, 30 and 365 days following hospitalisation, 2004–2012 *(Continued)*

SAH							
All cases	1753	26.9 %	-	35.6 %	-	40.4 %	-
Age							
<65y	1043	22.5 %	-	27.0 %	-	28.9 %	-
65–74y	317	29.7 %	-	41.0 %	-	47.3 %	-
75–84y	266	34.6 %	-	54.1 %	-	62.4 %	-
85y+	127	40.2 %	-	53.5 %	-	70.5 %	-
Gender							
Male	634	26.8 %	Ref	35.6 %	Ref	40.5 %	Ref
Female	1119	27.0 %	1.08 (0.85, 1.37)	35.6 %	1.03 (0.82, 1.29)	40.3 %	1.00 (0.80, 1.25)
Social deprivation							
I (Least deprived)	291	28.2 %	Ref	34.7 %	Ref	40.0 %	Ref
II	318	25.8 %	0.91 (0.62, 1.34)	35.5 %	1.09 (0.75, 1.56)	39.6 %	1.02 (0.71, 1.47)
III	366	26.0 %	0.99 (0.69, 1.44)	36.3 %	1.24 (0.88, 1.76)	41.5 %	1.25 (0.88, 1.77)
IV	355	27.0 %	1.10 (0.76, 1.59)	34.9 %	1.19 (0.83, 1.69)	39.4 %	1.13 (0.80, 1.61)
V (Most deprived)	369	27.4 %	1.09 (0.75, 1.58)	36.9 %	1.32 (0.93, 1.87)	42.5 %	1.32 (0.93, 1.88)

Ref = Reference category. Bold font denotes significance at the 5 % level
Gender for 1 case was not recorded for AMI. No WIMD score was available for 3.2 % of AMI cases, 2.4 % of stroke cases or 3.1 % of SAH cases
[a] denotes significance after applying a Bonferroni correction
[b] The OR for sex gender is adjusted for age group and comorbidities. All other facto's were adjusted for age group, gender and comorbidities

SAH was 9.2, 11.6 and 26.9 % and at 365 days it was 24.6, 37.7 and 40.4 % respectively.

Social deprivation was significantly associated with higher mortality at 30 days for AMI (deprivation quintile V = 25 % (95 % CI = 12 %, 40 %, when compared with quintile I), stroke (V = 24 %; 14 %, 34 %; III = 12 %; 4 %, 22 % and II = 9 %; 0 %, 19 %) and there was a non-significant increase for SAH (V = 32 %; −7 %, 87 % - see Table 1). There was also a significant association between social deprivation and mortality at 7 days for AMI (deprivation quintile IV = 23 %; 7 %, 40 % and V = 34 %; 17 %, 53 %), stroke (V = 17 %; 5 %, 30 %) and there was a non-significant increase for SAH (V = 9 %; −25 %, 58 % - see Table 1).

Table 2 shows the numbers of admissions and 30 day mortality rates for each condition and the least and most deprived quintiles (I and V) of patients according to each study each risk factors. For the majority of factors there was a higher 30 day mortality rate for the most deprived quintile compared to the most affluent quintile. The only exceptions were dementia, public holidays, winter and spring admissions and admissions to medium sized hospitals in AMI cases, COPD, diabetes, renal failure, male gender and community hospitals in stroke cases and asthma, diabetes, dementia, female gender, spring admissions and admissions during 2004–05 and 2009–11 for SAH. The data for all five deprivation quintiles can be found as an Additional file 1.

Effect of risk factors on the relationship between mortality and social deprivation

Patient demographics
The higher mortality among the most deprived quintile of patients V, compared with the least deprived quintile I, was most pronounced among patients aged "75–84y" admitted for AMI (32 %; 9 %, 59 %), and stroke (30 %; 13 %, 50 %), and among the 85y + group for SAH (138 %; −49 %, 1004 % - see Table 3). However, when interaction effects on mortality between social deprivation and age group were assessed, they were significant only for AMI ($p = 0.035$).

Mortality for deprivation quintile V compared with I was highest among females for AMI (26 %; 7 %, 49 %) and stroke (36 %; 21 %, 52 %) and among males for AMI (21 %; 3 %, 42 %) and SAH (145 %; 21 %, 395 % - see Table 3) but there were no significant interactions between gender and deprivation on mortality.

Timing of admission
Although mortality for deprivation quintile V versus I was highest for weekday admissions for AMI (27 %; 11 %, 45 %) and stroke (27 %; 15 %, 40 %), there were no significant interactions on mortality between week day of admission and social deprivation for SAH. Deprivation inequalities in mortality were highest for admissions during

the autumn for both AMI (57 %; 23 %, 101 %) and stroke (36 %; 14 %, 62 % - see Table 3) but there was no significant variation in mortality across seasons.

When analysing deprivation-related mortality over time, there was no clear trend for AMI, with inequalities in 2004–2005 and 2009–2011 of 25 % (2 %, 53 %) and 32 % (7 %, 63 %) respectively; see Table 3), or for stroke (31 %; 10 %, 55 % in 2004–2005 and 21 %;5 %, 40 % in 2009–2011). For SAH, there was significantly higher mortality in deprived cases for 2006–2008 (3.54 fold) which was significant ($p = 0.036$).

Hospital size
There was no significant variation in social inequalities in mortality among quintile V versus I according to the size of the admitting hospital for any of the three conditions (Table 3).

First admissions and their effect on mortality with social deprivation
When confining the study to first admissions for AMI, stroke and SAH during the study period, we excluded 1.3 % of AMI cases, 3.8 % of stroke cases and 0.3 % of SAH cases. The mortality rates at 30 days were unchanged at 14.3, 21.4 and 35.6 % respectively and for 7 days were marginally lower at 9.1, 11.5 and 26.9 %. There were no changes to the significance of the interaction effects on mortality between social deprivation and any of the study factors.

Discussion
We found that social deprivation was significantly associated with higher mortality following admissions for AMI and stroke and, although not significantly, for SAH. We also found that the higher mortality at 30 days with increased social deprivation varied significantly according to patient age for AMI patients and time period for SAH. It was also highest for both AMI and stroke patients, although not significantly, for female patients, for admissions on weekdays and during autumn months.

Major strengths of the study are its size, covering more than 30,000 cases of AMI, almost 38,000 cases of stroke and over 1700 cases of SAH. The methodology was based on systematic, validated record linkage of inpatient, death certificate and primary care data to identify all admissions and all deaths that occur during the impatient stay and following discharge from hospital.

As with other large-scale studies that used NHS administrative health data, this study lacked detailed information about stroke severity, patient disease history, treatment allocated and time to treatment. Our study investigated post-hospital mortality for AMI, stroke and SAH, so did not include deaths that occurred rapidly before admission to hospital.

Table 2 Admissions and 30 day mortality rates split by risk factors and social deprivation quintiles

Risk factors	AMI		Stroke		SAH	
	Admissions, % 30 days mortality		Admissions, % 30 days mortality		Admissions, % 30 days mortality	
	I	V	I	V	I	V
Comorbidities						
Ischaemic heart disease (I20–I25)	4776, 14.5 %	6342, 15.0 %	1873, 23.8 %	2726, 23.3 %	35, 45.7 %	83, 45.8 %
Other cardiovascular diseases (I00–I15, I26–I52)	3702, 16.0 %	4887, 16.3 %	5088, 20.3 %	6273, 21.8 %	161, 39.1 %	197, 41.1 %
Cerebrovascular disease (I60–I69)	521, 18.4 %	733, 24.0 %	6390, 20.9 %	7886, 22.0 %	291, 34.7 %	369, 36.9 %
Other circulatory diseases (I70–I99)	1391, 15.0 %	1827, 17.0 %	2289, 18.0 %	2780, 19.2 %	69, 36.2 %	88, 36.4 %
Malignancies (C00–C97)	634, 18.6 %	661, 19.5 %	986, 21.8 %	998, 24.4 %	22, 36.4 %	21, 47.6 %
Chronic obstructive pulmonary disease (J40–J44)	511, 17.6 %	1271, 18.7 %	581, 22.2 %	1433, 21.1 %	20, 40.0 %	43, 44.2 %
Asthma (J45–J46),	470, 12.3 %	864, 13.5 %	548, 17.9 %	994, 18.2 %	25, 44.0 %	53, 30.2 %
Diabetes (E10–E14)	912, 16.1 %	1492, 17.4 %	1089, 22.4 %	1857, 19.8 %	17, 52.9 %	35, 45.7 %
Dementia (F00–F03, F05.1, G30)	215, 29.8 %	318, 28.6 %	686, 25.1 %	945, 25.9 %	6, 66.7 %	12, 33.3 %
Liver disease (K70–K77)	64, 10.9 %	99, 22.2 %	101, 20.8 %	201, 23.4 %	6, 50.0 %	4, 50.0 %
Renal failure (N17–N19)	628, 25.2 %	830, 25.8 %	608, 27.3 %	824, 25.6 %	13, 61.5 %	13, 69.2 %
Age						
< 65y	1324, 3.6 %	2307, 4.9 %	871, 11.1 %	1791, 11.4 %	166, 28.3 %	228, 28.1 %
65–74y	1019, 10.2 %	1465, 13.4 %	1250, 12.8 %	1800, 15.2 %	52, 34.6 %	65, 41.5 %
75–84y	1428, 17.6 %	1576, 22.1 %	2357, 19.9 %	2587, 24.8 %	54, 50.0 %	45, 57.8 %
85 + y	1005, 28.9 %	994, 29.8 %	1912, 31.7 %	1708, 36.1 %	19, 47.4 %	31, 61.3 %
Gender						
Male	2976, 12.3 %	3680, 12.3 %	2996, 18.1 %	3761, 17.5 %	100, 30.0 %	131, 41.2 %
Female	1800, 18.2 %	2662, 18.9 %	3394, 23.4 %	4125, 26.1 %	191, 37.2 %	238, 34.5 %
Day type						
Weekdays (Mon–Fri)	3493, 14.5 %	4617, 15.4 %	4829, 20.3 %	5814, 21.7 %	213, 33.8 %	267, 33.3 %
Weekends (Sat–Sun)	1182, 13.8 %	1600, 14.1 %	1456, 22.7 %	1913, 23.0 %	74, 37.8 %	98, 45.9 %
Public holidays	101, 22.8 %	125, 14.4 %	105, 21.0 %	159, 22.0 %	4, 25.0 %	4, 50.0 %
Season						
Winter	1231, 15.5 %	1673, 15.1 %	1607, 23.1 %	1967, 23.0 %	77, 35.1 %	83, 36.1 %
Spring	1293, 16.9 %	1585, 15.0 %	1601, 20.8 %	2063, 22.4 %	70, 37.1 %	95, 31.6 %
Summer	1125, 13.1 %	1530, 15.0 %	1584, 19.3 %	1974, 20.4 %	70, 27.1 %	100, 38.0 %
Autumn	1127, 12.2 %	1554, 15.1 %	1598, 20.3 %	1882, 22.3 %	74, 39.2 %	91, 41.8 %
Year group						
2004–2005	1382, 16.4 %	1838, 16.9 %	1562, 20.8 %	2062, 23.3 %	69, 40.6 %	114, 33.3 %
2006–2008	1798, 15.2 %	2432, 15.1 %	2353, 22.2 %	3006, 22.6 %	112, 29.5 %	132, 45.5 %
2009–2011	1596, 12.1 %	2072, 13.4 %	2475, 19.7 %	2818, 20.5 %	110, 36.4 %	123, 30.9 %
Hospital size						
Small (100–399 beds)	277, 11.9 %	853, 16.5 %	288, 19.4 %	859, 21.9 %	10, 30.0 %	27, 44.4 %
Medium (400–599 beds)	2133, 15.1 %	3400, 14.3 %	2961, 21.3 %	4271, 22.9 %	102, 39.2 %	184, 38.6 %
Large (600+ beds)	2102, 14.4 %	1867, 15.4 %	2772, 21.7 %	2335, 22.4 %	173, 33.5 %	147, 36.1 %
Community hospitals	264, 14.0 %	222, 17.1 %	369, 12.2 %	421, 11.2 %	6, 0.0 %	11, 0.0 %

Our 30 day mortality rates were comparable with those reported by other NHS-based studies for AMI [28–30], stroke [1, 31, 32] and SAH [31–33]. The significant association between 30 day mortality and deprivation were also consistent with other similar studies of these conditions in the UK [2, 3, 6–8, 22, 23, 34, 35].

Table 3 Mortality rates and adjusted odds ratios at 30 days following hospitalisation for social deprivation quintiles I and V, 2004 to 2012

Risk factor	AMI			Stroke			SAH		
	Mortality rate (Quintile I)	Mortality rate (Quintile V)	30 days mortality OR (95 % CI) [b]	Mortality rate (Quintile I)	Mortality rate (Quintile V)	30 days mortality OR (95 % CI) [b]	Mortality rate (Quintile I)	Mortality rate (Quintile V)	30 days mortality OR (95 % CI) [b]
Age									
< 65y	3.6 %	4.9 %	1.35 (0.94, 1.94)	11.1 %	11.4 %	1.14 (0.88, 1.49)	28.3 %	28.1 %	1.20 (0.72, 2.02)
65–74y	10.2 %	13.4 %	1.28 (0.98, 1.67)	12.8 %	15.2 %	1.22 (0.98, 1.51)	34.6 %	41.5 %	2.03 (0.80, 5.13)
75–84y	17.6 %	22.1 %	**1.32[a] (1.09, 1.59)**	19.9 %	24.8 %	**1.30[a] (1.13, 1.50)**	50.0 %	57.8 %	1.33 (0.53, 3.38)
85+ y	28.9 %	29.8 %	1.06 (0.87, 1.29)	31.7 %	36.1 %	**1.19 (1.03, 1.37)**	47.4 %	61.3 %	2.38 (0.51, 11.04)
Gender									
Male	12.3 %	12.2 %	**1.21 (1.03, 1.42)**	18.1 %	17.5 %	1.11 (0.97, 1.27)	30.0 %	41.2 %	**2.45 (1.21, 4.95)**
Female	18.2 %	18.9 %	**1.26 (1.07, 1.49)**	23.4 %	26.1 %	**1.36[a] (1.21, 1.52)**	37.2 %	34.5 %	1.04 (0.66, 1.65)
Day of the week									
Weekdays (Mon–Fri)	14.5 %	15.4 %	**1.27[a] (1.11, 1.45)**	20.3 %	21.7 %	**1.27[a] (1.15, 1.40)**	33.8 %	33.3 %	1.18 (0.77, 1.82)
Weekends (Sat–Sun)	13.8 %	14.1 %	1.21 (0.96, 1.54)	22.7 %	23.0 %	1.16 (0.98, 1.38)	37.8 %	45.9 %	1.96 (0.86, 4.51)
Public holidays	22.8 %	14.4 %	0.72 (0.32, 1.63)	21.0 %	22.0 %	1.15 (0.59, 2.23)	25.0 %	50.0 %	NA
Season of admission									
Winter	15.5 %	15.1 %	1.09 (0.87, 1.36)	23.1 %	23.0 %	1.10 (0.93, 1.30)	35.1 %	36.1 %	0.98 (0.42, 2.28)
Spring	16.9 %	15.0 %	1.09 (0.87, 1.37)	20.8 %	22.4 %	**1.29 (1.09, 1.53)**	37.1 %	31.6 %	0.99 (0.43, 2.29)
Summer	13.1 %	15.0 %	**1.36 (1.07, 1.72)**	19.3 %	20.4 %	**1.27 (1.06, 1.51)**	27.1 %	38.0 %	2.26 (0.97, 5.24)
Autumn	12.2 %	15.1 %	**1.57[a] (1.23, 2.01)**	20.3 %	22.3 %	**1.36[a] (1.14, 1.62)**	39.2 %	41.8 %	1.76 (0.75, 4.09)
Year of admission									
2004–2005	16.4 %	16.9 %	**1.25 (1.02, 1.53)**	20.8 %	23.3 %	**1.31[a] (1.10, 1.55)**	40.6 %	33.3 %	0.67 (0.27, 1.65)
2006–2008	15.2 %	15.1 %	1.16 (0.96, 1.39)	22.2 %	22.6 %	**1.23[a] (1.07, 1.41)**	29.5 %	45.5 %	**3.54[a] (1.77, 7.07)**
2009–2011	12.1 %	13.4 %	**1.32 (1.07, 1.63)**	19.7 %	20.5 %	**1.21 (1.05, 1.40)**	36.4 %	30.9 %	0.75 (0.40, 1.43)
Hospital size									
Small (100–399 beds)	11.9 %	16.5 %	1.50 (0.96, 2.36)	19.4 %	21.9 %	1.27 (0.89, 1.82)	30.0 %	44.4 %	NA
Medium (400–599 beds)	15.1 %	14.3 %	1.11 (0.94, 1.31)	21.3 %	22.9 %	**1.25[a] (1.11, 1.42)**	39.2 %	38.6 %	1.28 (0.72, 2.29)
Large (600+ beds)	14.2 %	15.4 %	**1.28 (1.06, 1.55)**	21.7 %	22.4 %	**1.20 (1.04, 1.39)**	33.5 %	36.1 %	1.44 (0.84, 2.47)
Community hospitals	14.0 %	17.1 %	1.57 (0.92, 2.69)	12.2 %	11.2 %	1.10 (0.69, 1.76)	0.0 %	0.0 %	NA

Quintile I was used as the reference group. The ORs of quintile V are reported in the table
Bold font denotes significance at the 5 % level
NA The sample size was too small to perform logistic regression
[a] denotes significance after applying a Bonferroni correction
[b] The OR for age group was adjusted for gender and comorbidities; gender was adjusted for age group and comorbidities; all other factors were adjusted for age group, gender and comorbidities

The impact of social deprivation on mortality following acute myocardial infarction, stroke or subarachnoid...

29

Although not statistically significant we found indications of increased social inequalities in mortality among older age groups, which has been reported from a study of AMI patients aged over 65y in Scotland [36], whilst another study based in Wales reported no association between deprivation and mortality for males aged 50–59y [3], supportive of our study findings for our male group.

We found highest deprivation-related mortality for admissions in autumn for AMI and stroke and in summer for SAH. However, there was no significant overall interaction effect between season and social deprivation on mortality.

Our study found no significant change over time in deprivation-related mortality for AMI and stroke from 2004–05 to 2009–11 as most of the fixed year groups analysed showed increased mortality in deprived groups. For AMI the difference was 25 % in 2004–05 and 32 % in 2009–11, and for stroke it was 31 and 21 %. There was a significantly higher, social inequality in mortality for SAH for 2006–2008 than in the other year groups.

Previous studies have reported a reduced likelihood of receiving appropriate, timely treatment for more deprived cases, and therefore, poorer outcomes for stroke [37] and cardiovascular conditions [38, 39], particularly if patients are older [40]. Deprived patients are also known to be less likely to attend or complete rehabilitation following cardiovascular conditions [40–42], which may negatively impact on outcomes.

Admissions to small hospitals showed the highest social inequality in mortality although this was not significant. This finding is supported by an American study comparing mortality rates in large and small hospitals [43]. In some cases the most severe cases are triaged or transferred to the largest hospitals, which increases mortality risks in these hospitals. However, hospital size should be regarded only as a possible indicator, since there were only four 'large' hospitals in our study population.

When considering the findings of this study it is important to remember that any association between (postcode-based) deprivation and higher mortality can be subject to ecological fallacy - not everyone living in a deprived area is deprived - and that not all deprived people live in deprived areas. Our measure of area social deprivation is a mixed exposure that due to economic segregation is correlated with both individual and area characteristics. Social deprivation refers to problems caused by a general lack of resources and opportunities and not just money. The association between social deprivation and higher mortality is also multifaceted. Patient-based factors could include the person's health and wellbeing, with deprived people more likely to have single and multiple comorbidities compared with more affluent patients [44], reduced resources (car and home

ownership), lower education status and higher unemployment. Lower social class is associated with lifestyle factors such as smoking and poorer mental health [45] which can also affect prognosis following AMI, stroke and SAH. As such, a patient's baseline clinical and psychological status may largely contribute to any relationship between social deprivation and mortality. We found that the influence of patient demographics, timing of admission and hospital size on social inequalities in mortality are quite similar for AMI and stroke.

Conclusions

To conclude, we have demonstrated a clear association between social deprivation and higher mortality following emergency admission for AMI, stroke and SAH. The study findings also suggest that the influence of patient demographics, timing of admission and hospital size on social deprivation inequalities in mortality are quite similar for AMI and stroke.

Abbreviations
ALF: Anonymised linking field; AMI: Acute myocardial infarction; AR: Administrative Register; DGH: District General Hospital; ICD-10: International Classification of Diseases tenth revision; MACRAL: Matching Algorithm for Consistent Results in Anonymised Linkage; NHS: National Health Service; ONS: Office of National Statistics; PEDW: Patient Episode Database for Wales; SAH: Subarachnoid haemorrhage; SAIL: Secure Anonymised Information Linkage; WIMD: Welsh Index of Multiple Deprivation.

Competing interests
The authors declare that they have no competing interests.

Authors' contributions
KT performed the literature review, analysed the data, interpreted the findings and wrote and edited the manuscript. JGW advised on study design, interpreted the study findings and edited the manuscript. AA programmed and analysed the data, interpreted the study findings and edited the manuscript. SER initiated, designed and led the study, obtained funding, reviewed the literature, supervised the analyses, interpreted the findings and edited the manuscript. All authors approved the final version of the article.

Acknowledgements
This work was supported by the Wellcome Trust [Grant No: 093564/Z/10/Z]. The views expressed in this paper are those of the authors and not necessarily those of the funding body.
The authors are grateful to the Health Information Research Unit (HIRU), College of Medicine, Swansea University, for preparing and providing access to the project specific linked datasets from the SAIL databank, funded by the National Institute of Social Care and Health Research (NISCHR) of the Welsh Government.

References
1. Nichols M et al. Cardiovascular disease in Europe: epidemiological update. Eur Heart J. 2013;34(39):3028–34.

2. Capewell S et al. Age, sex, and social trends in out-of-hospital cardiac deaths in Scotland 1986–95: a retrospective cohort study. Lancet. 2001;358(9289):1213–7.

3. Vescio MF et al. Mortality at ages 50–59 and deprivation at early and late stages of the life course in Wales. J Epidemiol Community Health. 2009;63(1):56–63.

4. Bernheim SM et al. Socioeconomic disparities in outcomes after acute myocardial infarction. Am Heart J. 2007;153(2):313–9.

5. Chang WC et al. Effects of socioeconomic status on mortality after acute myocardial infarction. Am J Med. 2007;120(1):33–9.

6. Morrison C et al. Effect of socioeconomic group on incidence of, management of, and survival after myocardial infarction and coronary death: analysis of community coronary event register. BMJ. 1997;314(7080):541–6.

7. Chen R et al. Socioeconomic deprivation and survival after stroke: findings from the prospective South london stroke register of 1995 to 2011. Stroke. 2014;45(1):217–23.

8. Macleod MR, Andrews PJ. Effect of deprivation and gender on the incidence and management of acute brain disorders. Intensive Care Med. 2002;28(12):1729–34.

9. Macleod MR, Lewis SC, Dennis MS. Effect of deprivation on time to hospital in acute stroke. J Neurol Neurosurg Psychiatry. 2003;74(4):545–6.

10. Jakovljevic D et al. Socioeconomic status and ischemic stroke: The FINMONICA Stroke Register. Stroke. 2001;32(7):1492–8.

11. Kunst AE et al. Socioeconomic inequalities in stroke mortality among middle-aged men: an international overview. European Union Working Group on Socioeconomic Inequalities in Health. Stroke. 1998;29(11):2285–91.

12. Maheswaran R, Elliott P, Strachan DP. Socioeconomic deprivation, ethnicity, and stroke mortality in Greater London and south east England. J Epidemiol Community Health. 1997;51(2):127–31.

13. Ahacic K, Trygged S, Kareholt I. Income and education as predictors of stroke mortality after the survival of a first stroke. Stroke Res Treat. 2012;2012:983145.

14. Jakovljevic D et al. Socioeconomic differences in the incidence, mortality and prognosis of intracerebral hemorrhage in Finnish Adult Population. The FINMONICA Stroke Register. Neuroepidemiology. 2001;20(2):85–90.

15. Hawkins NM et al. The UK National Health Service: delivering equitable treatment across the spectrum of coronary disease. Circ Cardiovasc Qual Outcomes. 2013;6(2):208–16.

16. Picciotto S et al. Associations of area based deprivation status and individual educational attainment with incidence, treatment, and prognosis of first coronary event in Rome, Italy. J Epidemiol Community Health. 2006;60(1):37–43.

17. Fournier S et al. Influence of socioeconomic factors on delays, management and outcome amongst patients with acute myocardial infarction undergoing primary percutaneous coronary intervention. Swiss Med Wkly. 2013;143:w13817.

18. Weir NU et al. Study of the relationship between social deprivation and outcome after stroke. Stroke. 2005;36(4):815–9.

19. Wong KY et al. Effect of social deprivation on mortality and the duration of hospital stay after a stroke. Cerebrovasc Dis. 2006;22(4):251–7.

20. Aslanyan S et al. Effect of area-based deprivation on the severity, subtype, and outcome of ischemic stroke. Stroke. 2003;34(11):2623–8.

21. Barakat K et al. Socioeconomic differentials in recurrent ischaemia and mortality after acute myocardial infarction. Heart. 2001;85(4):390–4.

22. Davies CA, Leyland AH. Trends and inequalities in short-term acute myocardial infarction case fatality in Scotland, 1988–2004. Popul Health Metr. 2010;8:33.

23. Uren Z and Fitzpatrick J. Geographic variations in health (DS No. 16) - Chapter 11. Office of National Statistics; 2001. London: The Stationary Office p. 325–38. http://www.ons.gov.uk/ons/rel/subnational-health3/geographic-variations-in-health–ds-no-16-/2001/index.html

24. Ford DV et al. The SAIL Databank: building a national architecture for e-health research and evaluation. BMC Health Serv Res. 2009;9:157.

25. Lyons RA et al. The SAIL databank: linking multiple health and social care datasets. BMC Med Inform Decis Mak. 2009;9:3.

26. Welsh Assembly Government. Welsh Index of Multiple Deprivation 2008. Cardiff. Welsh Government; 2008. http://gov.wales/docs/statistics/2008/080609wimd2008leafleten.pdf

27. Roberts SE et al. Mortality following acute pancreatitis: social deprivation, hospital size and time of admission: record linkage study. BMC Gastroenterol. 2014;14:153.

28. Gale CP et al. Age-dependent inequalities in improvements in mortality occur early after acute myocardial infarction in 478,242 patients in the Myocardial Ischaemia National Audit Project (MINAP) registry. Int J Cardiol. 2013;168(2):881–7.

29. Chung SC et al. Acute myocardial infarction: a comparison of short-term survival in national outcome registries in Sweden and the UK. Lancet. 2014;383(9925):1305–12.

30. Smolina K et al. Incidence and 30-day case fatality for acute myocardial infarction in England in 2010: national-linked database study. Eur J Public Health. 2012;22(6):848–53.

31. Bamford J et al. A prospective study of acute cerebrovascular disease in the community: the Oxfordshire Community Stroke Project–1981-86. 2. Incidence, case fatality rates and overall outcome at one year of cerebral infarction, primary intracerebral and subarachnoid haemorrhage. J Neurol Neurosurg Psychiatry. 1990;53(1):16–22.

32. Syme PD et al. Community-based stroke incidence in a Scottish population: the Scottish Borders Stroke Study. Stroke. 2005;36(9):1837–43.

33. Pobereskin LH. Incidence and outcome of subarachnoid haemorrhage: a retrospective population based study. J Neurol Neurosurg Psychiatry. 2001;70(3):340–3.

34. Lovelock CE, Rinkel GJ, Rothwell PM. Time trends in outcome of subarachnoid hemorrhage: Population-based study and systematic review. Neurology. 2010;74(19):1494–501.

35. Macpherson KJ et al. Trends in incidence and in short term survival following a subarachnoid haemorrhage in Scotland, 1986–2005: a retrospective cohort study. BMC Neurol. 2011;11:38.

36. Macintyre K et al. Relation between socioeconomic deprivation and death from a first myocardial infarction in Scotland: population based analysis. BMJ. 2001;322(7295):1152–3.

37. Lazzarino AI et al. Inequalities in stroke patients' management in English public hospitals: a survey on 200,000 patients. PLoS One. 2011;6(3), e17219.

38. Taylor FC et al. Socioeconomic deprivation is a predictor of poor postoperative cardiovascular outcomes in patients undergoing coronary artery bypass grafting. Heart. 2003;89(9):1062–6.

39. MacLeod MC et al. Geographic, demographic, and socioeconomic variations in the investigation and management of coronary heart disease in Scotland. Heart. 1999;81(3):252–6.

40. Melville MR et al. Cardiac rehabilitation: socially deprived patients are less likely to attend but patients ineligible for thrombolysis are less likely to be invited. Heart. 1999;82(3):373–7.

41. Pell J et al. Retrospective study of influence of deprivation on uptake of cardiac rehabilitation. BMJ. 1996;313(7052):267–8.

42. Hippisley-Cox J, Pringle M. Inequalities in access to coronary angiography and revascularisation: the association of deprivation and location of primary care services. Br J Gen Pract. 2000;50(455):449–54.

43. Fareed N. Size matters: a meta-analysis on the impact of hospital size on patient mortality. Int J Evid Based Healthc. 2012;10(2):103–11.

44. Charlton J et al. Impact of deprivation on occurrence, outcomes and health care costs of people with multiple morbidity. J Health Serv Res Policy. 2013;18(4):215–23.

45. Fone DL, Dunstan F. Mental health, places and people: a multilevel analysis of economic inactivity and social deprivation. Health Place. 2006;12(3):332–44.

4

Atorvastatin treatment improves effects of implanted mesenchymal stem cells: meta-analysis of animal models with acute myocardial infarction

Guo Dai[1], Qing Xu[1], Rong Luo[1], Jianfang Gao[1], Hui Chen[1], Yun Deng[1], Yongqing Li[1], Yuequn Wang[1], Wuzhou Yuan[1] and Xiushan Wu[1,2]*

Abstract

Background: Previous studies reported that Atorvastatin (ATOR) can improve the efficacy of Mesenchymal stem cells (MSCs) transplantation after acute myocardial infarction (AMI). However, the results of those studies were inconsistent. To clarify the beneficial effects of atorvastatin added to the cell therapy with MSCs in animal model of acute myocardial infarction (AMI), we performed a systematic review and meta-analysis of case–control studies.

Methods: Searches were performed using the PubMed database, the Excerpta Medica Database (Embase), the Science Citation Index, the China National Knowledge Information database, the Wanfang database, and the Chinese Scientific and Technological Journal Database (VIP database). The search term included "Atorvastatin (or Ator)", "Mesenchymal Stem Cells (or Mesenchymal Stem Cell or MSC or MSCs)" and "Acute Myocardial Infarction (or Myocardial Infarction or AMI or MI)". The endpoints were the left ventricular ejection fraction (LVEF) in animal model with AMI.

Results: In total, 5 studies were included in the meta-analysis. Pooled analysis indicated a significant LVEF difference at 4 weeks follow-up between MSCs + ATOR combine group and MSCs alone group (95 % CI, 9.09–13.62 %; $P < 0.01$) with heterogeneity ($P = 0.28$; $P > 0.05$) and inconsistency (I^2: 22 %).

Conclusions: Atorvastatin can enhance the existing effects of MSCs transplantation, and this combinational therapy is a superior cell/pharmacological therapeutic approach that merits future preclinical and clinical studies.

Keywords: Meta-analysis, Acute myocardial infarction, Animal models, Cell therapy, Mesenchymal stem cells

Background

Acute myocardial infarction (AMI) is the leading cause of death among people in industrialized nations [1]. Although early revascularization can save part of ischemic myocardium, necrotic myocardial cells, which cannot regenerate, will gradually be replaced by scar tissue, leading to ventricular remodeling and heart failure, and thus seriously affect the survival rate and quality of life of survivors [2]. Despite the rapid development of therapeutic techniques and ideas, the treatments of heart failure secondary to AMI are still very limited, among which stem cell transplantation is one of the most promising [3].

Due to no strong differentiation of immune rejection and easy to get, the bone marrow-derived mesenchymal stem cells (MSCs) is one of the best sources of transplanted cells. Therefore, MSCs have been widely utilized as a result of their plasticity, availability, and lack of immunological rejection or ethical issues [4]. However, many studies have demonstrated the poor survival and retention of transplanted cells in vivo, whether this is due to properties of the cells themselves, the extremely hostile microenvironment in the per infarct region, or a combination of both [5]. For these reasons the focus has

* Correspondence: xiushanwu@yahoo.com
[1]The Center for Heart Development, Key Laboratory of MOE for Developmental Biology and Protein Chemistry, College of Life Sciences, Hunan Normal University, Changsha, Hunan 410081, P. R. China
[2]The Center for Heart Development, Hunan Normal University, Changsha 410081, Hunan, P. R. China

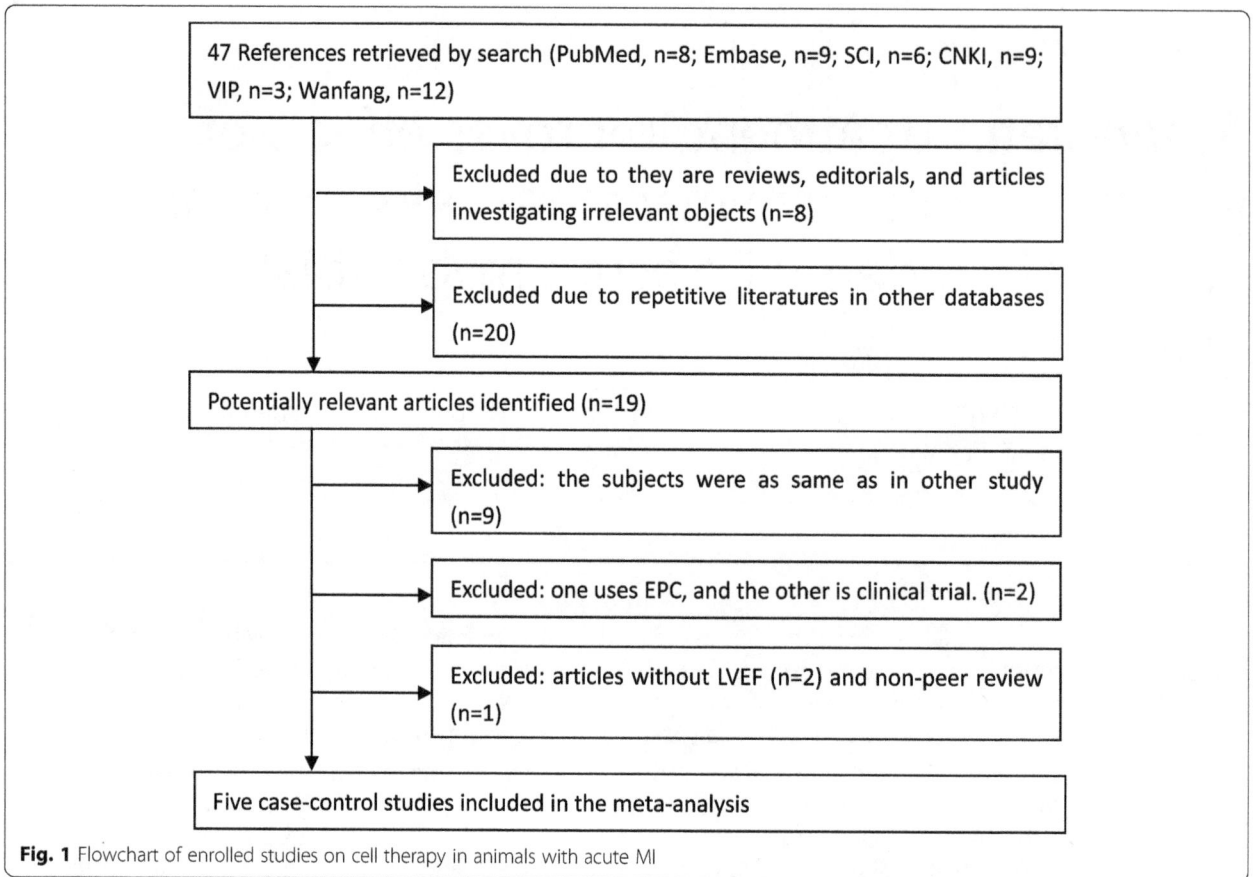

Fig. 1 Flowchart of enrolled studies on cell therapy in animals with acute MI

been on efforts to improve the tolerance of stem cells to the adverse microenvironment, which would hopefully lead to the development of a clinical approach to improve stem cell survival and tissue repair capacity [6].

Recent studies have demonstrated that combined therapy with MSCs and atorvastatin (ATOR), a blood cholesterol-lowering agent, produces synergistic beneficial effects in the treatment of AMI [7]. However, the number of experimental animals in most of studies selected is limited. In addition, many large animal studies in AMI and ischaemic

cardiomyopathy have been conflicting outcomes. We hypothesize that meta-analysis of these experimental data might be helpful to design future clinical studies similarly to the meta-analysis of human cardiac stem cell trials.

We performed a systematic overview of the pertinent literature including a quantitative meta-analysis to assess the effects of stem cell transplantation in animals with acute myocardial infarction. Combined MSCs therapy and pharmacotherapy is one of these proof-in-principle approaches.

Table 1 Characteristics of studies included in the Meta-Analysis

Author (year)	Language	Type of animal	Number of cells	Atorvastatin treatment	Route of delivery	Timing of cell therapy after MI
Zhang Q et al. (2014) [16]	English	Rat	5×10^6cells/animal	10 mg/kg/day	Intramuscularly injection	4 weeks
Qu Z et al. (2013) [17]	English	Rabbit	4×10^7cells/50uL	1.5 mg/kg/day	Intramuscularly injection	4 weeks
Song L et al. (2013) [18]	English	Swine	3×10^7cells/animal	0.25 mg/kg/day	Intramuscularly injection	4 weeks
Cai A et al. (2011) [19]	English	Rat	1×10^6cells /100uL	10 mg/kg/day	Intramuscularly injection	4 weeks
Yang YJ et al. (2008) [20]	English	Swine	3×10^7cells/animal	0.25 mg/kg/day	Intramuscularly injection	4 weeks

Table 2 Methodological quality of the included studies

Study	RCT	Adequate allocation	Method of randomization described	Operator blinded	Analyst blinded
Zhang Q et al. (2014) [16]	Y	N	N	N	N
Qu Z et al. (2013) [17]	Y	N	N	N	N
Song L et al. (2013) [18]	Y	N	N	N	N
Cai A et al. (2011) [19]	Y	N	N	N	N
Yang YJ et al. (2008) [20]	Y	N	N	N	N

RCT Randomized trial, *Y* Yes, *N* No

Methods

Search strategy

The following databases were searched in Dec 2014: PubMed database, the Excerpta Medica Database (Embase), the Science Citation Index, the China National Knowledge Information database, the Wanfang database, and the Chinese Scientific and Technological Journal Database (VIP database).

For the association of ATOR, Mesenchymal Stem Cells and Acute Myocardial Infarction, the following search term were used in searching the previous database: "Atorvastatin (or Ator)", "Mesenchymal Stem Cells (or Mesenchymal Stem Cell or MSC or MSCs)" and "Acute Myocardial Infarction (or Myocardial Infarction or AMI or MI)". No language is limited. In addition, the references of retrieved articles were also screened to find the related papers. In addition, we performed manual searches by scanning the reference lists of the selected articles to locate additional papers related to the topic.

Study selection

Two investigators independently reviewed all studies and extracted the data using a standard information extraction and reached consensus on all items. Only those articles that investigated the effect of ATOR combined with mesenchymal stem cell transplantation on cardiac function in animals with acute myocardial infarction were included. Reviews, editorials, comments, reports from scientific sessions and discussions were excluded. We obtained the full text of articles that were identified as either relevant or possibly relevant, based on their titles and abstracts.

Quality assessment and data extraction

The quality of studies was independently assessed by two reviewers using a risk of bias assessment by van der Spoel TI's studies [8]: including randomization (yes/no), adequate allocation (y/n), adequate method of randomization (y/n), blinding of the operator (y/n), and blinding of the functional analysis (y/n). The following information was extracted from the complete manuscripts of the qualified studies: basal characteristics of the study, the left ventricular ejection fraction (LVEF).

Statistical analysis

Our primary outcome was difference in mean LVEF (reported in %) at follow-up between mesenchymal stem cells transplantation group (MSCs group) and mesenchymal stem cells treated with ATOR transplantation group (MSCs + ATOR group). In case of multiple measurements over time, data measured at the longest duration of follow-up were used for analysis. A random-effect model was applied. Continuous variables were reported as weighted mean differences (WMD) with 95 % confidence intervals (CI) between the cell-treated animals and control groups. In case of data, the pooled estimate of effect was presented as odds ratio (OR) with 95 % CI [9]. Inconsistency was estimated by using the I^2 statistic; values of 25, 50, and 75 % were considered low, moderate, and high inconsistency, respectively [10]. Sensitivity analysis was also performed to test the robustness of the results by excluding a study one by one. All analyses were performed with Review Manager version 5 (The Nordic Cochrane Center, København, Denmark) and IBM SPSS Statistics 19 (SPSS, Chicago, IL, USA).

Table 3 Comparisons of cardiac function measured by echocardiography and hemodynamic examination in animal model of acute myocardial infarction

Study	Type of animal	Control LVEF (%)	Number	MSCs LVEF (%)	n	Ator + MSCs LVEF (%)	Number
Zhang Q et al. (2014) [16]	Rat	48.1 ± 5.2	10	51.9 ± 2.4	10	65.3 ± 5.3	10
Qu Z et al. (2013) [17]	Rabbit	48.67	8	59.14	9	67.32	9
Song L et al. (2013) [18]	Swine	43.16 ± 8.02	6	48.75 ± 12.64	6	49.76 ± 12.09	6
Cai A et al. (2011) [19]	Rat	44.63 ± 3.22	8	46.17 ± 2.03	7	56.78 ± 3.66	7
Yang YJ et al. (2008) [20]	Swine	42.0 ± 7.1	6	41.3 ± 8.8	6	49.7 ± 10.4	7

LVEF (%) The left ventricular ejection fraction, (mean ± SD)

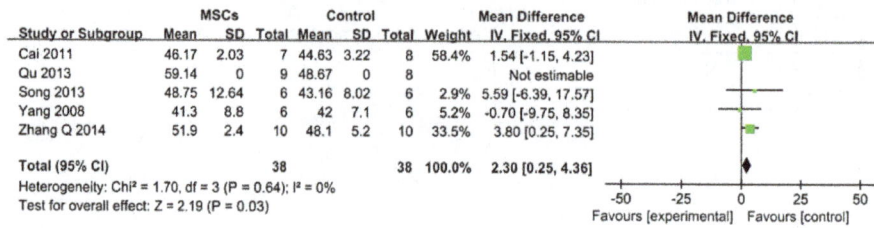

Fig. 2 Forest plot showing the impact of MSCs therapy on LVEF improvement compared with controls

Results

Search results

Totally forty-seven references were retrieved. Among them, twenty were repetitive literatures in other databases; eight literatures were excluded because they are reviews, editorials, and or comments. In the end, five case–control studies were included in the meta-analysis. Figure 1 showed the flow diagram of studies selection.

The quality of studies

The five studies all established an AMI animal model by performing thoracotomy and ligating the left descending coronary artery, and then randomly divided them into three groups: one group of AMI control group, one group of MSC transplantation group, and the third group conducted a joint ATOR and MSC transplantation group. Table 1 lists the eligible studies which included in as well as their main characteristics. Finally, within the four weeks after transplantation, five studies examined the left ventricular ejection fraction (LVEF) by echocardiography. Table 2 show the methodological quality of the enrolled studies. All studies reported the method of randomization, but did not indicate whether blinded analysis of LVEF. Table 3 shows the comparisons of cardiac function measured by echocardiography and hemodynamic examination in animal model of acute myocardial infarction of the enrolled studies.

Meta-analysis

Within the four weeks after transplantation, five studies examined LVEF, including thirty-eight cases in AMI control group, thirty-eight cases of MSC transplantation group, and thirty-nine cases which conducted a joint ATOR and MSC transplantation. Firstly, comparing

MSCs group and control group, it has been found a LVEF difference of 2.30 % at follow-up after MSCs group vs control (95 % CI, 0.25–4.36 %; $P > 0.01$) with inconsistency (I^2: 0 %; Fig. 2), implying that there is no significant difference between MSCs group and control group.

As shown in Fig. 3, pooled analysis showed a LVEF difference of 13.16 % at follow-up after MSCs + ATOR group vs. control (95 % CI, 10.55–15.78 %; $P < 0.01$) with heterogeneity ($P = 0.12$; $P > 0.05$) and inconsistency (I^2: 48 %). The results suggested that, compared with control, MSCs + ATOR contributes more to restoring myocardial infarction cardiac function. As shown in Fig. 4, pooled analysis showed a LVEF difference of 11.35 % at follow-up after MSCs + ATOR group vs. MSCs group (95 % CI, 9.09–13.62 %; $P < 0.01$) with heterogeneity ($P = 0.28$; $P > 0.05$) and inconsistency (I^2: 22 %). The results suggested that, compared with MSCs transplantation alone, MSCs + ATOR contributes more to restoring myocardial infarction cardiac function.

In addition, Sensitivity analysis demonstrated that the result is same as before, indicated that the pooled meta-analysis results is very robust. The funnel plot for LVEF suggests a lack of publication bias as values were evenly distributed around the overall estimate (Fig. 5).

Discussion

Although stem cells are studied clinically for cardiac repair, its effects are still controversial [11]. Some studies have shown that most stem cells were lost within 24 h of transplantation, only 15 % survived for 12 weeks. The quick loss after transplantation is mainly due to cell leakage out of the myocardium or wash-out through the vascular system [9]. Therefore, protection of graft cells from acute death in ischemic myocardium is important for

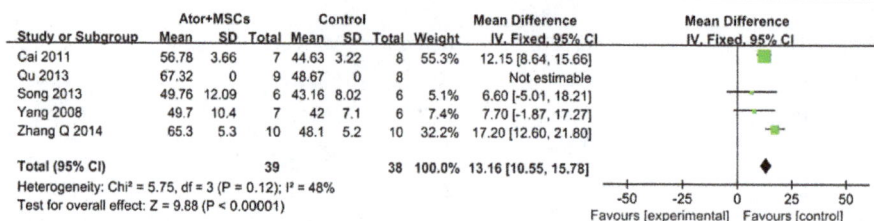

Fig. 3 Forest plot showing the impact of MSCs + Ator therapy on LVEF improvement compared with controls

Atorvastatin treatment improves effects of implanted mesenchymal stem cells: meta-analysis of animal...

35

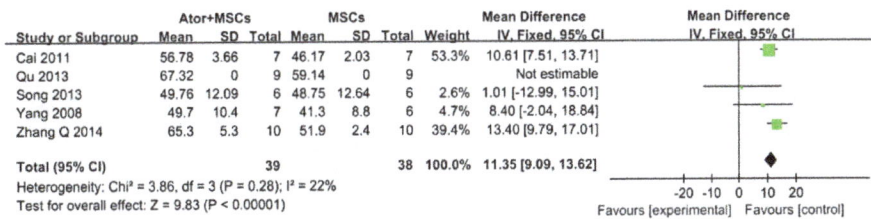

Study or Subgroup	Ator+MSCs			MSCs			Weight	Mean Difference IV, Fixed, 95% CI	Mean Difference IV, Fixed, 95% CI
	Mean	SD	Total	Mean	SD	Total			
Cai 2011	56.78	3.66	7	46.17	2.03	7	53.3%	10.61 [7.51, 13.71]	
Qu 2013	67.32	0	9	59.14	0	9		Not estimable	
Song 2013	49.76	12.09	6	48.75	12.64	6	2.6%	1.01 [-12.99, 15.01]	
Yang 2008	49.7	10.4	7	41.3	8.8	6	4.7%	8.40 [-2.04, 18.84]	
Zhang Q 2014	65.3	5.3	10	51.9	2.4	10	39.4%	13.40 [9.79, 17.01]	
Total (95% CI)			39			38	100.0%	11.35 [9.09, 13.62]	

Heterogeneity: Chi² = 3.86, df = 3 (P = 0.28); I² = 22%
Test for overall effect: Z = 9.83 (P < 0.00001)

Favours [experimental]   Favours [control]

Fig. 4 Forest plot showing the impact of MSCs + Ator therapy on LVEF improvement compared with that of MSCs therapy

clinical applications. Common statins include prava-statin, lovastatin, simvastatin and atorvastatin, which were used agents in patients with coronary heart disease owing to their superior ability to reduce blood choles-terols [12]. Previous studies showed that different types of statins play different roles in the induction of apop-tosis of MSC. Lovastatin and atorvastatin have protective effect [13], while simvastatin can promote apoptosis [14]. The properties of Ator are well predicted to offer improvement of the microenvironment for implanted stem cells [15]. Among them most articles have explored the combination of atorvastatin and MSC to treat myo-cardial infarction.

The current analysis comprises data of five published studies involving animals with AMI, which treated with mesenchymal stem cells or Atorstatin + MSCs [16–20]. We first analyzed the therapy of AMI by MSCs trans-plantation alone. However, it was found compared with the control group, the recovery of ventricular function is limited after transplantation, which might be related to insufficient MSC's survival rate. Subsequently, we ana-lyzed the transplantation of ATOR combined with MSC, it showed compared with both the control group and MSC group, the ventricular function was significantly improved as reflected by the magnified restoration of the enlarged LVEF in AMI. The study showed the

therapeutic effect of the transplantation of ATOR+ MSC is better than sole MSCs transplantation, which contrib-utes to further clinical application of MSCs. Our data have demonstrated that atorvastatin enhanced MSCs-induced improvement of ischemic cardiac dysfunction, as reflected by the magnified restoration of the enlarged LVEF in AMI. This is to say, Ator can exert protective effects on the myocardium undergoing infarction and reperfusion injury in conjunction with MSC transplantation.

Limitations of this paper are in the following aspects: 1) the sample size is still relatively small, only including approximately 80 animals of different species. It is hoped that more researches can be incorporated; 2) the study failed to analyze the appropriate dose of the drug. Dur-ing transplantation, different studies chose a different dose, but how much dose is the optimal needs further study. 3) The study didn't cover the mechanism of Ator. This study researched the impact of Ator to the therapy of AMI, but failed to provide data analysis of the causes of the impact, for example, whether it is anti-apoptotic, pro-differentiation, etc., which needs further study. 4) Other statins may also have a similar effect, which is yet to be explored. 5) D'Ascenzo F's study shows that remote ischaemic preconditioning (RIPC) can reduce the inci-dence of periprocedural myocardial infarction (PMI) fol-lowing percutaneous coronary intervention (PCI), especially when performed in the lower limb and for pa-tients with multivessel disease and complex lesions [21]. During the "ATOR + MSC" transplantation process, RIPC may have a synergistic effect, which needs to be further studied.

To the best of our knowledge, this is the first system-atic review and meta-analysis in large animal models to evaluate the effect of cell therapy in ischaemic heart dis-ease. This analysis showed that large animal models are valid to predict outcome of clinical trials. More-over, the results showed that cardiac cell therapy is safe, led to an improved LVEF, and revealed important clues for design-ing (pre-) clinical trials.

The reported benefits of stem cell therapy for cardiac function in clinical trials have been only modest. One of the unresolved issues is the rather rapid disappearance of cells after a few days, which is accompanied by the lack of any demonstrable regenerative effect.

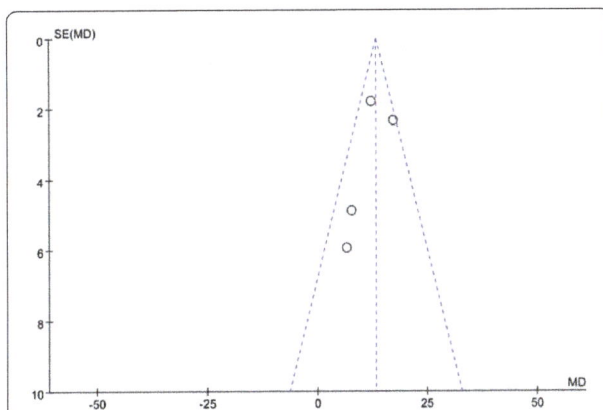

Fig. 5 Funnel plot for LVEF improvement between MSCs + ATOR group and MSCs group. No evidence for publication bias was found. SE, standard error; MD, mean difference

Conclusions

Atorvastatin can enhance the existing effects of MSCs transplantation, and this combinational therapy is a superior cell/pharmacological therapeutic approach that merits future preclinical and clinical studies.

Abbreviations

AMI: Acute myocardial infarction; ATOR: Atorvastatin; Embase: The Excerpta Medica Database; LVEF: The left ventricular ejection fraction; MSCs: Mesenchymal stem cells; VIP database: The Chinese Scientific and Technological Journal Database.

Competing interests

The authors declare that they have no competing interests.

Authors' contributions

GD, XQ and RL carried out searched the databases, extracted the data and drafted the manuscript. JG and HC carried out the statistical analysis. YD, YL, YW and WY participated in the design of the study and performed the statistical analysis. XW conceived of the study, and participated in its design and coordination and helped to draft the manuscript. All authors read and approved the final manuscript.

Acknowledgements

This study was supported by Hunan Province Science and Technology Plan Project fund (No: 2013RS403), Hunan Provincial Education Department-Sponsored Science Research Project fund (No: 15B141) and National Natural Science Foundation of China (81170229, 31171402, 81170088, 31172044, 31272396, 81270156, 31472060, 81270291, 81370451, 81400304, 81470377, 81470449), the Cooperative Innovation Center of Engineering and New Products for Developmental Biology of Hunan Province (2013-448-6).

References

1. Go AS, Mozaffarian D, Roger VL, Benjamin EJ, Berry JD, Blaha MJ, et al. Executive summary: heart disease and stroke statistics–2014 update: a report from the American Heart Association. Circulation. 2014;129(3):399–410.
2. Singh JA, Lu X, Ibrahim S, Cram P. Trends in and disparities for acute myocardial infarction: an analysis of Medicare claims data from 1992 to 2010. BMC Med. 2014;12(1):190.
3. Hsiao LC, Carr C, Chang KC, Lin SZ, Clarke K . Stem cell-based therapy for ischemic heart disease. Cell Transplant. 2013;22(4):663–75.
4. Samper E, Diez-Juan A, Montero JA, Sepúlveda P. Cardiac cell therapy: boosting mesenchymal stem cells effects. Stem Cell Rev. 2013;9(3):266–80.
5. Abdel-Latif A, Bolli R, Tleyjeh IM, Montori VM, Perin EC, Hornung CA, et al. Adult bone marrow-derived cells for cardiac repair: a systematic review and meta-analysis. Arch Intern Med. 2007;167(10):989–97.
6. Tang Y, Cai B, Yuan F, He X, Lin X, Wang J, et al. Melatonin pretreatment improves the survival and function of transplanted mesenchymal stem cells after focal cerebral ischemia. Cell Transplant. 2014;23(10):1279–91.
7. Mamidi MK, Pal R, Govindasamy V, Zakaria Z, Bhonde R. Treat the graft to improve the regenerative ability of the host. Med Hypotheses. 2011;76(4):599–601.
8. van der Spoel TI, Jansen of Lorkeers SJ, Agostoni P, van Belle E, Gyöngyösi M, Sluijter JP, et al. Human relevance of pre-clinical studies in stem cell therapy: systematic review and meta-analysis of large animal models of ischaemic heart disease. Cardiovasc Res. 2011;91(4):649–58.
9. Green S, Higgins JP, Alderson P. Cochrane Hand-book for Systematic Reviews of Interventions: Cochrane Book Series. Chichester: John Wiley & Sons, Ltd; 2008.
10. Higgins JPT, Thompson SG, Deeks JJ, Altman DG. Measuring inconsistency in meta-analyses. BMJ. 2003;327:557–60.
11. Matar AA, Chong JJ. Stem cell therapy for cardiac dysfunction. Springerplus. 2014;3:440.
12. Schaefer EJ, McNamara JR, Tayler T, Daly JA, Gleason JL, Seman LJ, et al. Comparisons of effects of statins (atorvastatin, fluvastatin, lovastatin, pravastatin, and simvastatin) on fasting and postprandial lipoproteins in patients with coronary heart disease versus control subjects. Am J Cardiol. 2004;93(1):31–9.
13. Xu R, Chen J, Cong X, Hu S, Chen X. Lovastatin protects mesenchymal stem cells against hypoxia- and serum deprivation-induced apoptosis by activation of PI3K/Akt and ERK1/2. J Cell Biochem. 2008;103:256–69.
14. Ghavami S, Mutawe MM, Hauff K, Stelmack GL, Schaafsma D, Sharma P, et al. Statin-triggered cell death in primary human lung mesenchymal cells involves p53-puma and release of smac and omi but not cytochrome c. Biochim Biophys Acta. 1803;2010:452–67.
15. Landmesser U, Engberding N, Bahlmann FH, Schaefer A, Wiencke A, Heineke A, et al. Statin-induced improvement of endothelial progenitor cell mobilization, myocardial neovascularization, left ventricular function, and survival after experimental myocardial infarction requires endothelial nitric oxide synthase. Circulation. 2004;110(14):1933–9.
16. Zhang Q, Wang H, Yang YJ, Dong QT, Wang TJ, Qian HY, et al. Atorvastatin treatment improves the effects of mesenchymal stem cell transplantation on acute myocardial infarction: The role of the RhoA/ROCK/ERK pathway. Int J Cardiol. 2014;176(3):670–9.
17. Qu Z, Xu H, Tian Y, Jiang X. Atorvastatin improves microenvironment to enhance the beneficial effects of BMSCs therapy in a rabbit model of acute myocardial infarction. Cell Physiol Biochem. 2013;32(2):380–9.
18. Song L, Yang YJ, Dong QT, Qian HY, Gao RL, Qiao SB, et al. Atorvastatin enhance efficacy of mesenchymal stem cells treatment for swine myocardial infarction via activation of nitric oxide synthase. PLoS One. 2013; 8(5):e65702.
19. Cai A, Zheng D, Dong Y, Qiu R, Huang Y, Song Y, et al. Efficacy of Atorvastatin combined with adipose-derived mesenchymal stem cell transplantation on cardiac function in rats with acute myocardial infarction. Acta Biochim Biophys Sin (Shanghai). 2011;43(11):857–66.
20. Yang YJ, Qian HY, Huang J, Geng YJ, Gao RL, Dou KF, et al. Atorvastatin treatment improves survival and effects of implanted mesenchymal stem cells in post-infarct swine hearts. Eur Heart J. 2008;29(12):1578–90.
21. D'Ascenzo F, Moretti C, Omedè P, Cerrato E, Cavallero E, Er F, et al. Cardiac remote ischaemic preconditioning reduces periprocedural myocardial infarction for patients undergoing percutaneous coronary interventions: a meta-analysis of randomised clinical trials. EuroIntervention. 2014;9(12): 1463–71.

Sex differences in in-hospital mortality following a first acute myocardial infarction: symptomatology, delayed presentation, and hospital setting

George Mnatzaganian[1*], George Braitberg[2,3], Janet E. Hiller[4,5], Lisa Kuhn[6] and Rose Chapman[7]

Abstract

Background: Women generally wait longer than men prior to seeking treatment for acute myocardial infarction (AMI). They are more likely to present with atypical symptoms, and are less likely to be admitted to coronary or intensive care units (CCU or ICU) compared to similarly-aged males. Women are more likely to die during hospital admission. Sex differences in the associations of delayed arrival, admitting ward, and mortality have not been thoroughly investigated.

Methods: Focusing on presenting symptoms and time of presentation since symptom onset, we evaluated sex differences in in-hospital mortality following a first AMI in 4859 men and women presenting to three emergency departments (ED) from December 2008 to February 2014. Sex-specific risk of mortality associated with admission to either CCU/ICU or medical wards was calculated after adjusting for age, socioeconomic status, triage-assigned urgency of presentation, blood pressure, heart rate, presenting symptoms, timing of presentation since symptom onset, and treatment in the ED. Sex-specific age-adjusted attributable risks were calculated.

Results: Compared to males, females waited longer before seeking treatment, presented more often with atypical symptoms, and were less likely to be admitted to CCU or ICU. Age-adjusted mortality in CCU/ICU or medical wards was higher among females (3.1 and 4.9 % respectively in CCU/ICU and medical wards in females compared to 2.6 and 3.2 % in males). However, after adjusting for variation in presenting symptoms, delayed arrival and other risk factors, risk of death was similar between males and females if they were admitted to CCU or ICU. This was in contrast to those admitted to medical wards. Females admitted to medical wards were 89 % more likely to die than their male counterparts. Arriving in the ED within 60 min of onset of symptoms was not associated with in-hospital mortality. Among males, 2.2 % of in-hospital mortality was attributed to being admitted to medical wards rather than CCU or ICU, while for females this age-adjusted attributable risk was 4.1 %.

Conclusions: Our study stresses the need to reappraise decision making in patient selection for admission to specialised care units, whilst raising awareness of possible sex-related bias in management of patients diagnosed with an AMI.

Keywords: Attributable risk, Hospital setting, In-hospital mortality, Myocardial infarction, Sex disparity

* Correspondence: George.Mnatzaganian@acu.edu.au
[1]School of Allied Health, Faculty of Health Sciences, Australian Catholic University, Fitzroy, Victoria 3065, Australia
Full list of author information is available at the end of the article

Background

Cardiovascular disease (CVD), of which coronary heart disease (CHD) accounts for more than half, is a global health problem that contributes considerably to global mortality and disease burden in men and women [1–5]. In the United States, it accounts for 1 in 2.8 deaths per year [2], while in the United Kingdom, approximately 1 in 6 deaths in men and 1 in 10 in women each year are from CHD [1, 3]. In 2005, from a total of 58 million deaths worldwide, 7.6 million (i.e., 13 %) were due to coronary heart disease [4]. Myocardial infarction (MI) is one of the manifestations of CHD and its incidence in a population is often used as a proxy for estimating the coronary heart disease burden for that country [4]. Each year, it is estimated that around 55,000 Australians suffer an acute myocardial infarction (AMI), on average claiming the lives of 27 individuals each day [5]. Notwithstanding, various reports over the past two decades suggest that mortality from a first AMI is steadily decreasing [6], mainly owing to new technologies, revascularisation, more effective drugs to control for heart related conditions and increased diagnosis of previously indeterminable AMI by high sensitivity blood tests [7]. Nonetheless, females hospitalised with AMI have well-documented higher rates of in-hospital mortality than males [8–10]; which is often attributed to the relatively older age of women at the time of diagnosis compared to men [9]. However, differences in in-hospital mortality following AMI have been mainly observed among younger women compared to their similarly aged male counterparts [10, 11]. Hochman and colleagues have suggested that this may be attributed to the different clinical presentation with which women arrive at hospital and the subsequent greater in-hospital complications [12]. Sex-based disparities have also been reported in the treatment of AMI, and it has been argued that such differences could be associated with sex bias in physicians' approach to treatment [13]. However, research findings are inconsistent with respect to whether females with AMI are more likely to be undertreated, including the implementation of revascularisation procedures [14–16].

In Australia, as in other countries [17–22], a considerable proportion of patients diagnosed with AMI is treated in medical wards rather than in coronary care units (CCU) or intensive care units (ICU). It has been reported that patients treated in CCU are less likely to die during hospital admission than those treated in medical wards [20, 21], although in some studies, these findings may have been confounded by the older age of patients treated in medical wards [17, 21]. Sex-specific risk of in-hospital mortality attributable to the hospital treatment setting is not known. Our study is unique in that it investigates sex differences in the associations of delayed arrival, admitting ward, and in-hospital mortality after being diagnosed with a first AMI in a large sample of men and women. The study also assesses the sex-specific age-adjusted risk of dying attributed to being admitted to CCU, ICU or medical wards.

Methods

Study population

All adult (18 years or older) patients hospitalised after being diagnosed with a first acute myocardial infarction (AMI) in the emergency department of three acute care Victorian teaching hospitals in Australia between 1st December 2008 and 28th February 2014 were eligible to participate in this study. The three participating hospitals serve a large catchment population with a total of approximately 170,000 presentations per annum. All repeat admissions following discharge from the index AMI admission were excluded. Patients were not eligible to participate if they were diagnosed with AMI after experiencing a trauma or any other injury.

Study variables

Case identification for AMI relied on recorded diagnoses in the emergency department electronic database (SYMPHONY Version 2.29, Ascribe plc, Bolton, UK) using codes from the International Classification of Diseases, 10th Revision, (Australian Modification) (ICD-10-AM). ICD-10-AM codes 121.0-121.9 were used to define AMI. These codes include all myocardial infarctions specified as acute or within a stated duration of 4 weeks or less from onset. These codes do not include old myocardial infarctions or recurrent myocardial infarctions. Data collected for each patient included age, sex, socio-economic status as defined by the Socio Economic Index For Areas (SEIFA) [23], country of birth, language spoken at home, symptoms and main cause of presentation, time from onset of symptoms to arrival to ED, arrival by ambulance, triage urgency score, systolic and diastolic blood pressures, heart rate, time from arrival to the ED to being seen by an attending physician, screening blood tests and electrocardiograms ordered in the ED, length of stay in the ED, hospital ward destination, and in-hospital mortality. All clinical variables relating to the presentation at the ED and the vital signs including blood pressure and pulse rate were measured and recorded by a triage nurse. Vital signs were measured once on arrival to the ED. Atypical symptoms were defined as dyspnoea, diaphoresis, nausea and vomiting, syncope, abdominal pain and musculoskeletal pain.

Socio Economic Index For Areas (SEIFA) is a composite index that ranks geographic areas across Australia according to their relative socio-economic advantage or disadvantage based on Australian Bureau of Statistic 2006 census data, with lower scores indicating more disadvantage.

Statistical analysis

Patients admitted to hospital were followed until they were discharged, died or were right censored at the end of study (February 28, 2014). The sex-specific analyses were conducted on all patients as a single group and separately on patients 50 years of age or younger and those 51 years of age or older. This cut-point was chosen to differentiate between pre and post-menopausal women in the multicultural Australian population where natural menopause occurs between 45 and 55 years of age [24]. Patients' characteristics were summarised using descriptive statistics. Pearson chi-square tests were used to compare groups of interest and Student's t-test or ANOVA were used to compare means. Sex differences in age-adjusted in-hospital mortality rates among patients admitted to CCU, ICU or medical wards were analysed using the direct adjustment method – a method that calculates a weighted average of the group's age-specific mortality rates where the weights represent the age-specific sizes of a standard population [25]. The sex-specific attributable risk (AR) of dying associated with the admitting hospital ward (i.e., CCU or ICU compared to medical wards) was calculated using the following formula:

Attributable risk

$$= \frac{(Incidence\ in\ total\ population) - (incidence\ in\ nonexposed\ populaiton)}{Incidence\ in\ total\ population}$$

The weighted-sum approach was utilised to calculate the age-adjusted attributable risk (AR) using the following formula [26]:

$$AR = \sum_j wj\ ARj$$

where AR_j and w_j, respectively, denote the AR value specific to different j age category levels and the corresponding weight. The weight was calculated as the inverse variance of the AR estimate in each age category over the sum of inverse variances over all age groups [26].

Furthermore, we constructed a multivariable logistic regression to analyse the association between the study variables and in-hospital mortality binary outcome.

Multiple imputation for missing data

Approximately 2 % of the patients had a missing value on time from onset of symptoms to arrival to the ED, while 39 % had a missing value on vital signs. Multiple imputation technique was used to estimate the missing data as suggested by Rubin [27]. The technique assigned twenty plausible values to the missing data representing the uncertainty about the true value. These multiple imputed datasets were then analysed. The *mi* Stata command was used to conduct the imputations.

Sensitivity analyses

Uncertainly levels of comorbidity in males and females were accounted for by using sensitivity analysis [28, 29]. Sex-specific uncertainty in the true prevalence of

comorbidity, which may differ by sex, was simulated by performing sensitivity analyses with a range of +/- 5 % in the group with AMI while keeping the prevalence of those without AMI constant.

Assumptions used in the sensitivity analyses

We assumed that the risk-adjusted odds ratio (OR) relating comorbidity (measured as Charlson Comorbidity Index) to in-hospital mortality in patients diagnosed with AMI was 1.17 (95 % CI, 1.11–1.23) as reported in a seven-year longitudinal study that assessed the impact of comorbidities on in-hospital mortality among a similar population of male and female patients diagnosed with AMI [30]. The risk-adjusted OR was derived from a multivariable regression model that accounted for age, sex, Charlson Comorbidity Index, and coronary revascularisation. Comorbidity prevalence in adult hospitalised patients with and without an AMI was set as 35 % [based on a multi-centre ten-year study] [31] and 32 % [based on data from six countries] [32].

All analyses were performed using Stata statistical program (version 13, StataCorp, College Station, TX, USA). Statistical significance was set at a P value of < 0.05 (two-sided).

Results

During the study's 63-month period, 4859 patients were diagnosed with their first AMI in the three emergency departments and were admitted to hospital, with 3293 (67.8 %) being male and 1566 (32.2 %) being female. Compared to males, females waited longer until they sought medical advice, were more likely to arrive to the ED by ambulance, presented with more atypical symptoms and were more likely to receive less acute triage urgency scores by the triage nurse (Table 1). Delayed arrival to the ED was observed for all female patients who presented with any symptom (i.e., chest pain, atypical symptoms) in any age category compared to their male counterparts (Table 2). Irrespective of age, females also waited significantly longer in the ED until they were examined by a physician [mean 63 min (SD 78) in females compared to mean 43 min (SD 64) in males, $P < 0.001$] and were less likely to be admitted to CCU or ICU compared to males (61 % in females compared to 72 % in males, $P < 0.001$) (Table 1). However, no sex-differences were observed in admission to CCU or ICU in those presenting with atypical symptoms (Table 3). Compared to those admitted to medical wards, patients admitted to CCU or ICU were also significantly younger and were assigned a higher urgency level by the triage nurse. Of those admitted to CCU or ICU, 2.5 % died during their index hospital admission compared to 5.2 % of those treated in medical wards ($P < 0.001$). Crude death rates in either CCU or ICU, or medical wards were significantly higher among females

Table 1 Characteristics of patients diagnosed with their first acute myocardial infarction in the emergency department by sex and age category

Characteristics	Age 50 years or younger		Age 51 years or older	
	Male N = 647	Female N = 175	Male N = 2646	Female N = 1391
Age, mean (SD)	43.4 (6.1)	43.6 (5.5)	67.9 (11.0)	73.8 (11.4)**
Socioeconomic status[a], %				
Low	43.0	42.3	38.4	37.8
Middle	28.7	26.3	28.5	26.7
High	28.3	31.4	33.1	35.5
Born in Australia, %	51.3	66.3**	43.6	48.2*
Arrived by ambulance, %	54.7	52.6	69.9	76.1**
Arrived within 60 min of onset of symptoms, %	21.2	10.3**	13.3	9.9*
Triage urgency[b], %				
Resuscitation /Emergency	77.1	65.1	67.0	53.0
All else	22.9	34.9**	33.0	47.0**
Presenting symptom, %				
Chest pain	86.2	84.0	80.1	71.2
Arrhythmia	6.0	5.1	7.4	7.6
Other (e.g., musculoskeletal, SOB)	5.6	9.1	10.7	18.8
Referred due to abnormal finding	2.2	1.7	1.8	2.4**
Pulse pressure, mean (SD)	67.5 (20.8)	63.1 (25.6)*	76.3 (25.2)	80.1 (28.0)**
Heart rate, mean (SD)	81.1 (14.4)	85.5 (17.4)**	81.9 (14.7)	85.0 (17.1)**
Time from arrival till examined by a physician in minutes, mean (SD)	30.9 (52.9)	49.1 (61.9)**	46.1 (65.9)	64.5 (79.4)**
Discharged from ED to: %				
CCU or ICU or operating theatre	78.8	69.1	70.7	60.3
Medical ward	21.2	30.9**	29.3	39.7**

Abbreviations: *CCU* coronary care unit, *ED* emergency department, *ICU* intensive care unit, *SD* standard deviation, *SOB* shortness of breath
**P value <0.001; * 0.001 < P value < 0.05
[a]The socioeconomic status was based on the Socio-Economic Index For Areas disadvantage score (SEIFA)
[b]The triage score is a ranking from one to five (one being the most urgent and five being non-urgent), given by a Triage nurse, used to prioritise or classify patients on the basis of illness or injury severity and need for medical and nursing care

Table 2 Percent arrived to emergency department within 60 min of onset of symptoms by presenting symptom, sex, and age category

	Age 50 years or younger		Age 51 or older	
	Male	Female	Male	Female
Chest pain	20.1	10.2	13.1	9.8
Arrhythmia	46.2	11.1	24.5	18.9
Atypical symptoms (e.g., musculoskeletal pain, shortness of breath)	16.7	12.5	8.2	7.3
Referred to emergency department due to abnormal findings	7.1	0.0	6.3	5.9
All	21.2	10.3	13.3	9.9

Table 3 Percent admitted to coronary care unit or intensive care unit by presenting symptom, sex, and age category

	Age 50 years or younger		Age 51 or older	
	Male	Female	Male	Female
Chest pain	79.0	70.1*	74.6	67.0**
Arrhythmia	87.2	66.7	68.9	43.4**
Atypical symptoms (e.g., musculoskeletal pain, shortness of breath)	63.9	56.3	44.7	43.3
Referred to emergency department due to abnormal findings	85.7	100.0[a]	60.4	50.0
All	78.7	69.1*	70.7	60.3**

[a]Less than 5 patients
**P value <0.001; * 0.001 < P value < 0.05

(3.3 % in females versus 2.1 % in males in CCU or ICU, $P = 0.03$; and 7.8 % in females versus 3.5 % in males in medical wards, $P < 0.001$). Adjusting for age did not eliminate the disparities in death rates as shown in Table 4.

A multivariable logistic regression that also adjusted for age, sex, socioeconomic status, country of birth, language spoken at home, symptoms and main cause of presentation, time from onset of symptoms to arrival to ED, arrival in ambulance, urgency level, heart rate, time from arrival in the ED until examination by attending physician, length of stay in the ED and hospital providing the service, showed that those admitted to CCU or ICU were significantly less likely to die than those admitted to medical wards (adjusted-OR = 0.5, 95 % CI 0.3–0.7, $P < 0.001$) (Table 5). This association was observed in both sexes (CCU/ICU adjusted-OR = 0.5, 95 % CI 0.3–0.9, $P = 0.013$ for males; and 0.4, 95 % CI 0.3–0.7, $P = 0.003$ for females). Compared to those experiencing any of the other presenting symptoms, those presenting with chest pain were 70 % less likely to die during their hospital admission (adjusted-OR = 0.3, 95 % CI 0.2–0.4, $P < 0.001$). Arriving in the emergency department within 60 min of onset of symptoms was not associated with in-hospital mortality (adjusted-OR = 0.9, 95 % CI 0.6–1.9, $P = 0.9$), also observed in both sexes.

Running separate multivariable models by hospital treating ward showed that females admitted to medical wards were 89 % more likely to die than their male counterparts (adjusted-OR = 1.89, 95 % CI 1.1–3.2, $P = 0.017$), but no statistically significant sex differences were observed in risk of dying in CCU or ICU (adjusted-OR = 1.5, 95 % CI 0.9–2.4, $P = 0.1$).

After adjusting for age, among males, 2.2 % of in-hospital mortality was attributed to being admitted to medical wards compared with admission to CCU or ICU, whereas in females, this age-adjusted attributable risk was 4.1 %. Accounting for various levels of comorbidity in males and females using sensitivity analyses did not eliminate gender differences in in-hospital mortality (Appendix).

Discussion

In this 5.3-year study, we have shown that a considerable amount of sex disparity in in-hospital mortality after being admitted with a first AMI is attributed to the hospital admitting ward. In medical wards, women in our study had worse short-term outcomes with higher in-hospital mortality rates than men, which could not be explained by their age, presenting symptoms, delayed arrival, or treating hospital. Sensitivity analyses that accounted for uncertainty in comorbidity also showed similar results. No such sex differences were observed among those admitted in coronary or intensive care units. Based upon our results, admitting patients who are diagnosed with AMI in the ED, to CCU or ICU instead of medical wards could prevent 2 to 4 % of in-hospital mortality.

Although men are more likely than women to be diagnosed with AMI during their lifespan, the short-term outcomes such as mortality are worse for some groups of women, particularly younger women relative to their similarly-aged male counterparts [10]. Some authors argue that the patients' risk factor profiles may account for much of the sex disparity in in-hospital mortality [9, 10], while others debate that under-treatment of women may be an independent contributor to the sex disparity in

Table 4 Age adjusted rates of in-hospital mortality among patients admitted to CCU or ICU versus medical hospital wards by sex: direct adjustment method[a]

| Age groups | Standard Population | Male | | | | Female | | | |
| | | CCU or ICU | | Medical ward | | CCU or ICU | | Medical ward | |
		Death rate %	Expected # death	Death rate %	Expected # death	Death rate %	Expected # death	Death rate %	Expected # death
All ages	4859								
18–54	1223	0.53	6.5	0.97	11.9	1.10	13.5	2.70	33.0
55–65	1245	1.78	22.2	1.84	22.9	1.72	21.4	1.52	18.9
66–78	1289	2.77	35.7	3.65	47.0	2.95	38.0	3.97	51.2
79 +	1102	5.80	63.9	6.67	73.5	7.08	78.0	12.03	132.6
Total number of deaths expected			128		155		151		236
Crude rates		2.1 %		3.5 %		3.3 %		7.8 %	
Age adjusted rates		128/4859 = 2.6 %		155/4859 = 3.2 %		151/4859 = 3.1 %		236/4859 = 4.9 %	

Abbreviations: *CCU* coronary care unit, *ICU* intensive care unit
[a]Direct adjustment method is one that calculates a weighted average of the group's age-specific mortality rates where the weights represent the age-specific sizes of a standard population

Table 5 Risk of in-hospital mortality following a diagnosis of first acute myocardial infarction: a multivariable logistic regression[a]

Covariate	Odds ratio, 95 % CI	P value
Age categories (tertiles)		
18–58 years (reference)	1.00	
59–74 years	2.3 (1.3–4.3)	0.006
75 year or more	5.0 (2.8–9.1)	<0.001
Female sex	1.6 (1.1–2.3)	0.007
Socioeconomic status[b]		
Low tertile (reference)	1.00	
Middle tertile	0.8 (0.5–1.3)	0.4
High tertile	0.8 (0.6–1.2)	0.3
Born in Australia	0.8 (0.6–1.1)	0.2
Chest pain as main presenting symptom	0.3 (0.2–0.4)	<0.001
Arrival in the ED within 60 min of onset of symptoms	0.9 (0.6–1.6)	0.9
Arrival in ambulance	3.9 (2.0–7.8)	<0.001
Triage classification of urgency		
Non-urgent presentations (reference)	1.00	
Emergency presentations/resuscitation needed	3.0 (1.8–4.9)	<0.001
Admitted to CCU or ICU	0.5 (0.3–0.7)	<0.001
Time from arrival in the ED to examination by physician (continuous variable)	1.0 (0.9–1.0)	0.9

Abbreviation: CCU coronary care unit, *CI* confidence interval, *ED* emergency department, *ICU* intensive care unit

[a]Also adjusted for hour of presentation, hospital type, length of stay in the ED, and language spoken at home

[b]The socioeconomic status was based on the Socio-Economic Index For Areas disadvantage score (SEIFA)

mortality [14]. Our study shows that the hospital setting to which the patient is admitted is an important contributor to the sex disparity in in-hospital deaths amongst those diagnosed with AMI. Although admission to CCU or ICU is not without risks [33, 34], we show that such an admission is beneficial to both young and older patients diagnosed with their first AMI, regardless of sex. Patients diagnosed with AMI may often suffer from life-threatening complications that require highly specialised care. Consequently, the standard of care for such patients is to treat them in either coronary or intensive care units, which have been shown to be cost-effective [35]. However, the cost-effectiveness of treatment in the CCU is debatable and less favourable among younger patients because of their relative lower underlying risk of life-threatening complications [36].

Similar to other researchers [37], we found that women with AMI were less often admitted to coronary or intensive care units than their male counterparts. This was mainly observed in those presenting with chest pain or arrhythmia. In the former, admission to these specialised units was less in both younger and older women. The reason for this is unclear, especially because all our patients were diagnosed with AMI before the decision was made about the admitting hospital setting. Furthermore, since the demand for intensive and coronary care unit beds far exceeds their availability [18], patients presenting with symptoms other than chest pain may be more likely to be admitted to medical wards, as was shown in our study. Our analysis indicates that due consideration of the impact of hospital setting must be given when deciding whether to admit a patient with an AMI to a coronary or intensive care unit bed versus a medical ward bed. Since increasing evidence indicates sex disparity in short-term outcomes following AMI, there is a need to re-assess the cost-effectiveness of treatment in specialised CCU and ICU wards, armed with the knowledge that sex and age are contributing factors to in-hospital mortality.

Timely treatment of men and women with acute myocardial infarction depends on symptom recognition and prompt presentation to the emergency department. Although the benefits of early treatment of AMI are clearly evident, only a small proportion of such patients receives treatment within evidence-based timeframes from symptom onset [38]. Our study did not show any significant association between a timely arrival to the hospital and in-hospital mortality. This may be explained by the fact that those who delayed seeking medical advice may have not arrived at the ED, as it has been shown that approximately half of those who have an AMI die before reaching a hospital within an hour of symptom onset [39].

Strengths of our large sample study include our ability to account for presenting symptoms and time to arrival to the ED since onset of symptoms – factors which are often not considered when assessing short-term outcomes following an AMI. The study has some limitations. We have not separately examined whether the effect of the hospital setting is related to the nature of the ward structure (including such factors as nurse-patient ratios, the skill set of the attendant nursing staff or the monitoring capability of the ward) or whether it is related to medical expertise or variation in clinical practices within each of these three hospitals. The physiologic and clinical data were collected once on arrival to the ED and these were not validated; however these were measured and recorded by a triage nurse. Case identification was retrospective being entirely based on the final diagnosis reached at discharge from the ED. Available data did not permit us to validate the ED diagnosis of AMI, as we did not have access to patients' hospital discharge charts. We also did not have information on patients' comorbidities. Nevertheless, age, which is often considered the simplest co-morbidity score [40–42], was accounted for over the study period. Similarly, using sensitivity analyses we accounted for various prevalence estimates of comorbidities among males and females, showing similar results in sex differences. Finally, we did not have information on the location (e.g., inferior versus anterior wall MI) or the nature of the myocardial infarction whether it was with ST segment elevation (STEMI) or without (NSTEMI)); however, there is no evidence to indicate that misclassifications of diagnoses such as AMI are sex specific.

Conclusion

Our study demonstrates that sex differences exist in frequency of admission to coronary or intensive care units among patients diagnosed with an acute myocardial infarction. However, among those admitted to these specialised units, no sex differences were observed in in-hospital mortality after accounting for age, presenting symptoms, delayed arrival and other risk factors. The disparity in this short-term outcome was prominent in the medical wards and was not explained by the patient age or other risk factors. This study calls for appropriate knowledge transfer while addressing decision making regarding admission to coronary or intensive care units while considering possible sex-related biases.

Abbreviations
AMI, acute myocardial infarction; AR, attributable risk; CCU, coronary care unit; CHD, coronary heart disease; CI, confidence interval; CVD, cardiovascular disease; ED, emergency department; ICD-10-AM, International Classification of Diseases (Australian Modification); ICU, intensive care unit; NSTEMI, Non-ST-segment elevation myocardial infarction; OR, odds ratio; SD, standard deviation; SEIFA, Socio Economic Index For Areas; STEMI, ST-segment elevation myocardial infarction.

Appendix

Table 6 Observed and expected gender-specific odds ratios of in-hospital mortality following acute myocardial infarction: sensitivity analysis accounting for sex-specific uncertainty in the prevalence of comorbidity

Level of uncertainty[a]	Comorbidity prevalence %, females : males	Odds ratio of females dying compared to males	Expected percent bias
		Observed unadjusted OR	–
–	–	2.1 (1.5–2.8)	
		Expected comorbidity adjusted OR: sensitivity analysis[b]	
5 %	40 : 35	2.06	1 %
10 %	45 : 35	2.05	2 %
25 %	60 : 35	2.00	4 %
45 %	80 : 35	1.94	7 %
65 %	100 : 35	1.88	10 %

[a]Uncertainty in the prevalence of comorbidity in females. The assumed prevalence of both females and males was set at 35 % (McManus et al. [31]). The prevalence of comorbidity in females was increased in accordance to the level of uncertainty
[b]The sensitivity analysis evaluated the odds ratio while accounting for unmeasured confounding by comorbidity

Funding
The study was supported by the Australian Catholic University.

Authors' contributions
GM, GB, and RC led the conceptual development of the manuscript. Subsequent study conception and design: GM, GB, JEH, LK, and RC; Data collection: GB and RC; Analysis of data: GM; Interpretation of findings: GM, GB, JEH, LK, and RC. All authors were involved in drafting the article and revising it critically for important intellectual content, and all authors approved the final version to be published. GM serves as the guarantor for the manuscript.

Competing interests
The authors declare that they have no competing interests.

Author details
School of Allied Health, Faculty of Health Sciences, Australian Catholic University, Fitzroy, Victoria 3065, Australia. [2]Department of Medicine, The University of Melbourne, Parkville, Victoria 3010, Australia. [3]Department of Emergency Medicine, Royal Melbourne Hospital, Parkville, Victoria 3010, Australia. [4]School of Health Sciences, Faculty of Health, Arts and Design, Swinburne University of Technology, Hawthorn, Victoria 3122, Australia. Discipline of Public Health, School of Population Health, The University of Adelaide, Adelaide, South Australia 5000, Australia. [6]School of Nursing and Midwifery, Faculty of Health, Deakin University, Geelong, Victoria 3220, Australia. [7]School of Physiotherapy and Exercise Science, Faculty of Health Sciences, Curtin University, Bentley, Western Australia 6102, Australia.

References
1. Scarborough P, Wickramasinghe K, Bhatnagar P, Rayner M. Trends in coronary heart disease 1961–2011. London: British Heart Foundation; 2011.
2. Roger VL, Go AS, Lloyd-Jones DM, Benjamin EJ, Berry JD, Borden WB, et al. Heart disease and stroke statistics 2012 update: A report from the American Heart Association. Circulation. 2012;125:e2–220. doi:10.1161/CIR. 0b013e31823ac046.
3. Greenlund K, Giles WH, Keenan NL, Malarcher AM, Zheng ZJ, Casper ML, et al. Heart disease and stroke mortality in the 20th century. Oxford: Oxford University Press; 2006. p. 1–6. doi:10.1093/acprof:oso/9780195150698.003.18. Accessed September 3, 2015.
4. World Health Organization. World Health Statistics 2008. Geneva: WHO; 2008.
5. Australian Bureau of Statistics. Causes of Death 2013. 2015. Retrieved from http://www.abs.gov.au/ausstats/abs@.nsf/mf/3303.0/. Accessed 30 August 2015.
6. Krumholz HM, Wang Y, Chen J, Drye EE, Spertus JA, Ross JS, et al. Reduction in acute myocardial infarction mortality in the United States: risk standardized mortality rates from 1995–2006. JAMA. 2009;302:767–73.
7. Lewis WR, Peterson ED, Cannon CP, Super DM, LaBresh KA, Quealy K, et al. An organized approach to improvement in guideline adherence for acute myocardial infarction: results with the get with the Guidelines Quality Improvement Program. Arch Intern Med. 2008;168:1813–9.
8. Gulati M, Shaw LJ, Bairey Merz CN. Myocardial ischemia in women: lessons from the NHLBI WISE study. Clin Cardiol. 2012;35:141–8.
9. Bairey Merz CN, Shaw LJ, Reis SE, Bittner V, Kelsey SF, Olson M, et al. Insights from the NHLBI-sponsored Women's Ischemia Syndrome Evaluation (WISE) study, part II: gender differences in presentation, diagnosis, and outcome with regard to gender-based pathophysiology of atherosclerosis, macro-, and microvascular coronary disease. J Am Coll Cardiol. 2006;47(Suppl A):21A–9.
10. Jneid H, Fonarow GC, Cannon CP, Hernandez AF, Palacios IF, Maree AO, et al. Sex differences in medical care and early death after acute myocardial infarction. Circulation. 2008;118:2803–10.

11. Kuhn L, Page K, Rahman MA, Worrall-Carter L. Gender differences in treatment and mortality of patients with ST-segment elevation myocardial infarction admitted to Victorian public hospitals: A retrospective database study. Aust Crit Care. 2015;28:196–202. doi:10.1016/j.aucc.2015.01.004.

12. Hochman JS, Tamis JE, Thompson TD, Weaver WD, White HD, Van de Werf F, et al. Sex, clinical presentation and outcome in patients with acute coronary syndromes. N Engl J Med. 1999;341:226–32.

13. Healy B. The Yentl syndrome. N Engl J Med. 1991;325:274–6.

14. Nauta ST, Deckers JW, Akkerhuis M, Lenzen M, Simoons ML, van Domburg RT. Changes in clinical profile, treatment, and mortality in patients hospitalised for acute myocardial infarction between 1985 and 2008. PLoS One. 2011;6:e26917.

15. Chandra NC, Ziegelstein RC, Rogers WJ, Tiefenbrunn AJ, Gore JM, French WJ, et al. Observations of the treatment of women in the United States with myocardial infarction: a report from the National Registry of Myocardial Infarction-I. Arch Intern Med. 1998;158:981–8.

16. Gan SC, Beaver SK, Houck PM, MacLehose RF, Lawson HW, Chan L. Treatment of acute myocardial infarction and 30-day mortality among women and men. N Engl J Med. 2000;343:8–15.

17. Karlson BW, Herlitz J, Wiklund D, Petterson P, Hallgren P, Hjalmarson A. Characteristics and prognosis of patients with acute myocardial infarction in relation to whether they were treated in the coronary care unit or in another ward. Cardiology. 1992;81:134–44.

18. Simchen E, Sprung CL, Galai N, Zitser-Gurevich Y, Bar-Lavi Y, Gurman G, et al. Survival of critically ill patients hospitalized in and out of intensive care units under paucity of intensive care unit beds. Crit Care Med. 2004;32:1654–61.

19. Simchen E, Sprung C, Galai N, Zitser-Gurevich Y, Bar-Lavi Y, Levi L, et al. Survival of critically ill patients hospitalized in and out of intensive care. Crit Care Med. 2007;35:449–57.

20. Rotstein Z, Mandelzweig L, Lavi B, Eldar M, Gottlieb S, Hod H. Does the coronary care unit improve prognosis of patients with acute myocardial infarction? Eur Heart J. 1999;20:813–8.

21. Reznik R, Ring I, Fletcher P, Siskind V. Differences in mortality from acute myocardial infarction between coronary care unit and medical ward: treatment or bias? Br Med J. 1987;295:1437–40.

22. Bain C, Siskind V, Neilson G. Site of care and survival after acute myocardial infarction. Med J Aust. 1981;22:185–8.

23. Australian Bureau of Statistics (ABS) 2006. 2039.0 – Information paper: An introduction to Socio-Economic Indexes for Areas (SEIFA), 2006. Retrieved from http://www.abs.gov.au/ausstats/abs@.nsf/mf/2039.0/. Accessed 30 August 2015.

24. Gold EB. The timing of the age at which natural menopause occurs. Obstet Gynecol Clin North Am. 2011;38:425–40.

25. Gordis L. Epidemiology. 5th ed. Philadelphia: Elsevier Saunders; 2014.

26. Benichou J. A review of adjusted estimators of attributable risk. Stat Methods Med Res. 2001;10:195–216.

27. Rubin DB. Multiple imputation for nonresponse in surveys. New York: John Wiley & Sons, Inc; 1987.

28. Orsini N, Bellocco R, Bottai M, Wolk A, Greenland S. A tool for deterministic and probabilistic sensitivity analysis of epidemiological studies. SJ. 2008;8:29–48.

29. Jurek AM, Maldonado G, Greenland S, Church TR. Exposure-measurement error is frequently ignored when interpreting epidemiological study results. Eur J Epidemiol. 2006;21:871–6.

30. Gili M, Sala J, López J, Carrión A, Béjar L, Moreno J, Rosales A, Sánchez G. Impact of comorbidities on in-hospital mortality from acute myocardial infarction, 2003–2009. Rev Esp Cardiol. 2011;64:1130–7.

31. McManus DD, Nguyen HL, Saczynski JS, Tisminetzky M, Bourell P, Goldberg RT. Multiple cardiovascular comorbidities and acute myocardial infarction: temporal trends (1990–2007) and impact on death rates at 30 days and 1 year. Clin Epidemiol. 2012;4:115–23.

32. Quan H, Li B, Couris CM, Fushimi K, Graham P, Hider P, Januel J-M, Sundararajan V. Updating and validating the Charlson comorbidity index and score for risk adjustment in hospital discharge abstracts using data from 6 countries. Am J Epidemiol. 2011;173:676–82.

33. Mnatzaganian G, Galai N, Sprung C, Zitser-Gurevich Y, Mandel M, Ben-Hur D, et al. Increased risk of bloodstream and urinary infections in intensive care unit (ICU) patients compared with patients fitting ICU admission criteria treated in regular wards. J Hosp Infect. 2005;59:331–42.

34. Mnatzaganian G, Sprung C, Zitser-Gurevich Y, Galai N, Goldschmidt N, Levi L, et al. Effect of infections on 30-day mortality among critically ill patients hospitalized in and out of the intensive care unit. Crit Care Med. 2008;36:1097–104.

35. Tosteson ANA, Goldman L, Udvarhelyi S, Lee TH. Cost-effectiveness of a coronary care unit versus an intermediate care unit for emergency department patients with chest pain. Circulation. 1996;94:143–50.

36. Cannon CP. Management of acute coronary syndromes. 2nd ed. New Jersey: Springer; 2003.

37. Valentine A, Jordan B, Lang T, Hiesmayr M, Metnitz PGH. Gender-related differences in intensive care: a multiple-center cohort study of therapeutic interventions and outcome in critically ill patients. Crit Care Med. 2003;31:1901–7.

38. Moser DK, Kimble LP, Alberts MJ, Alonzo A, Croft JB, Dracup K, et al. Reducing delay in seeking treatment by patients with acute coronary syndrome and stroke. Circulation. 2006;114:168–82.

39. American Heart Association. Heart disease and stroke statistics – 2005 updates. Dallas: American Heart Association; 2005.

40. Mnatzaganian G, Ryan P, Hiller JE. Does co-morbidity provide significant improvement on age adjustment when predicting medical outcomes? Methods Inf Med. 2014;53:115–20.

41. Mnatzaganian G, Ryan P, Norman PE, Hiller JE. Accuracy of hospital morbidity data and the performance of comorbidity scores as predictors of mortality. J Clin Epidemiol. 2012;65:107–15.

42. Schneeweiss S, Seeger JD, Maclure M, Wang PS, Avorn J, Glynn RJ. Performance of comorbidity scores to control for confounding in epidemiologic studies using claims data. Am J Epidemiol. 2001;154:854–64.

6

Relationship between fasting glucose levels and in-hospital mortality in Chinese patients with acute myocardial infarction and diabetes mellitus

Hao Liang[1], Yi Chen Guo[2], Li Ming Chen[2], Min Li[2], Wei Zhong Han[2], Xu Zhang[3] and Shi Liang Jiang[2]* ⓘ

Abstract

Background: Previous studies have demonstrated that elevated admission and fasting glucose (FG) is associated with worse outcomes in patients with acute myocardial infarction (AMI). However, the quantitative relationship between FG levels and in-hospital mortality in patients with AMI remains unknown. The aim of the study is to assess the prevalence of elevated FG levels in hospitalized Chinese patients with AMI and diabetes mellitus and to determine the quantitative relationship between FG levels and the in-hospital mortality as well as the optimal level of FG in patients with AMI and diabetes mellitus.

Methods: A retrospective study was carried out in 1856 consecutive patients admitted for AMI and diabetes mellitus from 2002 to 2013. Clinical variables of baseline characteristics, in-hospital management and in-hospital adverse outcomes were recorded and compared among patients with different FG levels.

Results: Among all patients recruited, 993 patients (53.5 %) were found to have FG ≥100 mg/dL who exhibited a higher in-hospital mortality than those with FG < 100 mg/dL ($P < 0.001$). Although there was a high correlation between FG levels and in-hospital mortality in all patients ($r = 0.830$, $P < 0.001$), the relationship showed a J-curve configuration with an elevated mortality when FG was less than 80 mg/dL. Using multivariate logistic regression models, we identified that age, FG levels and Killip class of cardiac function were independent predictors of in-hospital mortality in AMI patients with diabetes mellitus.

Conclusions: More than half of patients with AMI and diabetes mellitus have FG ≥100 mg/dL and the relationship between in-hospital mortality and FG level was a J-curve configuration. Both FG ≥ 100 mg/dL and FG <80 mg/dL were identified to be independent predictors of in-hospital mortality and thus the optimal FG level in AMI patients with diabetes mellitus appears to be 80–100 mg/dL.

Keywords: Myocardial infarction, Diabetes mellitus, Glucose, Mortality

* Correspondence: dcotorjsl@163.com
[2]Department of Cardiology, Shandong Provincial Hospital affiliated to Shandong University, No.324, Jing Wu Wei Qi Road, Jinan 250021, Shandong, People's Republic of China
Full list of author information is available at the end of the article

Background

Recent studies have shown that an elevated admission or fasting glucose (FG) level is common in patients with acute myocardial infarction (AMI) and is associated with an increased short-term mortality and a high incidence of congestive heart failure [1–5]. Among many clinical variables affecting short-term outcomes in patients with AMI, an elevated FG level, termed as stress hyperglycemia, has been identified as a new independent predictor of 30-day mortality in a group of patients with AMI and hyperglycemia [5]. This finding has important clinical significance because FG levels may serve as a simple marker to help clinicians stratify risk for optimal triage and management. Although hyperglycemia associated with AMI portends a gloomy short-term outcome in these patients, whether a low level of glucose would be a good omen for these subjects is unknown. Therefore, the quantitative relationship between FG levels across a wide range of values and the in-hospital mortality, and the optimal level of FG, in patients with AMI need to be clarified. The present study was carried out to assess the prevalence of elevated FG levels in hospitalized Chinese patients with AMI and diabetes mellitus and to determine the quantitative relationship between FG levels and the in-hospital mortality as well as the optimal level of FG in AMI patients with diabetes mellitus.

Methods

Patients

All patients who were admitted to our hospital between January 2002 and December 2013 with a definite diagnosis of AMI and diabetes mellitus and measurement of FG within 24 h of admission were included in the present study. The study was approved by the Medical Ethics Committee of Shandong Provincial Hospital Affiliated to Shandong University (NO.2015-034). No patients were directly involved in the study and no written informed consent was given by participants for their clinical records to be used in this study. All patients' records/information was anonymized and de-identified prior to analysis. The diagnosis of AMI was based the following criteria [6]: Detection of a rise and/or fall of cardiac biomarker values (preferably cardiac troponin) with at least one value above the 99th percentile upper reference limit and with at least one of the following: (1) Symptoms of ischaemia, (2) New or presumed new significant ST-segment–T wave changes or new left bundle branch block, (3) Development of pathological Q waves in the electrocardiogram, (4) Imaging evidence of new loss of viable myocardium or new regional wall motion abnormality, (5) Identification of an intracoronary thrombus by angiography or autopsy. Diabetes mellitus is diagnosed by demonstrating any one of the following [7]: (1) Fasting plasma glucose level ≥ 7.0 mmol/l (126 mg/dl), (2) Plasma glucose ≥ 11.1 mmol/l (200 mg/dl)

two hours after a 75 g oral glucose load as in a glucose tolerance test, (3) Symptoms of hyperglycemia and casual plasma glucose ≥ 11.1 mmol/l (200 mg/dl). The exclusion criteria included development of AMI after percutaneous coronary intervention or coronary artery bypass grafting (CABG) or other cardiac operations.

Data collection and definitions

A detailed review of the medical record for each patient was performed and clinical variables including baseline characteristics, in-hospital management, and incidence of adverse events during hospitalization were analyzed. Baseline characteristics consisted of age, gender, cigarette smoking, and history of angina pectoris, myocardial infarction, hypertension, family history of coronary artery disease, Killip class of cardiac function on admission, and FG and total cholesterol (TC) levels. The blood sample for FG and TC measurement was obtained after an overnight fast of ≥8 h within 24 h of admission and both FG and TC were determined enzymatically using an Auto Analyzer (Hitachi Inc). Patients were classified as normal FG group (FG <100 mg/dL) and elevated FG group (FG ≥100 mg/dL) according to the criteria of the 2003 follow-up report of the American Diabetes Association [8]. Analysis of in-hospital management involved application of reperfusion therapy with primary percutaneous coronary intervention or thrombolysis performed within 12 h of symptom onset, and medical therapy with the administration of β-receptor blockers, antiplatelets, heparins, angiotensin-converting-enzyme inhibitors (ACEI), angiotensin receptor blockers (ARB), statins and nitrates. Adverse outcomes of patients during hospitalization were defined as recurrent unstable angina pectoris, myocardial reinfarction, congestive heart failure and death. The diagnosis of unstable angina pectoris was established when patients had typical chest pain at rest with concomitant ischemic ST-T changes. Reinfarction was diagnosed based on the following criteria [6, 9]: (1) recurrent ST segment elevation or new pathognomonic Q waves appear, in at least two contiguous leads, particularly when associated with ischaemic symptoms for 20 min or longer, and (2) a second rise of CK-MB level to ≥2 times the upper normal limit, or an increase of >200 U/L of CK-MB level over the previous value if it had not dropped below the upper normal limit. Congestive heart failure was defined as Killip class of cardiac function ≥ II and a need for diuretic treatment at any time during hospitalization [10].

Statistical analysis

Continuous variables were presented as means ± standard deviation (SD) and categorical variables as numbers and percentages. Comparisons between groups categorized by FG levels were made by 2-tailed Student t test for continuous data and by chi-square analysis for categorical variables. Spearman rank correlation analysis was applied to examine the quantitative relationship between FG levels and in-hospital mortality and multivariate logistic regression analysis used to identify risk factors that were predictive of in-hospital death independently. P value <0.05 was considered statistically significant. All analyses were performed with SPSS 13.0 (SPSS, Inc., Chicago, Illinois).

Results
Basic characteristics
A total of 1856 AMI patients with diabetes mellitus and measurement of FG within 24 h of admission were enrolled and there were 1301 men and 555 women aged from 25 to 91 years (63.2 ± 11.5 years). The basic characteristics in two groups of patients with normal and elevated FG were listed in Table 1. Compared with patients with normal FG, a greater proportion of patients with elevated FG were old and female, had a history of documented hypertension, and exhibited a high level of TC and Killip class of cardiac function. There was no significant difference in the history of angina pectoris and prior myocardial infarction, and family history of coronary artery disease between the two groups. In contrast, cigarette smoking was more common in patients with normal FG than those with elevated FG.

In-hospital management
The difference in in-hospital management between the two groups of patients was given in Table 2. Among 1856 patients with AMI and diabetes mellitus, only 708 underwent reperfusion therapy (38.1 %). It is noteworthy that patients with elevated FG received even less reperfusion therapy than those with normal FG. However, if the two reperfusion strategies were analyzed separately, there was no significant difference in receiving primary

percutaneous coronary intervention, whereas the difference in receiving thrombolytic therapy was highly significant, between patients with normal and elevated FG. On the other hand, statins were used less frequently in patients with normal FG than those with elevated FG. There was no significant difference in the administration of other medications including antiplatelets, nitrates, β-receptor blockers, heparins, and ACEI or ARB between patients with normal and elevated FG.

In-hospital adverse events
The incidence of adverse events in the two groups of patients during hospitalization was presented in Table 3. A higher incidence of in-hospital death (10.8 % vs 5.6 %, $P < 0.001$) and congestive heart failure (21.7 % vs 16.1 %, $P = 0.002$) was observed in patients with elevated FG than those with normal FG. In contrast, there was no significant difference in the incidence of recurrent unstable angina pectoris or reinfarction between the two groups.

The in-hospital mortality among patients with different FG levels was 13.5 % (5/37 with FG <70 mg/dL), 7.0 % (14/199 with FG 70–79.9 mg/dL), 4.5 % (13/290 with FG 80–89.9 mg/dL), 4.7 % (16/337 with FG 90–99.9 mg/dL), 5.0 % (11/218 with FG100-109.9 mg/dL), 5.7 % (8/141 with FG 110–119.9 mg/dL), 6.8 % (8/118 with FG 120–129.9 mg/dL), 8.0 % (7/88 with FG 130–139.9 mg/dL), 11.3 % (9/80 with FG 140–149.9 mg/dL), 13.2 % (10/76 with FG 150–159.9 mg/dL), 15.9 % (7/44 with FG 160–169.9 mg/dL), 15.4 % (4/26 with FG 170–179.9 mg/dL), 17.5 % (10/57 with FG 180–199.9 mg/dL), 19.1 % (9/47 with FG 200–219.9 mg/dL), 15.4 % (4/26 with FG 220–239.9 mg/dL), 25.0 % (6/24 with FG 240–259.9 mg/dL), 29.2 % (14/48 with FG ≥260 mg/dL), respectively (Fig. 1). Spearman rank correlation analysis demonstrated a high positive correlation between FG levels and in-hospital mortality in all patients with AMI

Table 1 Baseline characters in patients with fasting glucose <100 mg/dL and ≥ 100 mg/dL

Variables	Normal FG ($n = 863$)	Elevated FG ($n = 993$)	P value
Age (y)	61.7 ± 11.6	64.5 ± 11.2	<0.001
hospital stays (d)	9.6 ± 3.4	9.5 ± 3.4	0.677
TC(mg/dl)	192.5 ± 40.9	197.6 ± 46.6	0.013
Females	192 (22.2)	363(36.6)	<0.001
Hypertension	347(40.2)	452 (45.5)	0.021
Cigarette smoking	509 (59.0)	416 (41.9)	<0.001
Previous angina pectoris	551(63.8)	660(66.5)	0.237
Previous myocardial infarction	78(9.0)	95 (9.6)	0.696
Family history of CAD	208 (24.1)	205 (20.6)	0.074
Patients with Killip class ≥ III	46(5.3)	89 (9.0)	0.003

Data are mean values ± SD or number (%)

FG fasting glucose, *TC* total cholesterol, *CAD* coronary artery disease

Table 2 In-hospital management in patients with fasting glucose <100 mg/dL and ≥ 100 mg/dL

In-hospital Management	Normal FG (n = 863)	Elevated FG (n = 993)	P value
Reperfusion therapy	359 (41.6)	349 (35.1)	0.004
Thrombolysis	158 (18.3)	132 (13.3)	0.003
Primary PCI	201 (23.3)	217 (21.9)	0.46
Antiplatelets	847 (98.1)	968 (97.5)	0.332
Nitrates	852 (98.7)	975 (98.2)	0.351
β-receptor blockers	610 (70.7)	664 (66.9)	0.077
ACEI or ARB	663 (76.8)	746 (75.1)	0.393
Statins	668 (77.4)	816 (82.2)	0.010
Heparins	787 (91.2)	900 (90.6)	0.676

PCI percutaneous coronary intervention, ACEI angiotensin-converting-enzyme inhibitor, ARB angiotensin receptor blocker, GIK glucose-insulin-potassium

($r = 0.830$, $P < 0.001$) (Fig. 2). However, the relationship between the two variables displayed a J-curve configuration and the lowest mortality occurred in patients with FG of 80–99.9 mg/dL. The in-hospital mortality showed a stepwise increase when FG was ≥ 100 mg/dL and tended to increase again when FG was < 80 mg/dL. Although there was no significant difference in mortality between patients with FG of 80–99.9 mg/dL and those with FG of 70–79.9 mg/dl ($P = 0.182$), there was significant difference in mortality between patients with FG of 80–99.9 mg/dL and those with FG <70 mg/dL ($P = 0.046$).

Predictors of in-hospital mortality

In order to identify clinical variables that can independently predict the occurrence of in-hospital death in patients with AMI and diabetes mellitus, a multivariate logistic regression model was used in which in-hospital death was the dependent variable and risk factors including age, gender, history of hypertension, level of FG and TC, cigarette smoking, Killip class of cardiac function on admission, and administration of reperfusion therapy and statins, all of which showed a significant difference between patients with normal and elevated FG, were entered as independent variables. The results demonstrated that age, levels of FG and Killip class of cardiac function, history of hypertension, and administration of reperfusion therapy were significant predictors of in-hospital death in all patients with AMI and diabetes mellitus (Table 4). However, when multivariate logistic regression analysis was performed in patients with elevated FG, the prognostic value of history of hypertension disappeared and age,

levels of FG, Killip class of cardiac function and administration of reperfusion therapy still were significant predictors (Table 5).

To further explore the prognostic value of a low level of FG, we performed multivariate logistic regression analysis in the subgroup of patients with FG <80 mg/dL. There were 236 patients in this subgroup with 193 men and 43 women aged 61.1 ± 11.7 years. The dependent and independent variables were the same as previous analysis. The result demonstrated that only age, FG levels and Killip class of cardiac function were identified as the independent predictors of in-hospital mortality in this subgroup of patients (Table 5). However, the level of FG lost its prognostic value in the subgroup of patients with normal FG (Table 5). As we mentioned above, age and Killip class of cardiac function on admission, FG levels were significant predictors of in-hospital mortality in patients with AMI and diabetes mellitus regardless of the FG level was low or high.

Hemoglobin A1c (HbA1c), an indirect measure of mean blood glucose over the previous 2–3 months, does not require fasting, and is more reproducible than FG and the American Diabetes Association (ADA) report in 2009 advocated the diagnosis of diabetes may be based on A1c ≥ 6.5 %. When we reviewed the medical record for each AMI patient we found that HbA1c was measured 439 patients and there were 332 men and 107 women aged from 27 to 91 years (63.1 ± 12.1 years). The mean HbA1c level of the study population was 5.73 ± 1.42 % (range: 3.81–11.35 %) and HbA1c level < 6.5 % was found in 328 patients. Compared with patients with

Table 3 In-hospital Adverse Events in Patients with Fasting Glucose <100 mg/dL and ≥ 100 mg/dL

In-hospital adverse events	Normal FG (n = 863)	Elevated FG (n = 993)	P value
Unstable angina pectoris	341 (39.5)	363 (36.6)	0.190
Reinfarction	15 (1.7)	24 (2.4)	0.309
Congestive heart failure	139 (16.1)	215 (21.7)	0.002
Total mortality	48 (5.6)	107 (10.8)	<0.001

Relationship between fasting glucose levels and in-hospital mortality in Chinese patients with acute...

49

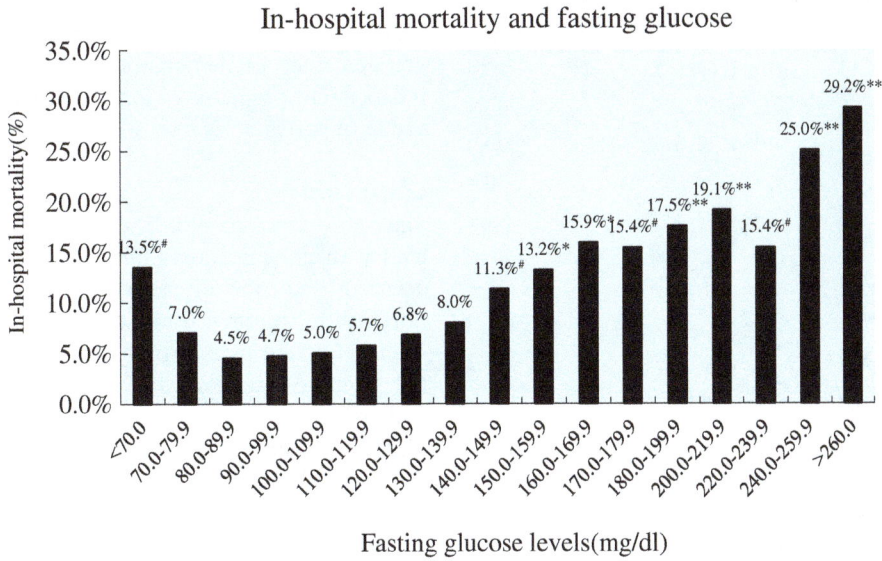

Fig. 1 In-hospital mortality and fasting glucose. Figure 1 showed the relationship between FG levels and in-hospital mortality in all patients with AMI and diabetes mellitus. Chi-square analysis was used to test the difference in mortality between patients with a FG level of 80–89.9 mg/dL and any of the other patient groups with different FG levels. The in-hospital mortality was the lowest in patients with a FG level of 80–89.9 mg/dL and increased continuously with the increase in FG levels when FG was ≥100 mg/dL. However, the mortality tended to increase again when FG was <80 mg/dL. # $P < 0.05$, * $P < 0.01$, ** $P < 0.001$. FG: fasting glucose; AMI: acute myocardial infarction

HbA1c level < 6.5 %, a greater proportion of patients with HbA1c level ≥ 6.5 % were old (64.9 ± 12.4 years vs 62.5 ± 11.9 years, $P = 0.067$) and female (39.6 % vs 19.2 %, $P < 0.001$), and exhibited a high level of FG (167.3 ± 47.4 mg/dL vs 92.0 ± 16.6 mg/dL, $P < 0.001$) and TC (223.0 ± 48.8 mg/dL vs 210.0 ± 38.5 mg/dL, $P = 0.004$). In contrast, cigarette smoking was more common

in patients with HbA1c level < 6.5 % than those with HbA1c level ≥ 6.5 % (60.7 % vs 45.0 %, $P = 0.004$). Among this study population, only 181 underwent reperfusion therapy (41.2 %). It is noteworthy that patients with HbA1c level ≥ 6.5 % received even less reperfusion therapy than those with HbA1c level < 6.5 % (26.1 % vs 46.3 %, $P < 0.001$). There was no significant difference in

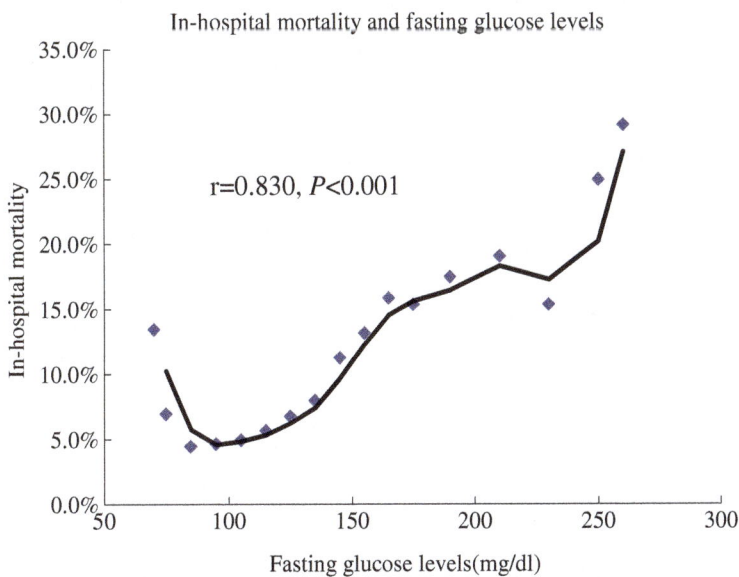

Fig. 2 In-hospital mortality and fasting glucose levels. Spearman rank correlation between FG levels and in-hospital mortality in all patients with AMI and diabetes mellitus. There was a high correlation between the two parameters ($r = 0.830$, $P < 0.001$). However, the relationship showed a J-curve configuration and the mortality rose again when FG was <80 mg/dL. FG: fasting glucose; AMI: acute myocardial infarction

Table 4 Results of logistic regression analysis in all patients

Factors	OR (95 % CI)	P value
Age	1.10 (1.08–1.13)	<0.001
Gender	0.79 (0.50–1.25)	0.307
Fasting glucose	1.19 (1.12–1.26)	<0.001
TC	1.14 (0.93–1.39)	0.204
Cigarette smoking	1.50 (0.97–2.33)	0.068
Hypertension	1.83 (1.23–2.73)	0.003
Killip classification	3.48 (2.80–4.32)	<0.001
Reperfusion therapy	0.59 (0.42–0.83)	0.003
Statins	1.04 (0.53–2.02)	0.918

OR odds ratio, CI confidence interval

receiving other life-saving therapies between the two groups of patients. A higher incidence of in-hospital death was observed in patients with HbA1c level ≥ 6.5 % than those with HbA1c level < 6.5 % (18.0 % vs 7.0 %, P < 0.001). In contrast, there was no significant difference in the incidence of congestive heart failure (17.1 % vs 13.7 %, $P = 0.381$), recurrent unstable angina pectoris (36.0 % vs 43.0 %, $P = 0.198$) and reinfarction (4.5 % vs 2.1 %, $P = 0.324$) between the two groups. Using multivariate logistic regression models, we identified that age, Killip class of cardiac function and reperfusion therapy were independent predictors of in-hospital mortality in this study population, fasting glucose concentration and HbA1c level were not independent predictors.

Up till now, only 835 patients have completed the follow-up which included 322 patients in the normal FG group and 513 patients in the elevated FG group. A higher incidence of death was observed in patients with elevated FG than those with normal FG during the long term follow-up (32.4 % vs 25.2 %, $P = 0.026$). Logistic regression showed that Killip class of cardiac function, age, gender, and fasting glucose levels were independent predictors of long term survival in the follow-up population.

Only 82 patients have completed the follow-up in the subgroup of patients with FG <80 mg/dL and logistic regression analysis demonstrated that FG levels was not independent predictor of long term mortality in the subgroup of patients.

Discussion

Since the occurrence of fasting hyperglycemia is associated with an untoward outcome in patients with AMI, accurate detection of this co-morbidity is of great importance for optimal triage and management. The major finding in the present study was that more than half of the Chinese patients with AMI and diabetes mellitus had an elevated FG level which was associated with higher in-hospital mortality than in those with a normal FG level. Although there was a high correlation between FG levels and in-hospital mortality in all patients, the relationship was a J-curve configuration with an increased mortality when FG was <80 mg/dL. Both FG ≥ 100 mg/dL and FG <80 mg/dL were identified to be independent predictors of in-hospitality and thus the optimal FG level in patients with AMI appears to be 80–100 mg/dL. To the best of our knowledge, this study is the first in the literature to report the J-curve relationship between FG levels and in-hospital mortality and define the optimal FG levels in Chinese patients with AMI and diabetes mellitus.

In the present study, a higher incidence of in-hospital death and congestive heart failure was found in AMI patients with elevated FG than those with normal FG. Although differences in baseline characteristics and management may contribute to the higher mortality in patients with elevated FG, the level of FG as a continuous variable remained a strong independent predictor of in-hospital death in this group of patients even after all risk factors were taken into account in our multivariate logistic regression model. It is noteworthy that the in-hospital mortality increased continuously with the increase

Table 5 Results of logistic regression analysis in patients with different fasting glucose levels

Factors	FG <80 mg/dL (n = 236) OR (95 % CI)	FG 80–100 mg/dL (n = 627) OR (95 % CI)	FG ≥ 100 mg/dL (n = 993) OR (95 % CI)
Age	1.08 (1.02–1.15)**	1.12 (1.06–1.18)**	1.11 (1.07–1.15)**
Gender	0.20 (0.02–1.82)#	076 (0.28–20.6)#	0.93 (0.52–1.67)#
Fasting glucose	0.13 (0.03–0.63)*	1.72 (0.46–6.50)#	1.25 (1.16–1.35)**
TC	1.08 (0.49–2.37)#	1.27 (0.80–2.00)#	1.11 (0.87–1.41)#
Cigarette smoking	2.22 (0.52–9.46)#	1.14 (0.46–2.81)#	1.56 (0.89–2.75)#
Hypertension	2.89 (0.88–9.51)#	2.47 (1.07–5.74)*	1.54 (0.92–2.57)#
Killip classification	4.93 (2.35–10.33)**	2.21 (1.37–3.56)**	4.06 (3.05–5.40)**
Reperfusion therapy	0.54 (0.20–1.48)#	0.66 (0.35–1.26)#	0.61 (0.38–0.98)*
Statins	1.11 (0.19–6.49)#	1.23 (0.30–4.94)#	1.08 (0.44–2.67)#

#P > 0.05, *P < 0.05, **P < 0.01

in FG across a wide range of FG measurements and there was a high correlation between FG levels and in-hospital mortality in all patients. It should also noted that the level of FG lost its prognostic value in patients with normal FG and the stepwise increase in mortality was not statistically significant until FG reached a level of ≥ 140 mg/dL (Fig. 1). These results suggest that FG <100 mg/dL may not be a risk factor of in-hospital death in patients with AMI, a finding similar to previous studies [5, 11]. However, the relationship between FG levels and in-hospital mortality revealed a J-curve configuration and the mortality tended to increase again when FG was < 80 mg/dL. Multivariate logistic regression analysis in this subgroup of patients demonstrated that FG < 80 mg/dL was also an independent predictor of in-hospital mortality in patients with AMI. This new finding indicates that a low albeit normal FG level may do harm to patients with AMI. Since both FG $\geq$ 100 mg/dL and FG <80 mg/dL were independent predictors of in-hospitality in patients with AMI and diabetes mellitus, it is logical to speculate that the optimal FG level in patients with AMI and diabetes mellitus should be 80–100 mg/dL.

The mechanisms underlying the relationship between FG levels and in-hospital mortality in patients with AMI and diabetes mellitus are not completely understood. It has been suggested that hyperglycemia is a marker of extensive myocardial damage and a consequence of excessive secretion of stress hormones that inhibit the action of insulin [12]. Alternatively, hyperglycemia may result from insulin resistance commonly seen in patients with coronary artery disease, which is aggravated by the onset of AMI. Insulin deficiency promotes lipolysis and increases circulating free fatty acids which may be toxic to ischemic myocardium. Recent studies have showed that insulin has a powerful anti-inflammatory effect, which is associated with improvements in morbidity and mortality [13], and these beneficial effects may have been reduced in patients with elevated FG. Moreover, fasting hyperglycemia per se may induce dysfunction of vascular endothelial cells, vascular smooth muscle cells and platelets [14], and cause hypercoagulability and impaired fibrinolysis [15]. The reason why a low-normal FG level carries a poor outcome in patients with AMI is not clear. The relatively low plasma glucose levels in these patients are probably be attributed to the administration of antidiabetic agents, insufficient food intake and/or excessive vomiting. When we reviewed the medical record we found the excessive administration of antidiabetic agents, insufficient food intake and/or excessive vomiting were seen in about one fourth of patients having low blood glucose levels. A low level of plasma glucose may reduce the glucose intake by the ischemic myocardium and impair remote ischemic preconditioning and further exacerbate myocardial damage [16].

Among 22 clinical parameters recorded in this study, we identified age, levels of FG and Killip class of cardiac function, history of hypertension, and administration of reperfusion therapy as significant predictors of in-hospital death in patients with AMI and diabetes mellitus. As mentioned in this study, compared with patients having lower FG levels, a greater proportion of patients with elevated FG were old and female, had a history of documented hypertension. Hemorrhage, especially cerebral hemorrhage was more common in old, female, hypertensive patients when thrombolytic therapy was administered. Thus patients with elevated FG received even less thrombolytic therapy than those having lower FG levels.

The odds ratio of FG was 1.19 in patients with elevated FG which is not as impressive as in the previous studies because FG levels were entered as the continuous variables in our multivariate logistic regression model whereas they were entered as categorical variables in previous studies [5]. However, as judged by their corresponding P values, the predictive power of FG levels was weaker than age and Killip class of cardiac function but stronger than the administration of reperfusion therapy and history of hypertension.

It is well known that HbA1c captures chronic hyperglycemia in the prior 2–3 months, is well correlated to chronic diabetes complications, and has less preanalytical problems and biological variability than plasma glucose, with a noninferior standardization. As shown in this study, high level of HbA1c is associated with an increased short-term mortality in patients with AMI and diabetes mellitus. However, multivariate logistic regression analysis demonstrated that HbA1c level was not an independent predictor of in-hospital mortality in the subgroup of patients whose HbA1c level and FG were all measured during hospital stay. The reason for this may be due the small sample size studied in this subgroup of patients because in contrast to seen in the whole population, like HbA1c level, FG was not an independent predictor in this subgroup of patients too.

Although most of patients lost to follow-up and we keep in touch with only 835 patients till now, high incidence of death was observed in patients with elevated FG during the long term follow-up and logistic regression showed that FG was also an independent predictor of long term survival in this subgroup population. This result showed that FG level was not only a short term but also a long term independent predictor of outcomes in patients with AMI and diabetes. This finding seems to be particularly important due to a limited number of proven predictors of mortality in these patients.

Study limitations

There were several important limitations in our study. First, this is a retrospective and observational study.

However, all the medical records were made by the same department of cardiology and laboratory of biochemistry and the quality control can thus be assured. Besides, our study provides unbiased data in real clinical practice. Second, the majority (61.9 %) of patients enrolled did not undergo reperfusion therapy because of late arrival at the hospital or economical restraint, which reflects the therapeutic situations in the past 12 years in Shandong Province of China. However, the in-hospital mortality in our patients was comparable to previous reports. Third, although all patients hospitalized between January 2002 and December 2013 were enrolled, patients who died before reaching the hospital may have been missed, which may have resulted in an underestimation of the mortality rate in patients with AMI and diabetes mellitus.

Conclusions

In conclusion, more than half of the Chinese patients with AMI and diabetes mellitus had elevated FG and there was higher in-hospital mortality in these patients than in those with AMI and a normal FG level. The in-hospital mortality in patients with AMI and diabetes mellitus increases continuously with the increase in FG and there was a high correlation between the two parameters. However, the relationship was a J-curve configuration with an increased mortality when FG was FG <80 mg/dL. Both FG ≥ 100 mg/dL and FG <80 mg/dL were identified to be independent predictors of in-hospitality and thus the optimal FG level in patients with AMI and diabetes mellitus appears to be 80–100 mg/dL. Long term follow-up study demonstrated that FG level was also a long term independent predictor of outcomes in patients with AMI and diabetes.

Abbreviations

ACEI, angiotensin-converting-enzyme inhibitors; AMI, acute myocardial infarction; ARB, angiotensin receptor blockers; CABG, coronary artery bypass grafting; CAD, coronary artery disease; CI, Confidence intervals; FG, fasting glucose; GIK, Glucose-Insulin-Potassium; OR, odds ratio; PCI, percutaneous coronary intervention; SD, standard deviation; TC, total cholesterol

Acknowledgments

This study was supported by the Shandong province science and technology research projects (No.2012GSF2180). We gratefully acknowledge the assistance provided by Dr. Li Hua Dai and Dr. Qing Bin Zhang in data collection.

Funding

This study was supported by the Shandong province science and technology research projects (No.2012GSF2180).

Authors' contributions

SLJ and HL designed and supervised the study and wrote the manuscript. YCG collected the data, LMC analyzed the data, ML and WZH participated in the study design and critical review of the study results, XZ helped to write and revised the manuscript. All authors listed in this paper had final approval of the submitted version.

Competing interests
The authors declare that they have no competing interests.

Author details
[1]The Ultrasonic Diagnosis and Treatment Department, Shandong Provincial Hospital affiliated to Shandong University, Jinan, Shandong, China. [2]Department of Cardiology, Shandong Provincial Hospital affiliated to Shandong University, No.324, Jing Wu Wei Qi Road, Jinan 250021, Shandong, People's Republic of China. [3]Department of Endocrinology, Shandong Provincial Hospital affiliated to Shandong University, Jinan, Shandong, China.

References
1. Chatterjee S, Sharma A, Lichstein E, Mukherjee D. Intensive glucose control in diabetics with an acute myocardial infarction does not improve mortality and increases risk of hypoglycemia-a meta-regression analysis. Curr Vasc Pharmacol. 2013;11(1):100–4.
2. Yang SW, Zhou YJ, Liu YY, Hu DY, Shi YJ, Nie XM, et al. Influence of abnormal fasting plasma glucose on left ventricular function in older patients with acute myocardial infarction. Angiology. 2012;63(4):266–74.
3. Hoebers LP, Damman P, Claessen BE, Vis MM, Baan J, van Straalen JP, et al. Predictive value of plasma glucose level on admission for short and long term mortality in patients with ST-elevation myocardial infarction treated with primary percutaneous coronary intervention. Am J Cardiol. 2012; 109(1):53–9.
4. Mazurek M, Kowalczyk J, Lenarczyk R, Zielinska T, Sedkowska A, Pruszkowska-Skrzep P, et al. The prognostic value of different glucose abnormalities in patients with acute myocardial infarction treated invasively. Cardiovasc Diabetol. 2012;11:78.
5. Suleiman M, Hammerman H, Boulos M, Kapeliovich MR, Suleiman A, Agmon Y, et al. Fasting glucose is an important independent risk factor for 30-day mortality in patients with acute myocardial infarction: a prospective study. Circulation. 2005;111(6):754–60.
6. Thygesen K, Alpert JS, Jaffe AS, Simoons ML, Chaitman BR, White HD. Third universal definition of myocardial infarction. Nat Rev Cardiol. 2012; 9(11):620–33.
7. Seino Y, Nanjo K, Tajima N, Kadowaki T, Kashiwagi A, Araki E, et al. Report of the committee on the classification and diagnostic criteria of diabetes mellitus. J Diabetes Investig. 2010;1(5):212–8.
8. Genuth S, Alberti KG, Bennett P, Buse J, Defronzo R, Kahn R, et al. Expert committee on the diagnosis and classification of diabetes mellitus. Follow-up report on the diagnosis of diabetes mellitus. Diabetes Care. 2003;26(11):3160–7.
9. Andersen HR, Nielsen TT, Vesterlund T, Grande P, Abildgaard U, Thayssen P, et al. DANAMI-2 Investigators. Danish multicenter randomized study on fibrinolytic therapy versus acute coronary angioplasty in acute myocardial infarction: rationale and design of the DANish trial in Acute Myocardial Infarction-2 (DANAMI-2). Am Heart J. 2003;146(2):234–41.
10. Abildstrom SZ, Ottesen MM, Rask-Madsen C, Andersen PK, Rosthøj S, Torp-Pedersen C, et al. Sudden cardiovascular death following myocardial infarction: the importance of left ventricular systolic dysfunction and congestive heart failure. Int J Cardiol. 2005;104(2):184–9.
11. Zeller M, Cottin Y, Brindisi M-C, Laurent Y, Janin-Manificat L, L'Huillier I, et al. Impaired fasting glucose and cardiogenic shock in patients with acute myocardial infarction. Eur Heart J. 2004;25(4):308–12.
12. Oliver MF, Opie LH. Effects of glucose and fatty acids on myocardial ischaemia and arrhythmias. Lancet. 1994;343(8890):155–8.
13. Hansen TK, Thiel S, Wouters PJ, Christiansen JS, Van den Berghe G. Intensive insulin therapy exerts antiinflammatory effects in critically ill patients and counteracts the adverse effect of low mannose-binding lectin levels. J Clin Endocrinol Metab. 2003;88(3):1082–8.
14. Creager MA, Luscher TF, Cosentino F, Beckman JA. Diabetes and vascular disease: pathophysiology, clinical consequences, and medical therapy: part I. Circulation. 2003;108(12):1527–32.
15. Beckman JA, Creager MA, Libby P. Diabetes and atherosclerosis: epidemiology, pathophysiology, and management. JAMA. 2002;287(19):2570–81.
16. D'Ascenzo F, Moretti C, Omedè P, Cerrato E, Cavallero E, Er F, et al. Cardiac remote ischaemic preconditioning reduces periprocedural myocardial infarction for patients undergoing percutaneous coronary interventions: a meta-analysis of randomised clinical trials. EuroIntervention. 2014;9(12):1463–71.

7

A comparative study of time-specific oxidative stress after acute myocardial infarction in patients with and without diabetes mellitus

Daisuke Kitano, Tadateru Takayama, Koichi Nagashima, Masafumi Akabane, Kimie Okubo, Takafumi Hiro and Atsushi Hirayama[*]

Abstract

Background: Oxidative stress is involved in the initiation and progression of atherosclerosis, and hyperglycemia is known to increase oxidative stress, which injures the endothelium and accelerates atherosclerosis. To clarify the relation between oxidative stress, diabetes mellitus (DM), and acute myocardial infarction (AMI), we evaluated and compared time-specific oxidative stress after AMI in patients with and without DM by simple measurement of derivatives of reactive oxygen metabolites (d-ROMs) levels as indices of reactive oxygen species production.

Methods: Sixty-eight AMI patients were enrolled (34 non-DM patients and 34 DM patients). Using the FRAS4 free radical analytical system, we measured d-ROMs levels in each patient at two time points: 1 and 2 weeks after AMI onset.

Results: d-ROM levels decreased significantly between week 1 and week 2 (from 475.4 ± 119.4 U.CARR to 367.7 ± 87.9 U.CARR, $p < 0.001$) in the non-DM patients but did not change in the DM patients (from 463.1 ± 109.3 U.CARR to 461.7 ± 126.8 U.CARR, $p = 0.819$). Moreover, significant correlation was found in the total patient group between d-ROMs levels at 1 week and N-terminal prohormone of brain natriuretic peptide ($r = 0.376$, $p = 0.041$) and between d-ROM levels at 2 weeks and 2-hour oral glucose tolerance test glucose levels ($r = 0.434$, $p < 0.001$).

Conclusions: Exposure to oxidative stress is greater in AMI patients with DM than AMI patients without DM. Our study results suggest that it is the continuous hyperglycemia that increases oxidative stress in these patients, causing endothelial dysfunction and accelerating atherosclerosis. However, long-term follow up study is needed to assess whether the increased oxidative stress affects patient outcomes.

Keywords: Derivatives of reactive oxygen metabolite, Oxidative stress, Acute myocardial infarction, Diabetes mellitus

Background

Oxidative stress, which is implicated in various disorders, especially lifestyle-related diseases such as diabetes mellitus (DM), is involved in the initiation and progression of atherosclerosis [1–3]. Biomarkers of oxidative stress, such as serum malondialdehyde measured as thiobarbituric acid-reactive substances, oxidized low-density lipoprotein, oxidative DNA damage byproduct 8-hydroxydeoxyguanosine, and urinary 8-iso-prostaglandin-F2α, are generally measured in research laboratories [4–7]. Indices of antioxidant potential, especially intracellular levels of superoxide dismutase and glutathione peroxidase, are also measured [8, 9]. However, the assay methods are complex and not suitable for large-scale analysis. Simpler means of detecting reactive oxygen species (ROS) by assay of derivatives of reactive oxygen metabolites (d-ROMs) and biological antioxidant potential have been developed, and reports of these methods and studies based on these methods have been increasing [10–19].

DM is a major risk factor for cardiovascular disease. Continuous hyperglycemia increases advanced glycation end products (AGEs) and induces ROS production [20]. ROS plays a pivotal role in the development of the

* Correspondence: hirayama.atsushi@nihon-u.ac.jp
Division of Cardiology, Department of Medicine, Nihon University School of Medicine, 30-1 Oyaguchi-kamicho, Itabashi-ku, Tokyo 173-8610, Japan

microvascular and cardiovascular complications of DM. The increased ROS in patients with type 2 DM and metabolic syndrome is a consequence of metabolic abnormalities, including hyperglycemia, insulin resistance, hyperinsulinemia, and dyslipidemia [21], each of which contributes to mitochondrial superoxide overproduction in endothelial cells of large and small vessels as well as the myocardium [22]. The atherosclerosis is accelerated and may induce acute coronary syndrome.

Thus, we are interested in the relations between oxidative stress, DM, and acute myocardial infarction (AMI), we evaluated and compared time-specific oxidative stress after AMI in patients with and without DM by simple measurement of d-ROMs levels as indices of ROS production.

Methods
Study patients
The study involved 68 consecutive patients who had suffered an ST-elevated AMI, admitted to the coronary care unit of Nihon University Itabashi Hospital between April 2010 and March 2011, and underwent successful primary percutaneous coronary intervention (PCI). Thirty-four had type 2 DM (DM group) and 34 did not (non-DM group). Patients with severe MI; those recovering from cardiopulmonary arrest or heart failure; and those with cardiomyopathy, severe valvular disease, atrial fibrillation, chronic kidney disease requiring hemodialysis, type 1 DM, type 2 DM requiring insulin or glucagon-like peptide-1 receptor agonists treatment, collagen disease, or malignant tumor were excluded from the study. Medications patients had been taking were not changed, and anti-diabetic agents were not given during the study period. We also collected d-ROM values in stable coronary artery disease (CAD) patients without DM (n = 40) and with DM (n = 28) as reference value, they had undergone coronary stenting for stable CAD except acute coronary syndrome more than 8 months before data collection.

The study was approved by the ethics committee of Nihon University Itabashi Hospital, and written informed consent was provided by each patient for participation.

Clinical evaluation and laboratory measurements
Patients' clinical characteristics, including age, sex, body mass index, smoking history, and history of hypertension and dyslipidemia were recorded, and blood samples were drawn 1 week after AMI onset for measurement of hemoglobin A1c (HbA1c), fasting glucose, total cholesterol, low-density lipoprotein-cholesterol, high-density lipoprotein-cholesterol, creatine phosphokinase (CPK), estimated glomerular filtration rate (eGFR), high-sensitivity C-reactive protein (hs-CRP) and N-terminal prohormone of brain natriuretic peptide (NT-proBNP). Insulin resistance was evaluated by means of homeostasis model assessment of insulin resistance (HOMA-IR), and an oral glucose tolerance test (OGTT) was given to evaluate glucose clearance.

Assay of oxidative stress
We quantified hydrogen peroxide levels by measuring d-ROMs using the FRAS4 Free Radical Analytical System (H&D srl, Parma, Italy). Hydrogen peroxides are converted into radicals that oxidize N, N-diethyl-para-phenylenediamine and can be detected spectrophotometrically with the use of an all-purpose automatic analyzer. The d-ROM levels are expressed in arbitrary units called Carratelli units (U.CARR) [10]. The normal reference level of d-ROMs is 250 to 300 U.CARR [23, 24]. We measured d-ROMs at 2 time points, 1 week and 2 weeks after AMI onset, to avoid the possible influence of AMI.

Statistical analysis
Continuous variables are expressed as mean ± SD values, and categorical variables are presented as numbers and percentages. Between-group differences were analyzed by one-way ANOVA with Tukey post-hoc honest significant difference test or by chi-square test, as appropriate. Differences between 1-week and 2-week values were analyzed by paired t-test, Wilcoxon signed-rank test, or unpaired t-test, as appropriate. Association between d-ROM levels and clinical variables was tested by linear regression analysis, and factors predictive of no or little change in the d-ROM level between 1 and 2 weeks after AMI were identified by multiple logistic regression analysis. Statistical analyses were performed with JMP ver. 9 (SAS Institute, Cary, NC, USA). A p value of 0.05 was considered significant.

Results
Patients' clinical characteristics and laboratory values
Clinical characteristics of the study patients are shown in Table 1. Only HbA1c, fasting plasma glucose, 2-h OGTT glucose, HOMA-IR, eGFR, and the use of nitrate differed significantly between the two patient groups. Additional file 1 shows clinical characteristics of reference patients.

Changes in oxidative stress
Shown in Fig. 1, the d-ROMs level 1 week after AMI did not differ significantly between the DM group and the non-DM group (463.1 ± 109.3 U.CARR vs. 475.4 ± 119.4 U.CARR, respectively, $p = 0.382$). At 2 weeks after AMI, the d-ROMs level had decreased significantly in the non-DM group (from 475.4 ± 119.4 U.CARR to 367.7 ± 87.9 U.CARR, $p < 0.001$) but remained unchanged in the DM group (from 463.1 ± 109.3 U.CARR to 461.7 ± 126.8

Table 1 Clinical characteristics of study patients upon enrollment[a], per study group

	non-DM	DM	p value[b]
	n = 34	n = 34	
Age (years)	62.1 ± 9.6	61.4 ± 9.9	0.739
Sex, male (%)	32 (94.1)	29 (85.3)	0.259
BMI	24.7 ± 2.5	25.3 ± 2.6	0.293
Risk factors			
Hypertension, n (%)	28 (82.4)	29 (85.3)	0.742
Dyslipidemia, n (%)	26 (76.5)	26 (76.5)	1.000
Smoking, n (%)	19 (55.9)	23 (67.6)	0.318
Biochemical markers			
HbA1c (%)	5.6 ± 0.3	6.6 ± 0.5	**<0.001**
Fasting plasma glucose (mg/dL)	97.5 ± 7.4	114.6 ± 18.6	**<0.001**
2 h OGTT plasma glucose (mg/dL)	119.8 ± 13.0	172.7 ± 33.7	**<0.001**
HOMA-IR	1.53 ± 0.81	2.73 ± 1.89	**<0.001**
eGFR (mL/min/1.73 m²)	63.2 ± 16.0	71.7 ± 16.5	**0.035**
CPK (maximum) (U/L)	3532.2 ± 3898.3	2360.6 ± 2181.8	0.247
hs-CRP (mg/dL)	0.654 ± 0.695	0.828 ± 0.712	0.311
Total cholesterol (mg/dL)	199.9 ± 35.3	196.0 ± 57.4	0.954
Triglyceride (mg/dL)	95.0 ± 55.2	127.6 ± 77.8	0.277
HDL cholesterol (mg/dL)	46.6 ± 12.3	45.8 ± 10.0	0.825
LDL cholesterol (mg/dL)	134.3 ± 29.5	116.7 ± 37.0	0.752
NT-proBNP (pg/mL)	804.8 ± 1057.8	645.1 ± 915.0	0.578
Medications			
Ca channel blocker, n (%)	9 (26.5)	6 (17.6)	0.470
Beta blocker, n (%)	19 (55.9)	18 (52.9)	0.924
ACE-I/ARB, n (%)	22 (64.7)	25 (73.5)	0.504
Nitrate, n (%)	30 (88.2)	18 (52.9)	**0.004**
Statin, n (%)	24 (70.6)	23 (67.6)	0.853

[a]At 1 week after AMI onset

Data are expressed as mean ± SD or number (%). [b]obtained by ANOVA or chi-square test. HbA1c, fasting plasma glucose, 2 h OGTT plasma glucose, HOMA-IR and eGFR levels were significantly higher and the use of nitrate was signifincatly lower in DM patients group. *DM* diabetes mellitus, *BMI* body mass index, *HbA1c* hemoglobin A1c, *OGTT* oral glucose tolerance test, *HOMA-IR* homeostatic model assessment-insulin resistance, *eGFR* estimated glomerular filtration rate, *CPK* creatine phosphokinase, *hs-CRP* high-sensitivity C-reactive protein, *HDL* high density lipoprotein, *LDL* low density lipoprotein, *NT-proBNP* N-terminal prohormone of brain natriuretic peptide, *ACE-I* angiotensin converting enzyme inhibitor, *ARB* angiotensin receptor blocker

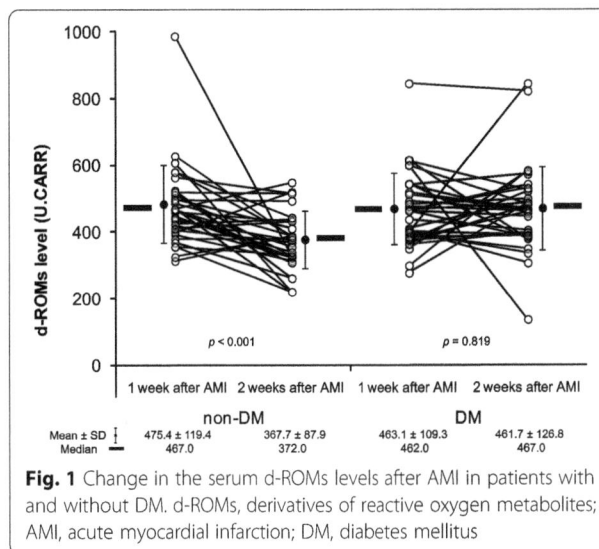

Fig. 1 Change in the serum d-ROMs levels after AMI in patients with and without DM. d-ROMs, derivatives of reactive oxygen metabolites; AMI, acute myocardial infarction; DM, diabetes mellitus

and NT-proBNP levels (r = 0.376, p = 0.041) (Fig. 2, left panel) and between d-ROMs levels at 2 weeks and 2-h OGTT glucose levels (r = 0.434, p < 0.001) (Fig. 2, right panel). There was no relation between the d-ROMs level and age, sex, BMI, glucose profiles except 2-h OGTT glucose level, renal function, CPK, lipids, or use of the various medications. Multivariate logistic regression analysis showed the presence of DM to be a significant predictor of little or no change in the d-ROMs level by 2 weeks after AMI (Table 2), after adjustment for significant factors identified by univariate analysis (odds ratio: 3.33, 95 % confidence interval: 1.15–10.48) (Table 2).

Discussion

Oxidative stress is implicated in various disorders and pathogeneses. Many studies have shown its involvement in the pathogeneses of lifestyle-related diseases. Previous clinical studies have made use of markers of ROS, such as 8-hydroxydeoxyguanosine and 8-iso-prostaglandin-F2α. However, it is difficult to measure these markers at health checkup facilities. Furthermore, superoxide dismutase, which can serve as an index of antioxidant potential, is also difficult to measure, even at research facilities. In this study, we used a simple assay method to examine the course of oxidative stress between 1 week and 2 weeks after AMI in patients with DM. This is the first study to observe time-specific change in oxidative stress in the early stage after AMI and to examine the difference in exposure to oxidative stress between patients with DM and those without DM.

Recent studies have shown the usefulness d-ROMs assay for evaluating oxidative stress [13–15, 17], and in such evaluation, Trotti et al. found no statistically significant difference between male and female Europeans [11], whereas Fukui et al. found the mean d-ROMs level

U.CARR, p = 0.819). Reference d-ROM values are shown in Additional file 2, the value in stable CAD patients without DM was 341.7 ± 101.7 U.CARR, and the value in those with DM was 377 ± 128.3 U.CARR. There was no signifincat difference between these values.

Major determinant of changes in oxidative stress

In the total patient group, significant positive correlation was found between d-ROMs levels 1 week after AMI

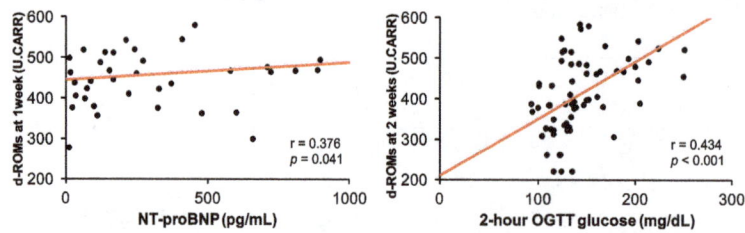

Fig. 2 Correlation between d-ROMs levels and NT-proBNP levels at 1 week after AMI (left) and between d-ROMs levels at 2 weeks after AMI and glucose levels at 2 h after OGTT (right). d-ROMs, derivatives of reactive oxygen metabolites; AMI, acute myocardial infarction; NT-proBNP, N-terminal prohormone of brain natriuretic peptide; OGTT, oral glucose tolerance test

in female Japanese to be significantly higher than that in male Japanese [25]. Moreover positive correlation between levels of hs-CRP and d-ROMs has been reported [14, 15, 17]. Nevertheless, we found that most clinical characteristics, including sex and hs-CRP, are not factors that significantly influence d-ROMs in

Table 2 Factors tested as predictors of lack of change in the d-ROMs level 2 weeks after AMI

Factor	Univariate analysis		Multivariate analysis	
	OR (95 % CI)	p value	OR (95 % CI)	p value
Age	1.01 (0.95–1.07)	0.677		
Sex	1.50 (0.31–10.87)	0.629		
BMI	1.09 (0.89–1.35)	0.396		
Diabetes mellitus	3.05 (1.07–9.34)	**0.037**	3.33 (1.15–10.48)	**0.027**
Fasting glucose level	1.01 (0.98–1.05)	0.363		
2 h OGTT glucose level	1.02 (1.00–1.03)	**0.032**	1.02 (1.00–1.04)	0.098
HOMA-IR	1.10 (0.79–1.51)	0.570		
eGFR	1.00 (0.98–1.04)	0.675		
CPK (maximum)	1.00 (1.00–1.00)	0.354		
LDL cholesterol	0.99 (0.97–1.01)	0.424		
hs-CRP	1.05 (0.48–2.13)	0.904		
NT-proBNP	1.00 (1.00–1.00)	0.147		
Ca channel blocker	0.18 (0.01–1.11)	0.122		
Beta blocker	3.35 (0.84–17.03)	0.105		
ACE-I/ARB	0.38 (0.02–3.38)	0.428		
Nitrate	0.20 (0.05–0.83)	**0.028**	0.36 (0.07–1.89)	0.216
Statin	0.39 (0.09–1.60)	0.180		

Multivariate logistic regression analysis showed the presence of diabetes mellitus was a significant predictor of no change in the d-ROMs level by 2 weeks after AMI. *d-ROMs* derivatives of reactive oxygen metabolites, *AMI* acute myocardial infarction, *OR* odds ratio, *CI* confidence interval, *BMI* body mass index, *OGTT* oral glucose tolerance test, *HOMA-IR* homeostatic model assessment-insulin resistance, *eGFR* estimated glomerular filtration rate, *CPK* creatine phosphokinase, *LDL* low density lipoprotein, *hs-CRP* high-sensitivity C-reactive protein, *NT-proBNP* N-terminal prohormone of brain natriuretic peptide, *ACE-I* angiotensin converting enzyme inhibitor, *ARB* angiotensin receptor blocker

patients with AMI. However, we did find that the NT-proBNP level was a significant predictor of the d-ROMs level at 1 week after AMI. This is consistent with the previously reported correlation between BNP and post-MI remodeling [26–28]. Furthermore, DM and hyperglycemia were identified as predictors of non-suppression of ROS production after AMI. Thus, it appears that the d-ROMs level at 1 week is influenced by the effect of MI on the heart itself, whereas the d-ROMs level at 2 weeks is the result of the continuous DM-induced hyperglycemia.

Continuous hyperglycemia increases production of AGEs and high levels of AGEs have been found in the cardiac tissue of diabetic patients [29]. AGEs induce oxidative stress and activate the protein kinase C/diacylglycerol signaling pathway, which is one of the mechanisms by which hyperglycemia exerts adverse cardiovascular effects. In addition, AGEs activate ROS production in mitochondria [20]. Increases in ROS cause cardiac dysfunction by directly damaging proteins and DNA and by inducing apoptosis [30]. We have reported a study in which we treated patients with alpha-glucosidase inhibitor (α-GI) from 1 week to 2 weeks after AMI [31]. In that study, we found that the d-ROMs level in patients treated with α-GI tended to decrease and that endothelial function improved. Thus, oxidative stress plays a pivotal role in the development of the microvascular and cardiovascular complications of DM.

There are some limitations to the present study. First, this was an association study using a case–control design and not randomized, however, the patient characteristics were well matched between groups (Table 1). Second, sample size was small and this was a single-center study. Therefore, we are not able to apply our result to the general population. Third, although we showed reference d-ROM values in stable CAD patients (Additional file 2: Table S1), this was a very short-term follow-up study, and because we did not record d-ROMs levels before AMI or primary PCI and after PCI or more than 2 weeks after AMI, any difference in d-ROMs levels after primary PCI and any progressive change in oxidative stress after AMI in patients with DM remain unknown. Fourth, we excluded patients with heart failure resulting from severe MI, first, because it has been reported that DM can lead to heart failure after MI, and second, because oxidative stress may be high in patients with heart failure [32, 33].

Conclusions

Our study showed that patients with DM are subject to clinically significant oxidative stress during the first 2 weeks after AMI. Although long-term changes in oxidative stress after AMI in patients with DM remain unknown, results of this short-term follow-up study imply that continuous hyperglycemia drives oxidative stress after AMI, leading to endothelial dysfunction, and progression of atherosclerosis.

Additional files

Additional file 1: Clinical characteristics of reference patients with stable CAD, per group. (DOCX 21 kb)

Additional file 2: d-ROM levels in stable CAD patient with DM and without DM. These data were collected from stable CAD patients with DM and without DM, who had undergone coronary stenting for stable CAD except ACS more than 8 months before data collection. Values are expressed as mean ± SD, and boxes show median and interquartile ranges between the 25th and the 75th percentiles. d-ROM, derivatives of reactive oxygen metabolites; CAD, coronary artery disease; DM, diabetes mellitus; ACS, acute coronary syndrome. (DOCX 385 kb)

Abbreviations

AGE: advanced glycation end product; AMI: acute myocardial infarction; CAD: coronary artery dieease; CPK: creatine phosphokinase; DM: diabetes mellitus; d-ROM: derivatives of reactive oxygen metabolite; eGFR: estimated glomerular filtration rate; HbA1c: hemoglobin A1c; HOMA-IR: homeostasis model assessment of insulin resistance; hs-CRP: high-sensitivity C-reactive protein; NT-proBNP: N-terminal prohormone of brain natriuretic peptide; OGTT: oral glucose tolerance test; PCI: percutaneous coronary intervenetion; ROS: reactive oxygen species.; α-GI: alpha-glucosidase inhibitor.

Acknowledgements

We sincerely thank all CCU staff at Nihon University Itabashi Hospital.

Authors' contributions

DK contributed to the study design, collected the data, and drafted the manuscript. KN, MA, and KO contributed to the study design and data collection. TT, TH, and AH contributed to the study design and reviewed and edited the manuscript. All authors critically reviewed the draft and approved the final manuscript.

Competing interests

The authors declare that they have no competing interests.

References

1. Aviram M. Review of human studies on oxidative damage and antioxidant protection related to cardiovascular diseases. Free Radic Res. 2000; 33(Suppl):85–97.

2. Griendling KK, FitzGerald GA. Oxidative stress and cardiovascular injury: Part II: animal and human studies. Circulation. 2003;108:2034–40.

3. Harrison D, Griendling KK, Landmesser U, Hornig B, Drexler H. Role of oxidative stress in atherosclerosis. Am J Cardiol. 2003;91:7A–11A.

4. Walter MF, Jacob RF, Jeffers B, Ghadanfar MM, Preston GM, Buch J, et al. Serum levels of thiobarbituric acid reactive substances predict cardiovascular events in patients with stable coronary artery disease: a longitudinal analysis of the PREVENT study. J Am Coll Cardiol. 2004;44:1996–2002.

5. Schwedhelm E, Bartling A, Lenzen H, Tsikas D, Maas R, Brümmer J, et al. Urinary 8-iso-prostaglandin F2alpha as a risk marker in patients with coronary heart disease: a matched case–control study. Circulation. 2004;109:843–8.

6. Shimada K, Mokuno H, Matsunaga E, Miyazaki T, Sumiyoshi K, Miyauchi K, et al. Circulating oxidized low-density lipoprotein is an independent predictor for cardiac event in patients with coronary artery disease. Atherosclerosis. 2004;174:343–7.

7. Wu LL, Chiou CC, Chang PY, Wu JT. Urinary 8-OHdG: a marker of oxidative stress to DNA and a risk factor for cancer, atherosclerosis and diabetics. Clin Chim Acta Int J Clin Chem. 2004;339:1–9.

8. Faraci FM, Didion SP. Vascular protection: superoxide dismutase isoforms in the vessel wall. Arterioscler Thromb Vasc Biol. 2004;24:1367–73.

9. Pyne-Geithman GJ, Caudell DN, Prakash P, Clark JF. Glutathione peroxidase and subarachnoid hemorrhage: implications for the role of oxidative stress in cerebral vasospasm. Neurol Res. 2009;31:195–9.

10. Cesarone MR, Belcaro G, Carratelli M, Cornelli U, De Sanctis MT, Incandela L, et al. A simple test to monitor oxidative stress. Int Angiol. 1999;18:127–30.

11. Trotti R, Carratelli M, Barbieri M. Performance and clinical application of a new, fast method for the detection of hydroperoxides in serum. Panminerva Med. 2002;44:37–40.

12. Lubrano V, Vassalle C, L'Abbate A, Zucchelli GC. A new method to evaluate oxidative stress in humans. Immuno-Anal Biol Spéc. 2002;17:172–5.

13. Atabek ME, Vatansev H, Erkul I. Oxidative stress in childhood obesity. J Pediatr Endocrinol Metab. 2004;17:1063–8.

14. Kamezaki F, Yamashita K, Kubara T, Suzuki Y, Tanaka S, Kouzuma R, et al. Derivatives of reactive oxygen metabolites correlates with high-sensitivity C-reactive protein. J Atheroscler Thromb. 2008;15:206–12.

15. Sakane N, Fujiwara S, Sano Y, Domichi M, Tsuzaki K, Matsuoka Y, et al. Oxidative stress, inflammation, and atherosclerotic changes in retinal arteries in the Japanese population; results from the Mima study. Endocr J. 2008;55:485–8.

16. Pasquini A, Luchetti E, Marchetti V, Cardini G, Iorio EL. Analytical performances of d-ROMs test and BAP test in canine plasma. Definition of the normal range in healthy Labrador dogs. Vet Res Commun. 2008;32:137–43.

17. Hirose H, Kawabe H, Komiya N, Saito I. Relations between serum reactive oxygen metabolites (ROMs) and various inflammatory and metabolic parameters in a Japanese population. J Atheroscler Thromb. 2009;16:77–82.

18. Kotani K, Tsuzaki K, Taniguchi N, Sakane N. Correlation between reactive oxygen metabolites & atherosclerotic risk factors in patients with type 2 diabetes mellitus. Indian J Med Res. 2013;137:742–8.

19. Hirata Y, Yamamoto E, Tokitsu T, Kusaka H, Fujisue K, Kurokawa H, et al. Reactive oxygen metabolites are closely associated with the diagnosis and prognosis of coronary artery disease. J Am Heart Assoc. 2015;4: e001451.

20. Santilli F, Lapenna D, La Barba S, Davì G. Oxidative stress-related mechanisms affecting response to aspirin in diabetes mellitus. Free Radic Biol Med. 2015;80:101–10.

21. Vazzana N, Santilli F, Sestili S, Cuccurullo C, Davi G. Determinants of increased cardiovascular disease in obesity and metabolic syndrome. Curr Med Chem. 2011;18:5267–80.

22. Giacco F, Brownlee M. Oxidative stress and diabetic complications. Circ Res. 2010;107:1058–70.

23. Iamele L, Fiocchi R, Vernocchi A. Evaluation of an automated spectrophotometric assay for reactive oxygen metabolites in serum. Clin Chem Lab Med. 2002;40:673–6.

24. Palmieri B, Sblendorio V. Oxidative stress tests: overview on reliability and use. Part II. Eur Rev Med Pharmacol Sci. 2007;11:383–99.

25. Fukui T, Yamauchi K, Maruyama M, Yasuda T, Kohno M, Abe Y. Significance of measuring oxidative stress in lifestyle-related diseases from the viewpoint of correlation between d-ROMs and BAP in Japanese subjects. Hypertens Res. 2011;34:1041–5.

26. Hirayama A, Yamamoto H, Sakata Y, Asakura M, Sakata Y, Fuji H, et al. Usefulness of plasma brain natriuretic peptide after acute myocardial infarction in predicting left ventricular dilatation six months later. Am J Cardiol. 2001;88:890–3.

27. Hirayama A, Kusuoka H, Yamamoto H, Sakata Y, Asakura M, Higuchi Y, et al. Serial changes in plasma brain natriuretic peptide concentration at the infarct and non-infarct sites in patients with left ventricular remodelling after myocardial infarction. Heart. 2005;91:1573–7.

28. Hirayama A, Kusuoka H, Yamamoto H, Sakata Y, Asakura M, Higuchi Y, et al. Usefulness of plasma brain natriuretic peptide concentration for predicting subsequent left ventricular remodeling after coronary angioplasty in patients with acute myocardial infarction. Am J Cardiol. 2006;98:453–7.

29. Willemsen S, Hartog JWL, Hummel YM, van Ruijven MH, van der Horst IC, van Veldhuisen DJ, et al. Tissue advanced glycation end products are associated with diastolic function and aerobic exercise capacity in diabetic heart failure patients. Eur J Heart Fail. 2011;13:76–82.

30. Liu Q, Wang S, Cai L. Diabetic cardiomyopathy and its mechanisms: role of oxidative stress and damage. J Diabetes Investig. 2014;5:623–34.

31. Kitano D, Chiku M, Li Y, Okumura Y, Fukamachi D, Takayama T, et al. Miglitol improves postprandial endothelial dysfunction in patients with acute coronary syndrome and new-onset postprandial hyperglycemia. Cardiovasc Diabetol. 2013;12:92.

32. Von Bibra H, St John Sutton M. Impact of diabetes on postinfarction heart failure and left ventricular remodeling. Curr Heart Fail Rep. 2011;8:242–51.

33. Dennis KE, Hill S, Rose KL, Sampson UK, Hill MF. Augmented cardiac formation of oxidatively-induced carbonylated proteins accompanies the increased functional severity of post-myocardial infarction heart failure in the setting of type 1 diabetes mellitus. Cardiovasc Pathol. 2013;22:473–80.

8

Long-term secondary prevention of acute myocardial infarction (SEPAT) – guidelines adherence and outcome

Constantinos Ergatoudes[1] ⓘ, Erik Thunström[1], Annika Rosengren[1], Lena Björck[1,2], Kristina Bengtsson Boström[3], Kristin Falk[2] and Michael Fu[1,4*]

Abstract

Background: A number of registry studies have reported suboptimal adherence to guidelines for cardiovascular prevention during the first year after acute myocardial infarction (AMI). However, only a few studies have addressed long-term secondary prevention after AMI. This study evaluates prevention guideline adherence and outcome of guideline-directed secondary prevention in patients surviving 2 years after AMI.

Methods: Patients aged 18–85 years at the time of their index AMI were consecutively identified from hospital discharge records between July 2010 and December 2011 in Gothenburg, Sweden. All patients who agreed to participate in the study (16.2%) were invited for a structured interview, physical examinations and laboratory analysis 2 years after AMI. Guideline-directed secondary preventive goals were defined as optimally controlled blood pressure, serum cholesterol, glucose, regular physical activity, smoking cessation and pharmacological treatment.

Results: The mean age of the study cohort ($n = 200$) at the index AMI was 63.0 ± 9.7 years, 79% were men. Only 3.5% of the cohort achieved all six guideline-directed secondary preventive goals 2 years after infarction. LDL < 1.8 mmol/L was achieved in 18.5% of the cohort, regular exercise in 45.5% and systolic blood pressure <140 mmHg in 57.0%. Anti-platelet therapy was used by 97% of the patients, beta-blockers by 83.0%, angiotensin-converting enzyme inhibitors/angiotensin receptor blockers by 76.5% and statins by 88.5%. During follow-up, non-fatal adverse cardiovascular events (cardiac hospitalization, recurrent acute coronary syndrome, angina pectoris, new percutaneous coronary intervention, new onset of atrial fibrillation, post-infarct heart failure, pacemaker implantation, stroke/transient ischemic attack (TIA), cardiac surgery and cardiac arrest) occurred in 47% of the cohort and readmission due to cardiac causes in 30%.

Conclusions: Our data showed the failure of secondary prevention in our daily clinical practice and high rate of non-fatal adverse cardiovascular events 2 years after AMI.

Keywords: Secondary prevention, Cardiovascular disease, Myocardial infarction, Long-term

* Correspondence: Michael.fu@vgregion.se
[1]Department of Molecular and Clinical Medicine, Institute of Medicine, Skövde, Sweden
[4]Department of Medicine, Section of Cardiology, Sahlgrenska University Hospital/Östra, 41651 Göteborg, Sweden
Full list of author information is available at the end of the article

Background

The main purpose of secondary prevention after acute myocardial infarction (AMI) is to reduce recurrence, decrease morbidity and mortality and improve quality of life. To achieve these goals, available guidelines for cardiovascular prevention worldwide uniformly recommend lifestyle interventions: smoking cessation, increased physical activity, maintaining a healthy body mass index (BMI), optimal control of risk factors (blood pressure, cholesterol and glucose control) and optimal use of cardio protective drug therapies (aspirin, beta-blockers, angiotensin-converting enzyme (ACE) inhibitors/angiotensin II receptor blockers (ARBs), lipid-lowering drugs) [1–5].

During the past decades, several studies have repeatedly demonstrated suboptimal adherence to guidelines in patients after AMI. EUROASPIRE (European Action on Secondary and Primary Prevention by Intervention to Reduce Events) I–IV surveys showed that a large majority of coronary artery disease patients did not achieve the standard of secondary prevention stipulated by the guidelines (1–5). The prevalence of smoking, poor diet and physical inactivity remains high and most patients remain overweight or obese with a high prevalence of diabetes. Moreover, despite increasing use of medications, risk factor control remains suboptimal [6–8]. A recent Swedish study showed that risk factor control has improved slightly over time after AMI, but improvement was mainly seen in control of blood pressure, indicating substantial potential for improvement in other preventive goals [9, 10].

Persistent secondary prevention is warranted after AMI for long-term cardiovascular protection. However, available studies that have evaluated secondary prevention have mainly been done up to within 1 year post AMI. Moreover, most studies have been registry-based, where data are often restricted and less detailed. Consequently, knowledge about secondary prevention 2 years post-AMI is limited. The main objectives of the current study were therefore to evaluate adherence to secondary prevention guidelines and outcome 2 years after AMI.

Methods

Patients

We included consecutive men and women who had undergone AMI, were aged ≥18 years and <85 years at the time of their index event and who were still alive 2 years post-AMI. The patients were identified retrospectively from hospital discharge lists. All participants were living in the catchment area of Gothenburg and had been hospitalized for AMI at Sahlgrenska University Hospital Östra or Sahlgrenska University Hospital/Sahlgrenska between July 2010 and December 2011. The diagnosis of AMI was based on the following criteria: at least one value of troponin level >15 ng/L and at least one of the following: chest pain,

newly discovered ECG changes (pathological ST/T-wave, left bundle branch block or a pathological Q-wave), regional wall motion abnormality in the left ventricle discovered by echocardiography or MRI or proven intracoronary thrombosis or stenosis by coronary angiography [11]. Patients unable to speak or understand Swedish were excluded.

Structured interview

A personal interview was conducted by experienced nurses at a minimum of 2 years after the index AMI event. A detailed questionnaire containing pre-defined questions was used that included information on marital status, living situation, education, occupation, past illnesses, chest pain and shortness of breath, depression, medication, smoking, use of Swedish snus, alcohol use, stress and exercise. The questionnaire was completed under supervision of the research staff.

Higher education was defined as having a university degree. Employment was coded dichotomously (working or not working). Smoking was defined as never smoked; yes, regularly; yes, sometimes; no, quit smoking. Quit smoking was defined as trying to quit during the 2 weeks preceding the interview. Depression was defined as feeling depressed for more than 2 consecutive weeks during the past 12 months. Self-perceived stress was defined as permanent stress during the last 5 years [12] Self-reported physical activity during leisure time was categorized into four levels according to a modified version of Saltin-Grimby Physical Activity Level Scale (SGPALS) [13]: sedentary; moderate physical activity at least 2 h per week (without sweating); regular physical activity (1–2 times per week); vigorous physical activity for at least 3 times per week.

Structured examinations

A variety of variables were measured, including height, weight, waist circumference, hip circumference, blood pressure and ECG. Body height was measured to the nearest ½ cm and weight to 0.1 kg (Tanita Corporation, Tokyo, Japan), with the subjects in light clothing and without shoes. BMI was calculated as weight (kg)/height (m) squared. Waist was defined as the area between the iliac crest and to the approximate area of the lowest rib. Hip circumference was measured as the widest circumference around the hips. Resting ECG was taken with a 12-lead ECG (Cardiolex, Solna, Sweden). Blood pressure was measured twice for each person after a 5-min rest with the person in a sitting position using the Omron HEM-907 IntelliSense professional digital blood pressure monitor (Omron Corporation, Omuro, Kyoto, Japan).

Laboratory analyses

Fasting blood samples were collected for analysis of hemoglobin, low-density lipoprotein (LDL) cholesterol, high-density lipoprotein (HDL) cholesterol, total triglycerides, total serum cholesterol, ApoB/ApoA1 ratio, glycated hemoglobin HbA1c, blood glucose, potassium, sodium and creatinine. HbA1c was measured in all participants because HbA1C is widely accepted as one of diagnostic criteria for diabetes. As long as patients have HbA1c < 48 mmol/mol they have achieved goals regardless of diabetes or not. Serum and plasma were aliquoted and stored at a −80 °C until analysed. All laboratory analyses were done at the Department of Clinical Chemistry, Sahlgrenska University Hospital, Gothenburg, Sweden.

Data from medical records
A retrospective review of medical records was conducted to collect data on demographic details, medical history, diagnostic test results (e.g., ECG, echocardiography and coronary angiogram), treatments and outcome data.

Outcome measures
The primary outcome measure was the proportion of patients with AMI who achieved the stipulated secondary preventive guideline recommendations, categorized as six variables (Table 1). The secondary outcome measure was non-fatal adverse cardiovascular events 2 years after AMI.

The definitions for achieving a guideline standard are presented in Table 1 [3]. Non-fatal cardiovascular events were defined as all cardiovascular events that occurred after the index AMI, including recurrent acute coronary syndrome, angina pectoris, new onset of atrial fibrillation, post-MI heart failure, percutaneous coronary intervention (PCI), cardiac arrest, stroke/TIA and any readmission secondary to cardiac disease. Post-MI heart failure was defined as a newly developed clinical manifestation of heart failure based on heart failure symptoms in combination with either increased NT pro BNP >300 pg/ml or LVEF <40% after AMI. Angina pectoris was defined as ≥ class 2 based on the Canadian Cardiovascular Society Angina Grading Scale (CCS

Angina Grading Scale) [14]. Cardiac readmissions were all readmissions due to any cardiac cause (according to The International Classification of Diseases ICD-10).

Statistical analyses
Data are reported as frequency and percentage for categorical variables and mean with standard deviation for quantitative variables. Data were analysed using IBM SPSS Statistics 22.0 (IBM Corp., Chicago, ILL, USA).

Ethics
This study complies with the Declaration of Helsinki [15] and the study protocol was approved by the Ethics Committee of the Medical Faculty of the University of Gothenburg. Written informed consent was obtained from each participant by the principal investigator. The research assistants signed the Case Report Form to confirm that informed consent was obtained.

Results
Study cohort
In total, 1234 patients were hospitalized with an AMI in the area of Gothenburg between July 2010 and December 2011. Of those 1234 patients, 860 were excluded from the study because of various reasons (Fig. 1). After excluding all participants that either did not meet the inclusion criteria, or who could not be accessed, 374 patients were eligible. Of those, 56 patients did not sign the informed consent form or declined further participation and 118 did not respond to the invitation. Thus, the final sample included 200 patients (Fig. 1).

Table 1 Secondary prevention guidelines after AMI

1	Optimally controlled blood pressure, defined as SBP <140 mmHg
2	Optimally controlled cholesterol levels, defined as LDL cholesterol <1.8 mmol/L
3	Optimally controlled glucose, defined as HbA1c <48 mmol/mol
4	Regular physical activity that caused sweating at least two times a week
5	Smoking cessation, defined as non-smoking at the time of the interview
6	Pharmacological treatment with ACE inhibitors or ARBs

AMI acute myocardial infarction, *SBP* systolic blood pressure, *LDL* low-density lipoprotein, *ACE* angiotensin-converting enzyme, *ARB* angiotensin II receptor blockers

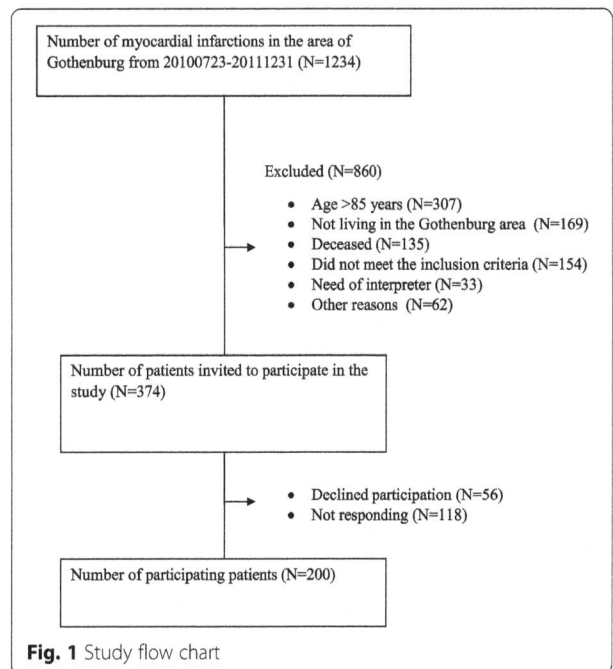

Fig. 1 Study flow chart

Number of myocardial infarctions in the area of Gothenburg from 20100723-20111231 (N=1234)

Excluded (N=860)
- Age >85 years (N=307)
- Not living in the Gothenburg area (N=169)
- Deceased (N=135)
- Did not meet the inclusion criteria (N=154)
- Need of interpreter (N=33)
- Other reasons (N=62)

Number of patients invited to participate in the study (N=374)

- Declined participation (N=56)
- Not responding (N=118)

Number of participating patients (N=200)

Baseline characteristics at the time of the index AMI

At the time of the index AMI, 69% of the patients had ST-segment elevation myocardial infarction (STEMI), 31% a non–STEMI (NSTEMI). Mean heart rate was 75.6 (SD ±18.8) beats/min, mean systolic blood pressure (SBP) 146.1 (SD ±25.7) mmHg and mean diastolic blood pressure (DBP) 91.3 (SD ±15.0) mmHg. Almost everyone that was included (96%) underwent a percutaneous coronary intervention (PCI) or a coronary artery bypass grafting (CABG) in association with the index event.

Demographic characteristics at interview

The mean age of the study cohort at follow-up ($n = 200$) was 65.5 (SD ±9.8) years and 79% were male (Table 2). Moreover, 79.3% were born in Sweden, 23.5% had a higher education and 34.4% were still actively working.

Lifestyle characteristics and psychological conditions at interview

As shown in Table 2, a minority of the patients were still smokers (12.5%) regularly or occasionally; however, most of these patients had smoked at some time in their life (69%). Only one of seven patients reported a sedentary lifestyle 2 years after their index AMI, whereas 40.5% claimed to engage in moderate physical exercise without sweating, 25% did moderate exercise with sweating and 20.5% participated in regular physical exercise and training. Concerning psychological factors, 15% of the patients had been depressed during the past year and almost 10% had felt constantly stressed during the past 5 years. Feeling stressed and depressed were more common in those aged <65 years. Almost 20% of the patients <65 years of age had been constantly stressed for the past 5 years, whereas only 2% of those aged >65 years had felt stressed during the same period.

Clinical characteristics based on interview, review of medical records and physical examinations

The two most common comorbidities were hypertension (63.4%) and hyperlipidemia (63.9%), followed by diabetes mellitus (21.8%) and atrial fibrillation (14.8%). Medical records showed that 22.5% of the patients were still smoking at the time of the index AMI, 13% had at least one previous myocardial infarction and 11.5% underwent PCI (Table 2).

At the physical examination, which was given during the interview, mean SBP was 137.5 mmHg and mean DBP 79.6 mmHg respectively (Table 3). Sinus rhythm constituted 93% with a mean heart rate at approximately 59.0 beats/minute. 17.5% of the study population had a BMI over 30 kg/m^2

Table 2 Social and clinical characteristics of patients at the time of the interview 2 years after AMI

Variables	Groups		
	All $N = 200$	Men $N = 158$	Women $N = 42$
Age, years, mean ± SD	65.5 ± 9.8	64.7 ± 9.5	68.2 ± 10.2
Social factors			
Born in Sweden[a] $n = 199$ (%)	158 (79.3)	123 (77.8)	35 (83.3)
Higher education[a] $n = 200$ (%)	47 (23.5)	35 (22.2)	12 (28.6)
Currently working[a] $n = 199$ (%)	72 (34.4)	62 (39.2)	10 (23.8)
Smoking[a] $n = 200$			
Never (%)	62 (31.0)	45 (28.5)	17 (40.5)
Regularly (%)	13 (6.5)	13 (8.2)	0 (0.0)
Sometimes (%)	12 (6.0)	11 (7.0)	1 (2.4)
Quit (%)	113 (56.5)	89 (56.3)	24 (57.1)
Exercise[a] $n = 200$			
Sedentary n (%)	28 (14)	18 (11.4)	10 (23.8)
Moderate activity n (%)	81 (40.5)	63 (39.9)	18 (42.9)
Regular activity n, (%)	50 (25.5)	41 (35.9)	9 (21.4)
Vigorous activity n, (%)	41 (20.5)	36 (22.8)	5 (11.9)
Cardiovascular diseases			
Atrial fibrillation[a] $n = 196$ (%)	29 (14.8)	19 (12.3)	10 (24.4)
Known heart failure[a] $n = 193$ (%)	16 (8.3)	10 (6.5)	6 (15.8)
Hypertension[a] $n = 194$ (%)	123 (63.4)	93 (61.2)	30 (71.4)
Diabetes[a] $n = 197$ (%)	43 (21.8)	37 (23.6)	6 (15)
Stroke/TIA[a] $n = 198$ (%)	14 (7.2)	12 (7.7)	2 (4.9)
Hyperlipidemia[a] $n = 180$ (%)	115 (63.9)	90 (63.4)	25 (65.8)
Previous MI $n = 200$ (%)	26 (13.0)	19 (12.0)	8 (19.0)
Previous PCI $n = 200$ (%)	23 (11.5)	18 (11.4)	5 (11.9)
Non-cardiovascular disease			
Cancer[a] $n = 200$ (%)	31 (15.5)	22 (13.9)	9 (21.4)
COPD $n = 193$ (%)	39 (20.2)	29 (19.1)	10 (24.4)
OSA $n = 162$ (%)	48 (29.6)	37 (29.6)	11 (29.7)
Renal failure GFR < 60 $n = 200$ (%)	55 (27.5)	33 (20.1)	18 (42.9)
Renal failure GFR < 30 $n = 200$ (%)	4 (2)	4 (2.5)	0 (0.0)
Depressed for at least 2 consecutive weeks in the past 12 months[a] $n = 200$ (%)	30 (15)	20 (12.7)	10 (23.8)

Data were presented as n (%)
TIA transient ischemic attack, *MI* myocardial infarction, *PCI* percutaneous coronary intervention, *COPD* chronic obstructive pulmonary disease, *OSA* obstructive sleep apnea
[a]Self-specified answers to questions in the SEPAT questionnaire

Table 3 Physical examination and laboratory analysis at the time of the interview 2 years after the index AMI event

| | Groups | | |
	All N = 200	Men N = 158	Women N = 42
SBP (mmHg)	137.5 (18)	138.3 (18.3)	134.2 (16.4)
DBP (mmHg)	79.6 (10.3)	80.7 (10.0)	75.5 (10.5)
HR (beats/minute)	59.7 (10.7)	59.1 (10.8)	61.9 (10.2)
Weight (Kg)	84.7 (16.2)	86.9 (15.4)	76.4 (16.3)
BMI			
25 kg/m^2 < BMI ≤30 kg/m^2 (%)	47.0	50.6	35.7
> 30 kg/m^2 (%)	25.5	20.9	40.5
Waist (cm)	100.2 (12.4)	101.4 (11.0)	95.7 (16.1)
Lab			
HbA1c (mmol/L)	40.5 (9.3)	39.8 (8.8)	43.0 (10.5)
Cholesterol (mmol/L)	4.1 (1.0)	4.1 (0.9)	4.5 (1.2)
LDL (mmol/L)	2.4 (0.9)	2.4 (0.8)	2.6 (1.1)
HDL (mmol/L)	1.4 (0.6)	1.4 (0.4)	1.6 (0.5)
ApoB/ApoA1 quote	0.6 (0.2)	0.6 (0.2)	0.5 (0.2)
Triglycerides (mmol/L)	1.3 (0.6)	1.3 (0.6)	1.3 (0.5)
P-glucose (mmol/L)	5.7 (1.3)	5.7 (1.3)	5.7 (1.3)
NTproBNP (pg/ml)	396.8 (750.7)	344.1 (682.3)	594.9 (949.6)
NTproBNP > 300 pg/ml (%)	31.5	25.3	44.2

Data were presented as n (%), otherwise in mean (SD). *SBP* systolic blood pressure, *DBP* diastolic blood pressure, *HR* heart rate, *BMI* body mass index, *LDL* low density lipoprotein, *HDL* high density lipoprotein

Non-fatal cardiovascular events
During the 2-year study period non-fatal cardiovascular events occurred in 46.5% of the participants. Readmissions due to all causes were 50.5% and due to cardiac disease 30%. Among them, new AMIs constituted 8%, new PCIs 11.5%, atrial fibrillation 7.5%, TIA/stroke 6%, cardiac arrest 1%, post-infarction heart failure 19.5% and cardiac surgery 9.5% (Table 4). It is noteworthy to mention that the number of cardiac events may outnumber readmission rate since several events may occur during the same readmission. Our study was not powered to assess the causal relation between increased non-fatal cardiovascular events and suboptimal secondary prevention.

Achievements of guideline standards in secondary prevention
As shown in Table 5, the goal of SBP was achieved in 57% of the patients, 18.5% had LDL of <1.8 mmol/L, 87.5% did not smoke, 45.5% achieved the goal defined by regular exercise with sweating. The goal for HbA1c was achieved in almost 90% of the patients; however, most of these patients did not have diabetes. ACE inhibitor/ARB

Table 4 Non-fatal cardiovascular events during the 2-year follow-up after the index AMI event

Readmissions, all cause, n (%)	101 (50.5)
Readmissions, cardiac, n (%)	60 (30.0)
Recurrent myocardial infarction, n (%)	16 (8.0)
Unstable angina, n (%)	8 (4.0)
PCI, n (%)	23 (11.5)
Cardiac surgery, n (%)[a]	19 (9.5)
Cardiac arrest, n (%)	2 (1.0)
Stroke/TIA, n (%)	9 (4.5)
Post-MI heart failure, n (%)	40 (20.0)
Post-MI atrial fibrillation, n (%)	15 (7.5)
Angina pectoris CCS ≥2, n (%)	34 (17.0)

AMI acute myocardial infarction, *PCI* percutaneous coronary intervention, *TIA* transient ischemic attack, *MI* myocardial infarction, *CCS* Canadian Cardiovascular Society
[a]cardiac surgery: all surgical procedure related to heart except percutaneous coronary intervention

medication was administered to 75% of the patients. For other medications, 96% of the patients were treated with antiplatelet medicines, 83.0% with beta-blockers and 88.5% with statins. Only 3.5% of the whole study cohort achieved all six secondary preventive goals 2 years after AMI (Tables 5, 6, and Fig. 2).

Development of risk profile 2 years after AMI
As shown in Table 5, there were more individuals that reached the goals of secondary prevention 2 years after the index AMI than at the time of AMI in terms of smoking, LDL reduction, blood pressure control and physical activity (Table 5). Moreover, there was a tendency towards increased BMI 2 years after the index AMI. The proportion of patients with BMI >30 kg/m^2 increased from 17.5% at the time of the index AMI to 25.5% 2 years later.

Discussion
In the present study the six secondary preventive goals were achieved by only 3.5% of the patients 2 years after the AMI event. Adherence to cardio-protective

Table 5 Development of a risk profile at the time of AMI and at the 2-year follow-up interview

	At AMI	At the 2-year follow-up interview
No smoking n (%)	155 (77.5)	175 (87.5)
LDL cholesterol <1.8 mmol/L n (%)	8 (4)	37 (18.5)
HbA1C <4.8 mmol/mol n (%)	NA	177 (88.5)
SBP <140 mmHg n (%)	152 (76)	114 (57)
Regular exercise training n (%)	NA	90 (45.5)

NA not available, *AMI* acute myocardial infarction, *LDL* low density lipoprotein, *SBP* systolic blood pressure

Table 6 Comparison of pharmacological treatments at the time of the index AMI event and at interview 2 years after AMI

	At AMI	At interview
Aspirin *n* = 200 (%)	199 (99.5)	183 (91.5)
Beta-blocker *n* = 200 (%)	187 (93.5)	166 (83.0)
ACE-inhibitor or Angiotensin receptor blocker *n* = 200 (%)	177 (88.5)	153 (76.5)
Statin *n* = 200 (%)	193 (96.5)	177 (88.5)
Clopidogrel/prasugrel *n* = 200 (%)	179 (89.5)	11 (5.5)

AMI acute myocardial infarction, *ACE* angiotensin-converting enzyme

medications, however, was generally good. Still, non-fatal cardiovascular events occurred in 46.5% of the cohort and cardiac readmissions in 30% at the 2-year follow-up.

Our study is an extension of the EUROASPIRE survey and the Secondary Prevention after Heart Intensive Care Admission (SEPHIA) Registry in Sweden. EUROASPIRE IV was a cross-sectional study carried out in 24 European countries. Patients included in that study were those with either acute coronary syndrome or elective revascularization in the form of balloon angioplasty or coronary artery surgery. The starting date for identification of an event was ≥ 6 months and < 3 years before the expected date of the study interview [8]. The SEPHIA Registry is an on-going Swedish quality registry of AMI patients that focuses on four preventive goals (smoking cessation, optimal control of blood pressure, cholesterol and glucose) and data on the patients are collected during the first year after an AMI. Patients older than 75 years of age are not included in the Registry. Patients are invited to be interviewed by either a registered nurse or physician during an outpatient visit or via a telephone call on two occasions: 4–10 weeks (mean 56 days) and 12–14 months (mean 399 days) after myocardial infarction [9].

Our findings extended available observations by showing divergent development of risk factors from short-term to long-term time frame after AMI. Firstly, our study confirmed some observations from previous short-term studies. For instance, regular physical activity is a

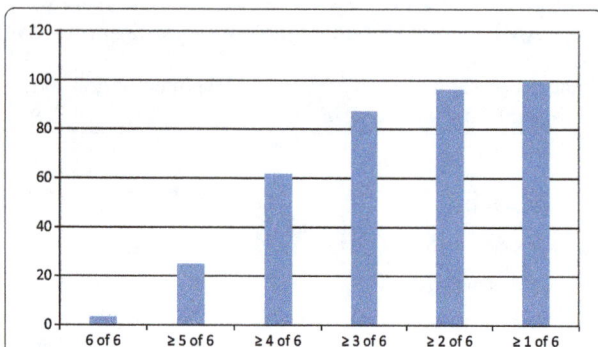

Fig. 2 Number of achieved goals (%) of guideline standard secondary prevention two years post AMI

secondary preventive goal that may be hard to achieve. In the EUROASPIRE IV survey only 40% of the participants attained a physical vigorous intensity level for at least 20 min one or more times per week [8]. In Sweden, the overall participation rate in exercise training within cardiac rehabilitation programs 1 year post-AMI is 51% [9]. Two years after AMI, 45.5% of our patients reported participating in moderate regular exercise that caused them to perspire. Thus, it appears that, as in the rest of Europe, a comparable number of our Swedish patients with coronary artery disease participate in cardiac rehabilitation. Furthermore, in our study physical exercise during leisure activity was comparable with that observed in the EUROASPIRE IV. Another example is smoking habit. Regrettably, despite that smoking cessation reduces the risk of a new myocardial infarction [16], about one third of the patients still smoked in EUROASPIRE IV survey study [8]. A similar trend was seen in the Swedish myocardial infarct registry [9] 1 year after the index AMI. Our study suggests that there is an improvement in the number of patients who quit smoking from the index AMI, since 87.5% of the study participants were classified as non-smokers 2 years after AMI. However, it is not clear whether the improved smoking cessation rate observed in our cohort could be attributed to an increase in the death rate in those patients that did continue smoking but did not survive long enough to be invited. The better results could therefore simply reflect a selection bias in our cohort because participation rates were low. Finally, guideline-directed medical therapy and glucose control 2 years after AMI were in accordance with those reported in EUROASPIRE IV [8] and SEPHIA [9], except that double anti-platelet therapy was indicated only 1 year after AMI and thus could not be adequately evaluated after 2 years.

Secondly, our study provided new information about negative developments in some risk factors from previous short-term studies. Compared with SEPHIA (9), our findings demonstrated failure of long-term secondary prevention as shown by decreased goal achievement in LDL <1.8 mmol/L from 51% in SEPHIA to 18,5% in our study, and in blood pressure control with SBP of <140 mmHg from 73% in SEPHIA to 57% in our study, notwithstanding that guideline-directed medical therapy were similar regardless of short or long term after AMI. However, caution must be taken because two studies are not fully comparable.

Limitations

Our study has some limitations. Patients who were too sick or disabled to attend the study visits could not participate. Moreover, patients who did not speak or understand Swedish were excluded. It is possible that this category of patients may show less compliance and thus if they had been included, the goal achievements might have been even lower. Furthermore, in our study, more STEMI than NTSEMI were included despite NSTEMI constitutes the majority of ACS. There are two possible explanations: 1) the majority of the participants (87%) in our study were hospitalized at Sahlgrenska University Hospital at the time of their index event, the only hospital in Gothenburg with round-the-clock service for PCI, thus more STEMI than NTSEMI were included 2) many patients with NSTEMI have more co-morbidity and thus more hospital visits. This might explain why they were less interested in participating in the study since it means additional hospitals visits. Finally, we could not interview the patients who died during the 2 years that passed between the index AMI and the study inclusion stage. These patients were probably less compliant with the secondary prevention interventions than those who were included in the study. Thus, our results, if anything, may exaggerate the number of persons who potentially achieve secondary prevention goals, further underlining the fact that much could be gained in this area with better adherence to guidelines. Finally, this study was not powered to investigate cause-effect relationship between cardiovascular events and secondary prevention.

Conclusion

Secondary prevention 2 years after AMI proved suboptimal in our cohort of patients. Only 3.5% of our patients attained all six secondary prevention goals. Therefore, there is considerable potential to raise the standard of preventive cardiology care through more effective lifestyle intervention and to more rigorously control of risk factors. Perhaps most importantly we need to increase awareness of the current situation and improve regular follow up. Such an effort should help to reduce cardiovascular morbidity and mortality in this patient group.

Abbreviations

ACE: Angiotensin-converting enzyme; AMI: Acute myocardial infarction; ARB: Angiotensin II receptor blockers; BMI: Body mass index; CABG: Coronary artery bypass grafting; DBP: Diastolic blood pressure; HDL: High-density lipoprotein; ICD-10: The International Classification of Diseases; LDL: Low-density lipoprotein; PCI: Percutaneous coronary intervention; SBP: Systolic blood pressure; STEMI: ST-segment elevation myocardial infarction; TIA: Transient ischemic attack

Acknowledgements
None.

Funding

This is an investigator-initiated study supported by the Swedish Heart-Lung Foundation, the Swedish agreement between the government and the county councils concerning economic support for providing an infrastructure for research and education of doctors, the Regional Development Fund, Västra Götaland County, Sweden (FOU-VGR).

Authors' contributions
CE engaged in followings: study design, discussion of protocol, statistical analyses, result interpretation, discussion, writing manuscript. ET engaged in followings: study design, ethical application, discussion of protocol, participation of examinations and interview, statistical analyses, discussion, writing manuscript. AR engaged in followings: study design, ethical application, discussion of protocol, result interpretation, discussion, writing manuscript. LB engaged in followings: study design, ethical application, discussion of protocol, result interpretation, discussion, writing manuscript. KBB engaged in followings: study design, ethical application, discussion of protocol, result interpretation, discussion, writing manuscript. KF engaged in followings: study design, ethical application, discussion of protocol, result interpretation, discussion, writing manuscript. MF study design, ethical application, discussion of protocol, result interpretation, discussion, writing manuscript.

Competing interests
The authors declare that they have no competing interests.

Author details
[1]Department of Molecular and Clinical Medicine, Institute of Medicine, Skövde, Sweden. [2]Institute of Health and Care Sciences, Sahlgrenska Academy, University of Gothenburg, Skövde, Sweden. [3]R & D Centre Skaraborg Primary Care, Skövde, Sweden. [4]Department of Medicine, Section of Cardiology, Sahlgrenska University Hospital/Östra, 41651 Göteborg, Sweden.

References

1. Graham I, et al. European guidelines on cardiovascular disease prevention in clinical practice: full text. Fourth Joint Task Force of the European Society of Cardiology and other societies on cardiovascular disease prevention in clinical practice (constituted by representatives of nine societies and by invited experts). Eur J Cardiovasc Prev Rehabil. 2007;14 Suppl 2:S1–S113.
2. Smith Jr SC, et al. AHA/ACC guidelines for secondary prevention for patients with coronary and other atherosclerotic vascular disease: 2006 update: endorsed by the National Heart, Lung, and Blood Institute. Circulation. 2006;113(19):2363–72.
3. Perk J, et al. European Guidelines on cardiovascular disease prevention in clinical practice (version 2012). The Fifth Joint Task Force of the European Society of Cardiology and Other Societies on Cardiovascular Disease Prevention in Clinical Practice (constituted by representatives of nine societies and by invited experts). Eur Heart J. 2012;33(13):1635–701.
4. Bauters C, et al. Prognostic impact of ss-blocker use in patients with stable coronary artery disease. Heart. 2014;100(22):1757–61.
5. Berger JS, Brown DL, Becker RC. Low-dose aspirin in patients with stable cardiovascular disease: a meta-analysis. Am J Med. 2008;121(1):43–9.
6. Cooney MT, et al. Determinants of risk factor control in subjects with coronary heart disease: a report from the EUROASPIRE III investigators. Eur J Prev Cardiol. 2013;20(4):686–91.
7. Kotseva K, et al. Cardiovascular prevention guidelines in daily practice: a comparison of EUROASPIRE I, II, and III surveys in eight European countries. Lancet. 2009;373(9667):929–40.
8. Kotseva K, et al. EUROASPIRE IV: A European Society of Cardiology survey on the lifestyle, risk factor and therapeutic management of coronary patients from 24 European countries. Eur J Prev Cardiol. 2015;23(6):636–48.
9. Hambraeus K, Tyden P, Lindahl B. Time trends and gender differences in prevention guideline adherence and outcome after myocardial infarction: Data from the SWEDEHEART registry. Eur J Prev Cardiol. 2015;23(4):340–8.
10. Jernberg T, et al. Cardiovascular risk in post-myocardial infarction patients: nationwide real world data demonstrate the importance of a long-term perspective. Eur Heart J. 2015;36(19):1163–70.
11. Thygesen K, et al. Third universal definition of myocardial infarction. Eur Heart J. 2012;33(20):2551–67.
12. Rosengren A, Tibblin G, Wilhelmsen L. Self-perceived psychological stress and incidence of coronary artery disease in middle-aged men. Am J Cardiol. 1991;68(11):1171–5.
13. Saltin B, Grimby G. Physiological analysis of middle-aged and old former athletes. Comparison with still active athletes of the same ages. Circulation. 1968;38(6):1104–15.

9

Risk factors of acute myocardial infarction in middle-aged and adolescent people (< 45 years) in Yantai

Hong Du[1], Chang-yan Dong[2*] and Qiao-yan Lin[3]

Abstract

Background: Yantai is a developed medium-sized coastal city in Eastern China, having a population of 1.6845 million. With the development of economy, some middle-aged and adolescent people (< 45 years) devote themselves to work and suffer from greater stress, which makes them ignore their own health. Moreover, they have unhealthy lifestyles and lack the knowledge of cardiovascular risk factors.

Objectives: To identify the risk factors for first acute myocardial infarction in middle-aged and adolescent people in Yantai, a developed medium-sized coastal city in Eastern China.

Methods: A total of 154 consecutive patients with first acute myocardial infarction (< 45 years), were enrolled in case group, and 462 patients without myocardial infarction were enrolled in control group. Three controls with the same sex and age were matched to each case. The risk factors were identified with univariate and multivariate analysis.

Results: Unhealthy food habit (eating seafood and meanwhile drinking beer), hypertension, current smokers, self-perceived stress, diabetes mellitus, obesity, sleep insufficience, hypercholesterolaemia and fatigue were independent risk factors for first acute myocardial infarction ($P < 0.05$).

Conclusions: Besides those recognized risk factors for cardiovascular disease (hypertension, hypercholesterolemia, diabetes mellitus and smoking), eating seafood and meanwhile drinking beer, self-perceived stress, sleep insufficience, obesity and fatigue were also the risk factors for first acute myocardial infarction in middle-aged and adolescent people in Yantai.

Keywords: Risk factors, Acute myocardial infarction, Middle-aged and adolescent people, Developed medium-sized coastal city, China

Background

As a leading cause of death in developed countries [1], cardiovascular disease (CVD) has an elevating incidence and prevalence in developing countries in recent years [2], which may be caused by urbanization, adoption of western life styles and aging of population. China has the biggest CVD burden as the biggest developing country [3]. In 2010, Chinese population with an age greater than 40 years has about 8 million of myocardial infarction (MI) patients, and the number will increase persistently in the next two decades. Moreover, the age of onset is younger for first acute myocardial infarction (AMI) in Chinese population [4]. However, younger patients with first AMI have rarely been researched.

Yantai is a developed medium-sized coastal city in Eastern China, having a population of 1.6845 million. With the development of economy, some middle-aged and adolescent people (< 45 years) devote themselves to work and suffer from greater stress, which makes them ignore their own health. Moreover, they have unhealthy lifestyles and lack the knowledge of cardiovascular risk factors (CVRF). Especially, many middle-aged and adolescent people like to eat seafood and meanwhile drink beer with the improvement of living standard in Yantai, which was uncommon in the before. Besides, we observed that the number of middle-aged and adolescent patients with

* Correspondence: dongchangyan666@126.com
[2]Chinese and Western Medicine Ward, the Yantai Yuhuangding Hospital, No. 20, Yuhuangding Eastern Road, Yantai 264000, Shandong Province, China
Full list of author information is available at the end of the article

primary AMI had an annual increase in our hospital in recent years. If the risk factors for first AMI could be identified in middle-aged and adolescent people, early prevention would be able to be administered.

The objective of the paper was to identify the risk factors for first AMI in middle-aged and adolescent people in Yantai, and then provide useful information for the prevention of primary AMI among middle-aged and adolescent people in the cities similar to Yantai.

Methods
Participants
A total of 154 consecutive patients with first AMI (< 45 years), including 127 males and 27 females, were enrolled in case group in the Yantai Yuhuangding Hospital from June 2005 to June 2013. A total of 462 patients without MI were enrolled in control group, including 381 males and 81 females. Three controls with the same sex and age were matched to each case. All the participants provided written informed consent, and the study was approved the Ethical Committee of the Yantai Yuhuangding Hospital.

Diagnostic criteria
1. Cardiac biomarkers had a rise (to at least one time of the upper normal value) or fall after rise (to at least one time of the upper normal value). 2. At least one of the following characteristics presented: [1] The patient had clinical symptoms of myocardial ischemia. [2] ECG showed new ST segment change or left bundle-branch block. [3] ECG showed pathological Q wave. [4] Imaging evidence showed new loss of myocardial activity or regional wall motion abnormality.

Variables and measurement
The selected factors in the study were as follows: self-perceived stress, physical activity, sleep, fatigue, smoking status, alcohol consumption, food habit, family history of coronary heart disease (CHD), body mass index (BMI), occupation, family income, education, blood pressure, blood glucose, and cholesterol. The information about the selected factors was collected by interview, physical examinations and referring to medical records.

Self-perceived stress was defined as yes or no according to the question "how many days have you felt stressful or depressive in a week?" Yes was determined if participants have felt stressful or depressive on three or more days, and no was determined if participants have felt stressful or depressive on two or less days. Physical activity was defined as active or inactive according to the question "have you had an activity of 30 min on five or more days in a week?" Sleep was defined as sufficient or insufficient according to the question "how many days have you had at least six hours of sleep duration in a week?" Sufficient was determined if participants had at least six hours of sleep

duration on five or more days, and insufficient was determined if participants had at least six hours of sleep duration on four or less days. Fatigue was defined as yes or no according to the question "have you experienced fatigue on three or more days in a week?" Smoking status was defined as current smokers, ex-smokers or non-smokers according to the question "how many cigarettes have you smoked per day?" The people that answered at least one cigarette per day were defined as current smokers, and the people that answered at least one year of smoking cessation was defined as ex-smokers. Alcohol consumption was defined as yes or no according to the question "have you drunk at least 100 g of distillate spirit or 500 g of beer on three or more days in a week?" Food habits were defined as unfavorable or favorable according to the question "how many times have you eaten seafood and meanwhile drunk beer in a meal in a week?" Unfavorable was determined if participants had at least two times of eating seafood and meanwhile drinking beer in a meal, and favorable was determined if participants had at most once. Family history of CHD was defined as yes or no according to the question "have you had one more parent or sibling with diagnosed CHD?" BMI was calculated according to the formula that weight (kg) was divided by squared height (m^2). BMI (18.5-24.9 kg/m^2) was defined as normal, (25–29 kg/m^2) was defined as overweight, and (≥30 kg/m^2) was defined as obesity. Occupation was defined as physical work or intellectual work. According to family income, all the participants were categorized into three groups: low income group (< 10,000 RMB/year), middle income group (10,000–20,000 RMB/year) and high income group (> 20,000 RMB/year). According to the time of education completed, all the participants were categorized into three groups: primary (1–8 years), secondary (9–12 years), and postsecondary (≥13 years).

Hypertension was determined if blood pressure was ≥140/90 mmHg [5] and/or the patient was receiving antihypertensive drugs. Diabetes mellitus was determined if fasting plasma glucose was ≥7.0 mmol/L or 2 h oral glucose tolerance test (OGTT) glucose was ≥11.1 mmol/L [6] and/or the patient was receiving antidiabetic drugs. Hypercholesterolaemia was determined if total serum cholesterol was ≥ 5.16 mmol/L (200 mg/dl) [7] and/or the patient was receiving cholesterol lowering treatment.

Statistical analysis
All the statistical analyses were carried out with the SPSS version 17.0 for Windows (SPSS Inc., USA). The quantitative variables were expressed as mean ± SD, and the qualitative variables were expressed as percentage. The quantitative variables were analyzed with Student's t test. The qualitative variables were analyzed with chi-square test or Fisher exact test. The variables with a P value less than 0.10 in univariate

analysis were included in the multivariate analysis with a backward stepwise logistic regression model. Multivariate logistic regression analyses were then performed to determine the risk factors correlated with the death of the elderly patients with AOSC. Significance was set at $P < 0.05$.

Results and discussion

The average age was 36.8 ± 5.2 years for the cases, and men accounted for 82.5 %. The difference was not significant in the age of first onset between men and women (36.5 ± 5.1vs37.7 ± 5.5 years, $P > 0.05$). Coronary catheterization was performed in all the cases.

According to the results of univariate analysis, the variables correlated with first AMI were as follows: self-perceived stress, sleep, fatigue, smoking status, food habit, BMI, blood pressure, blood glucose and cholesterol (Table 1). Multivariate analysis showed that unhealthy food habit (eating seafood and meanwhile drinking beer), hypertension, current smokers, self-perceived stress, diabetes mellitus, obesity, sleep insufficience, hypercholesterolaemia and fatigue were independent risk factors for first AMI (Table 2). The OR ranged from 1.70 to 3.18 among these risk factors, and the OR was highest for unhealthy food habit and lowest for fatigue (Table 2).

As a coastal city in Eastern China, Yantai had a rapid development of economy in the past two decades, which led to dietary and lifestyle changes [8], especially in middle-aged and adolescent people. These changes could increase the risk for CVD. In our study, other factors were associated with first AMI in middle-aged and adolescent people in Yantai, except for physical activity, alcohol consumption,

Table 1 Results of univariate analysis of the risk factors for first AMI

Variables	AMI	Non-AMI	χ^2/t	P
Self-perceived stress (yes)	36	60	9.477	0.002
Physical inactivity	36	79	2.997	0.083
Sleep insufficience	52	100	9.13	0.003
Fatigue (yes)	40	79	5.863	0.016
Current smokers	95	193	18.495	<0.001
Alcohol consumption (yes)	61	150	2.617	0.106
Eating seafood and meanwhile drinking beer	71	98	35.947	<0.001
Family history of CHD	19	46	0.694	0.405
Obesity	42	89	11.064	0.004
Physical work	67	208	0.107	0.743
Low family income	23	84	2.586	0.274
Education (none)	43	98	3.758	0.153
Hypertension	49	86	11.766	0.001
Diabetes mellitus	23	34	7.894	0.005
Hypercholesterolaemia	42	83	6.186	0.013

Table 2 Results of multivariate analysis of the risk factors for first AMI

Risk factors	Wald	P value	OR	95 % CI
Eating seafood and meanwhile drinking beer	20.537	<0.001	3.18	1.647-4.893
Hypertension	8.026	0.009	2.42	1.315-3.652
smoking status (compared with non-smokers)				
Current smokers	9.875	0.001	2.36	1.429-3.477
ex-smokers	2.238	0.073	1.21	0.736-1.704
Self-perceived stress	6.182	0.013	2.29	1.302-3.315
Diabetes mellitus	5.329	0.018	2.21	1.211-3.289
BMI (compared with normal)				
Obesity	4.251	0.024	2.04	1.192-3.024
Overweight	1.404	0.142	1.54	0.891-2.213
Sleep insufficience	4.832	0.021	1.85	1.105-2.758
Hypercholesterolaemia	3.006	0.041	1.71	1.048-2.396
Fatigue	2.817	0.043	1.70	1.034-2.282
Physical inactivity	1.327	0.159	1.50	0.863-2.206

family history of CHD, occupation, family income and education.

We found that eating seafood and meanwhile drinking beer was positively associated with first AMI. Firstly, consumption of seafood can increase the prevalence of hyperuricemia, which possibly results from the high content of purine in seafood [9]. Secondly, a recent study shows that heavy alcohol consumption of wine can increase the prevalence of hyperuricemia [10], and another study shows that alcohol consumption is directly associated with hyperuricemia [11]. Thirdly, drinking beer and spirits can increase the risk for gout, whereas a moderate consumption of wine cannot [12]. Eventually, hyperuricemia is associated with severity of coronary artery disease (CAD) [13]. However, our study showed that alcohol consumption was not associated with first AMI. The possible reason is that moderate alcohol consumption can reduce the risk for CVD [14] and people tend to drink heavily when they eat seafood.

It is reported that hypertension [15-17], hypercholesterolemia [18], diabetes mellitus [17, 19] and smoking [17] are the risk factors for CVD. Our study showed that hypertension, current smoking, diabetes mellitus and hypercholesterolemia were the risk factors for first AMI in middle-aged and adolescent people in Yantai. Moreover, we found that smoking cessation could reduce the risk for first AMI compared with current smoking, but the result needed to be further confirmed by a larger sample.

A study shows that work stress is a risk factors for CVD [20], and another study shows that stress is directly associated with coronary heart disease [21].We found that self-perceived stress was positively associated with first AMI. However, some studies show that stress is not associated with CVD [22-24]. We found that sleep insufficience was associated with first AMI, which was consistent with the previous study [25]. We also found that obesity and fatigue were associated with first AMI, but overweight was not.

The limitations of the study included: [1] The participants were chose from a small population (inpatients); [2] The relationship was not studied between HIV infection and first AMI because only 5 participants had HIV infection among all the participants; [3] The risk factors of first AMI were not studied in the population > 45 years.

Conclusions

In conclusion, besides those recognized risk factors for CVD (hypertension, hypercholesterolemia, diabetes mellitus and smoking), eating seafood and meanwhile drinking beer, self-perceived stress, sleep insufficience, obesity and fatigue were also the risk factors for first AMI in middle-aged and adolescent people (< 45 years) in Yantai. In a next study, the risk factors of first AMI will be comprehensively studied for inhabitants in Yantai, and a prospective cohort study will be performed, aiming to assess the outcome associated with these emerging risk factors.

Competing interest
The authors declare that they have no competing interests.

Authors' contributions
DH was responsible for collecting the data and writing the manuscript. DCY conceived of the study, and participated in its design and coordination and helped to draft the manuscript. LQY was responsible for analyzing the data. All authors read and approved the final manuscript.

Acknowledgements
None.

Author details
[1]Cardiology Ward, the Yantai Yuhuangding Hospital, No. 20, Yuhuangding Eastern Road, Yantai 264000Shandong Province, China. [2]Chinese and Western Medicine Ward, the Yantai Yuhuangding Hospital, No. 20, Yuhuangding Eastern Road, Yantai 264000, Shandong Province, China. [3]Cardiology in Intensive Care Unit, the Yantai Yuhuangding Hospital, No. 20, Yuhuangding Road, Yantai 264000Shandong Province, China.

References
1. Roger VL, Go AS, Lloyd-Jones DM, Adams RJ, Berry JD, Brown TM, et al. Heart disease and stroke statistics 2011 update: a report from the American Heart Association. Circulation. 2011;123:e18–e209.
2. Yusuf S, Reddy S, Ounpuu S, Anand S. Global burden of cardiovascular diseases, part I: general considerations, the epidaemiologic transition, risk factors, and impact of urbanization. Circulation. 2001;104:2746–53.
3. Zhai F, Wang H, Du S, He Y, Wang Z, Ge K, et al. Prospective study on nutrition transition in China. Nutr Rev. 2009;67 Suppl 1:S56–61.
4. Cao CF, Ren JY, Zhou XH, Li SF, Chen H. Twenty-year trends in major cardiovascular risk factors in hospitalized patients with acute myocardial infarction in Beijing. Chin Med J. 2013;126:4210–5.
5. National High Blood Pressure Education Program Coordinating Committee. Seventh report of the Joint National Committee on Prevention, Detection, Evaluation, and Treatment of High Blood Pressure. Hypertension. 2003;42:1206–52.
6. American Diabetes Association. Standards of medical care in diabetes-2008. Diabetes Care. 2008;31(1):S12–54.
7. National Cholesterol Education Program (NCEP) Expert Panel on Detection, Evaluation, and Treatment of High Blood Cholesterol in Adults (Adult Treatment Panel III). Third Report of the National Cholesterol Education Program (NCEP) Expert Panel on Detection, Evaluation, and Treatment of High Blood Cholesterol in Adults (Adult Treatment Panel III) final report. Circulation. 2002;106:3143–421.
8. Miao ZM, Li CG, Chen Y, Zhao SH, Wang YG, Wang ZC, et al. Dietary and lifestyle changes associated with high prevalence of hyperuricemia and gout in the Shandong coastal cities of Eastern China. J Rheumatol. 2008;35:1859–64.
9. Choi HK, Atkinson K, Karlson EW, Willett W, Curhan G. Purine-rich foods, dairy and protein intake, and the risk of gout in men. N Engl J Med. 2004;350:1093–103.
10. Guasch-Ferré M, Bulló M, Babio N, Martínez-González MA, Estruch R, Covas M, et al. Mediterranean diet and risk of hyperuricemia in elderly participants at high cardiovascular risk. J Gerontol A Biol Sci Med Sci. 2013;68:1263–70. doi:10.1093/gerona/glt028.
11. Nakamura K, Sakurai M, Miura K, Morikawa Y, Yoshita K, Ishizaki M, et al. Alcohol intake and the risk of hyperuricaemia: a 6-year prospective study in Japanese men. Nutr Metab Cardiovasc Dis. 2011;22:989–96.
12. Choi HK, Atkinson K, Karlson EW, Willett W, Curhan G. Alcohol intake and risk of incident gout in men: a prospective study. Lancet. 2004;363:1277–81.
13. Qureshi AE, Hameed S, Noeman A. Relationship of serum uric acid level and angiographic severity of coronary artery disease in male patients with acute coronary syndrome.Pak J Med Sci 2013; 29:1137–41.doi: http://dx.doi.org/10.12669/pjms.295.4029
14. Estruch R. Anti-inflammatory effects of the Mediterranean diet: the experience of the PREDIMED study. Proc Nutr Soc. 2010;69:333–40.
15. Centers for Disease Control and Prevention. Million hearts: strategies to reduce the prevalence of leading cardiovascular disease risk factors - United States, 2011. MMWR Morb Mortal Wkly Rep. 2011;60:1248–51.
16. Centers for Disease Control and Prevention. Vital signs: awareness and treatment of uncontrolled hypertension among adults - United States, 2003–2010. MMWR Morb Mortal Wkly Rep. 2012;61:703–9.
17. Teo KK, Liu L, Chow CK, Wang X, Islam S, Jiang L, et al. Potentially modifiable risk factors associated with myocardial infarction in China: the INTERHEART China study. Heart. 2009;95:1857–64.
18. Centers for Disease Control and Prevention. Prevalence of cholesterol screening and high blood cholesterol among adults-United States, 2005, 2007, and 2009. MMWR Morb Mortal Wkly Rep. 2012;61:697–702.
19. American Diabetes Association. Diagnosis and classification of diabetes mellitus. Diabetes Care. 2010;33 Suppl 1:S62–9.
20. Li Y, Cao J, Lin H, Li D, Wang Y, He J. Community health needs assessment with precedeproceed model: a mixed methods study. BMC Health Serv Res. 2009;9:181.
21. Chandola T, Britton A, Brunner E, Hemingway H, Malik M, Kumari M, et al. Work stress and coronary heart disease: what are the mechanisms? Eur Heart J. 2008;29:640–8.
22. Folta SC, Goldberg JP, Lichtenstein AH, Seguin R, Reed PN, Nelson ME. Factors related to cardiovascular disease risk reduction in midlife and older women: a qualitative study. Prev Chronic Dis. 2008;5:A06.
23. Gillison F, Greaves C, Stathi A, Ramsay R, Bennett P, Taylor G, et al. Waste the Waist': the development of an intervention to promote changes in diet and physical activity for people with high cardiovascular risk. Br J Health Psychol. 2012;17:327–45.
24. Kiawi E, Edwards R, Shu J, Unwin N, Kamadjeu R, Mbanya JC. Knowledge, attitudes, and behavior relating to diabetes and its main risk factors among urban residents in Cameroon: a qualitative survey. Ethn Dis. 2006;16:503–9.
25. Xie DF, Li W, Wang Y, Gu HQ, Teo K, Liu LS, et al. Sleep duration, snoring habits and risk of acute myocardial infarction in China population: results of the INTERHEART study. BMC Public Health, 2014; 14: 531. http://www.biomedcentral.com/1471-2458/14/531.

10

Regional wall function before and after acute myocardial infarction

Ulrika S Pahlm[1], Joey FA Ubachs[2], Einar Heiberg[1,3,4], Henrik Engblom[1], David Erlinge[5], Matthias Götberg[5] and Håkan Arheden[1*]

Abstract

Background: Left ventricular function is altered during and after AMI. Regional function can be determined by cardiac magnetic resonance (CMR) wall thickening, and velocity encoded (VE) strain analysis. The aims of this study were to investigate how regional myocardial wall function, assessed by CMR VE-strain and regional wall thickening, changes after acute myocardial infarction, and to determine if we could differentiate between ischemic, adjacent and remote segments of the left ventricle.

Methods: Ten pigs underwent baseline CMR study for assessment of wall thickening and VE-strain. Ischemia was then induced for 40-minutes by intracoronary balloon inflation in the left anterior descending coronary artery. During occlusion, ^{99m}Tc tetrofosmin was administered intravenously and myocardial perfusion SPECT (MPS) was performed for determination of the ischemic area, followed by a second CMR study. Based on ischemia seen on MPS, the 17 AHA segments of the left ventricle was divided into 3 different categories (ischemic, adjacent and remote). Regional wall function measured by wall thickening and VE-strain analysis was determined before and after ischemia.

Results: Mean wall thickening decreased significantly in the ischemic (from 2.7 mm to 0.65 mm, $p < 0.001$) and adjacent segments (from 2.4 to 1.5 mm $p < 0.001$). In remote segments, wall thickening increased significantly (from 2.4 mm to 2.8 mm, $p < 0.01$). In ischemic and adjacent segments, both radial and longitudinal strain was significantly decreased after ischemia ($p < 0.001$). In remote segments there was a significant increase in radial strain ($p = 0.002$) while there was no difference in longitudinal strain ($p = 0.69$). ROC analysis was performed to determine thresholds distinguishing between the different regions. Sensitivity for determining ischemic segments ranged from 70-80%, and specificity from 72%-77%. There was a 9% increase in left ventricular mass after ischemia.

Conclusion: Differentiation thresholds for wall thickening and VE-strain could be established to distinguish between ischemic, adjacent and remote segments but will, have limited applicability due to low sensitivity and specificity. There is a slight increase in radial strain in remote segments after ischemia. Edema was present mainly in the ischemic region but also in the combined adjacent and remote segments.

* Correspondence: hakan.arheden@med.lu.se
[1]Department of Clinical Physiology, Clinical Sciences, Lund University Hospital, SE-22185 Lund, Sweden
Full list of author information is available at the end of the article

Background

Acute myocardial infarction (AMI) is a major cause of death worldwide despite diagnostic and therapeutic improvements [1]. Mortality is especially high in patients with AMI and out of hospital cardiac arrest.

Regional left ventricular function is altered during and after AMI. This includes changes in the infarcted and ischemic regions as well as stunning in adjacent and remote areas of the myocardium [2-6]. Most studies describe changes in the infarcted myocardium while there is less information about changes in remote myocardium. It is still somewhat controversial whether remote myocardium after AMI is hypo-functioning [6] or hyper-functioning [7]. This has not been well studied in the hyper acute setting.

Cardiac magnetic resonance (CMR) is a comprehensive diagnostic tool that can provide accurate and reproducible measurements of cardiac volumes [8], dimensions [8], regional cardiac function [9,10] and infarct size [11,12]. It has emerged as the gold standard for assessing systolic wall thickening [10]. Studies have shown that regional wall function can be assessed using CMR strain analysis [13,14]. Strain is a measure of the change in size and shape of an object and can be derived from CMR by using grid-tagging [15], displacement encoding with stimulated echoes (DENSE) [16] or velocity-encoded (VE) imaging [14,17].

Myocardial function in patients with AMI reaching the hospital has been well studied [5,6,18]. Without knowledge of the pre-AMI function it precludes a detailed quantitative analysis of absolute and relative changes in function. The function in the superacute stage (hours) of infarction and in those suffering out of hospital cardiac death is also unknown.

Therefore, the aim of this study was to investigate how regional myocardial wall function, assessed by CMR velocity encoded strain and regional wall thickening, changes after acute myocardial infarction. In order to quantify absolute and relative regional changes we used an experimental pig model with induced ischemia and reperfusion using each animal as its own control. We also aimed to find out if we could differentiate between ischemic, adjacent and remote myocardium as determined by myocardial perfusion MPS by looking at regional myocardial function.

Methods

Animal preparation

The study conforms to the Guide for the Care and Use of Laboratory Animals, US National Institute of Health (NIH Publication No. 85-23, revised 1996) and was approved by the Ethics Committee of Lund University, Sweden.

Ten domestic pigs weighing 40-50 kg were fasted overnight with free access to water and all were premedicated with 2 mg/kg azaperone (Stresnil; Leo, Helsingborg, Sweden) administered intramuscularly 30 minutes before the procedure. Induction of anesthesia was performed with 5-25 mg/kg of thiopental (Pentothal; Abbott, Stockholm, Sweden). Administration of the anaesthetic was complemented with intermittent doses of meprobamat (Mebumal; DAK, Copenhagen, Denmark) and thiopental, if needed. Prior to inducing ischemia all pigs underwent a baseline CMR for assessment of wall thickening and velocity encoded strain. Ischemia was induced with inflation of an angioplasty balloon in the left anterior descending coronary artery distal to the first diagonal branch for 40 minutes. An angiogram was performed after inflation of the balloon and before deflation of the balloon in order to verify total occlusion of the coronary vessel and correct balloon positioning. After deflation of the balloon, a second angiogram was performed to verify restoration of blood flow in the previously occluded artery. During occlusion of the artery, ^{99m}Tc tetrofosmin was administered intravenously prior to reperfusion and MPS was performed 2-3 hours after occlusion for determination of the area subjected to ischemia. A second CMR examination was performed approximately 3-4 hours after reperfusion. After the second CMR examination the animals were euthanized.

CMR imaging and analysis

Magnetic resonance imaging was performed on a Philips Intera CV 1.5 T (Philips, Best, the Netherlands) with a five element cardiac synergy coil before and after ischemia. All pigs were placed in supine position and scout images in the three orthogonal planes were acquired as guidance for determination of the standard imaging planes.

Wall thickening

For assessment of regional wall thickening steady state free precession (SSFP) cine images were acquired in the short-axis plane covering the entire left ventricle from base to apex. Images were also acquired in the 2, 3 and 4 chamber imaging planes. Image parameters were: repetition time 3.2 ms, echo time 1.6 ms, flip angle 60°, image resolution 1.36 × 1.36, slice thickness 8 mm, retrospective ECG gated reconstruction.

From the short-axis cine images systolic wall thickness, wall thickening, and fractional wall thickening (defined as wall thickening divided by end diastolic wall thickness) were assessed before and after ischemia by manual tracing of the endocardial and epicardial borders. The left ventricle was divided in the American Heart Association 17 segment model. Papillary muscles were excluded from the myocardium. The most basal slice included in the analysis was the most basal short-axis slice containing myocardium in 360° of the left ventricular myocardial circumference in end-systole.

Myocardial strain

All 2D in-plane velocity encoded data was acquired in the 2, 3 and 4 chamber imaging planes. Imaging parameters were: repetition time 23.4 ms echo time 4.6 ms, velocity encoding gradient 20 cm/s, flip angle 15°. Image resolution was typically 1.6 × 1.6 mm, and slice thickness 7 mm with 18–22 time frames per cardiac cycle, retrospective ECG gating.

We used a previously validated method for VE strain analysis [14]. In short, the myocardium was manually segmented in the 2, 3 and 4 chamber SSFP cine images in end-diastole. Thereafter, the segmentation was exported to the 2D in-plane velocity encoded images and endocardial and epicardial borders were tracked in each time frame throughout the cardiac cycle using the acquired velocity information using an optimization scheme (Figure 1). In one dimension, strain is defined as the fractional change in length of an object. In two dimensions, strain is represented as a 2-dimensional tensor. As the myocardium deforms during the cardiac cycle, a particular myocardial region may be lengthening in the radial direction, while shortening in the circumferential or longitudinal directions. The radial and longitudinal strain directions are depicted in Figure 1 panel C. In the current study, the 2D in-plane velocity data was used to obtain longitudinal and radial strain for assessment of regional myocardial function on a per pixel basis. Strain for each pixel in the myocardium was then colour coded and transformed into colour coded polar plots using the AHA 17 segment model [19].

Late gadolinium enhancement (LGE)

An extracellular contrast agent (gadopentetate dimeglumine, Bayer Pharma, Berlin, Germany) was administered intravenously at 0.2 mmol/kg 15 minutes before late gadolinium enhancement (LGE) images were acquired. Standard clinical imaging parameters were used for LGE imaging covering the left ventricle from base to apex by using an inversion-recovery gradient-echo sequence (slice thickness, 8 mm; field of view, 340 mm; repetition time, 3.14 ms; echo time, 1.58 ms), with manually adjustment of the inversion time to null the signal from viable myocardium.

The area of hyperenhancement was defined on the LGE short-axis images and was quantified using a previously described and validated semi-automatic algorithm [20] incorporating manual adjustments. Finally, all LGE data was transformed into polar plots according to a 17 segment model [21].

MPS imaging and analysis

Five hundred MBq of ^{99m}Tc tetrofosmin (Amersham Health, Buckinghamshire, UK) was administered intravenously ten minutes before deflation of the angioplasty balloon. The pigs were then imaged in a supine position using a dual head camera (ADAC Vertex, Milpitas, CA, USA) at 32 projections (40s per projection) with a 64 × 64 matrix yielding a digital resolution of 5 x 5 x 5 mm. Short- and long-axis images, covering the left ventricle, gated to ECG, were then reconstructed.

For MPS analysis, automatic segmentation of the LV was performed [22]. In short, the automatic segmentation finds the centerline through the LV wall and identifies the endocardium and epicardium based on an individually estimated wall thickness and signal intensity values within the image. Following delineation, the ischemic area was assessed in contiguous short-axis slices from base to apex using a method for semi-automatic quantification [23]. All myocardium below a threshold of 50 percent of the maximum counts was considered ischemic and expressed as a percentage of the LV volume. Manual adjustment of the automatic delineation was sometimes required in the LV outflow region. Finally, the MPS delineations with ischemia were transformed into colour coded blacked-out polar plots.

All image analyses were performed using an in-house developed freely available software (Segment v1.8 R2860; http://segment.heiberg.se) [24].

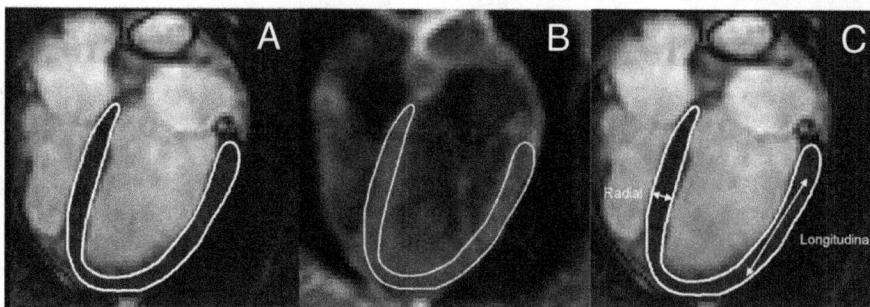

Figure 1 Outlining the left ventricle. A. Cine 4 chamber view of the heart before occlusion of LAD. The left ventricle is delineated in white in end-diastole. **B**. Velocity-encoded strain image of the heart in end-diastole, where the white line represents the left ventricle delineation as exported from the cine 4 chamber view. **C**. Illustration of radial and longitudinal strain directions.

Definition of left ventricular areas: ischemic, adjacent and remote myocardium

In this study, the left ventricle was divided in the AHA 17-segment model for analysis [19]. The 17 segments of the myocardium were divided into 3 groups according to the amount of ischemia seen on MPS. 1) Segments where >50% of the myocardium was ischemic where considered ischemic segments, 2) segments where 1–50% of the myocardium was ischemic were considered adjacent segments and 3) segments with no ischemia were considered remote. The 50% threshold was determined after a consensus discussion. If a segment contained more ischemic than non-ischemic myocardium it was considered ischemic and otherwise it was considered adjacent. Sectors that contained no ischemia were considered remote. The process is illustrated in Figure 2. Myocardial salvage index (MSI) was defined as MSI = 1-(infarct size by LGE)/(ischemic volume by MPS) in a similar fashion as described earlier [25].

Statistical methods

Wilcoxon Sign Rank test was used to assess changes in volumes, ejection fraction, cardiac output and heart rate. For changes in regional CMR wall thickening and VE strain we used a paired t-test. For all analysis, a p-value below 0.05 was considered significant. Values are expressed as mean ± SEM. To find thresholds to be able to discriminate between ischemic, adjacent and remote areas ROC analysis was performed. The ROC analysis was performed by evaluating sensitivity and specificity for different thresholds of wall thickening, radial strain, and longitudinal strain, respectively. The thresholds was tested in 1000 steps from minimum value to maximum value for each parameter.

Results

Table 1 shows the CMR measurements for all 10 pigs before and after induced ischemia. After ischemia, there was a significant decrease in stroke volume and ejection fraction associated with a significant increase in heart

rate, preserving the cardiac output. The mean myocardial salvage index was 25 ± 15%.

There was a significant increase in left ventricular mass from 86 ± 7 ml to 94 ± 15, an increase in 9% (p = 0.01) after ischemia. The increase in mass was not homogenous, and the increase in ischemic areas was 38% ± 3% (mean ± SEM) (p < 0.01), adjacent was 4% ± 2% (mean ± SEM) (p = ns), and in remote areas the increase was 7% ± 3% (mean ± SEM) (p = ns). When combining the results from remote and adjacent areas there was an increase in mass of 6% ±2% (p = ns).

There was no statistically significant difference in wall thickening between the ischemic, adjacent and remote groups before induced ischemia.

After reperfusion, the mean wall thickening decreased significantly in the ischemic (from 2.7 mm before ischemia to 0.65 mm, p < 0.001) and adjacent segments (from 2.4 to 1.5 mm p < 0.001). In remote myocardium, however, wall thickening increased significantly (from 2.4 mm to 2.8 mm, p < 0.01). Figure 3 shows wall thickening before and after ischemia. Fractional wall thickening was 8% in ischemic, 22% in adjacent, and 36% in remote sectors, respectively. Mean end-diastolic thickness was 10.5 mm in ischemic, 9.4 mm in adjacent, and 8.7 mm in remote sectors, respectively. Mean end-systolic thickness was 11.1 mm in ischemic, 11.4 mm in adjacent, and, 11.8 mm in remote sectors, respectively.

Figure 4 shows polar plots indicating ischemia by MPS, myocardial infarction by LGE, and wall thickening by cine-CMR for each study subject. Dysfunctional myocardium as assessed by CMR absolute wall thickening after ischemia was mainly present in the myocardial region supplied by the left anterior descending artery, similar to MPS and LGE. In the majority of the pigs, however dysfunctional myocardium extended to the adjacent and remote regions of the myocardium.

Before ischemia there was no statistically significant difference in radial or longitudinal strain in the later ischemic, adjacent and remote regions (p > 0.05).

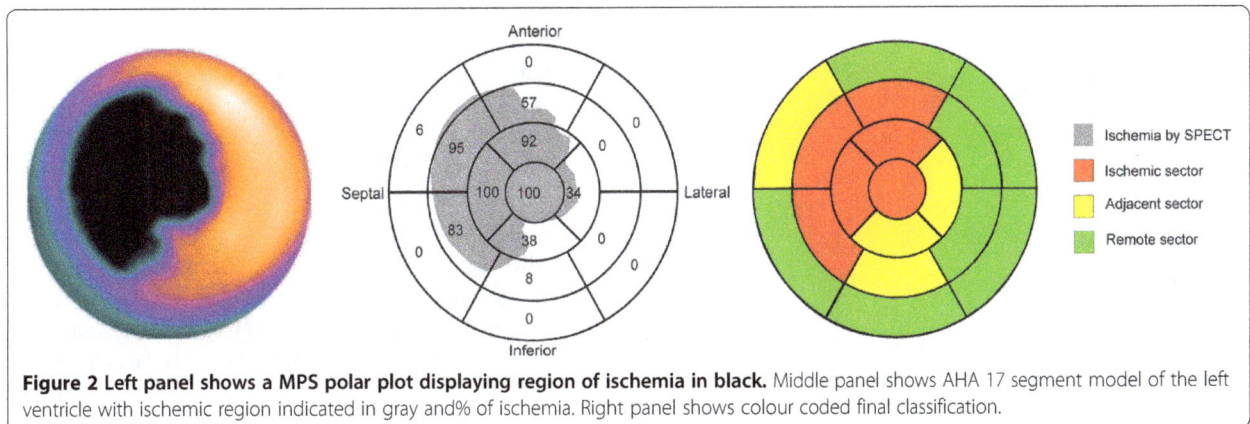

Figure 2 Left panel shows a MPS polar plot displaying region of ischemia in black. Middle panel shows AHA 17 segment model of the left ventricle with ischemic region indicated in gray and% of ischemia. Right panel shows colour coded final classification.

Table 1 Heart rate, cardiac volumes, ejection fraction (EF) and cardiac output (CO) before and after ischemia

	Before ischemia	After ischemia	p-value
Heart rate [bpm]	81 ± 21	113 ± 30	0.03
Left ventricular mass [ml]	86 ± 7	94 ± 15	0.01
End diastolic volume [ml]	82 ± 11	71 ± 10	0.04
End systolic volume [ml]	47 ± 7	48 ± 9	0.50
Stroke volume [ml]	36 ± 8	23 ± 5	0.01
Ejection fraction [%]	44 ± 7	32 ± 6	0.01
Cardiac output [l/min]	2.8 ± 0.7	2.6 ± 0.8	0.56

Figure 5 shows radial and longitudinal strain before and after ischemia. There was a strong correlation between global wall thickening and global radial strain ($r = 0.86$, $p < 0.001$). In ischemic and adjacent areas, both radial and longitudinal strain was significantly decreased after ischemia ($p < 0.001$). In remote myocardium, there was a significant increase in radial strain ($p = 0.002$), while there was no difference in longitudinal strain ($p = 0.69$).

There was a significant decrease in both radial and longitudinal strain between the ischemic and remote myocardium (both $p < 0.0001$) and between the ischemic and adjacent myocardium (radial $p < 0.001$, longitudinal $p = 0.03$) between adjacent and remote myocardium (radial $p < 0.0001$, longitudinal $p < 0.001$).). The regional function expressed as radial strain in sectors defined as salvaged (i.e. containing any ischemic myocardium but no infarct) was $12 ± 10\%$. There was no significant difference between regional strain in salvaged sectors versus adjacent sectors ($p = 0.79$).

Figure 6 shows that regional function measured by radial and longitudinal strain decreases most significantly in left ventricular areas supplied by the left anterior descending artery.

Figure 7 shows ROC curves for thresholds. Ischemic sectors were compared to adjacent and remote sectors combined, and remote sectors were compared to ischemic and adjacent sectors combined. The results of the ROC analysis are presented in Table 2.

Discussion

In this study we found that there is a significant decrease in regional wall function in the ischemic and adjacent segments of the left ventricle measured by CMR wall thickening and VE-strain after induced myocardial infarction. There is a slight increase in regional wall function seen by wall thickening and VE radial strain in remote myocardium. The non-significant increase in longitudinal strain seen in the remote myocardium was likely attributed to the limited number of subjects.

The decreased function in the ischemic region is well known and has obvious causes.

The reduced regional function in adjacent areas have been described previously [2] and represents myocardial stunning as described by Braunwald et al. [3,4]. This prolonged dysfunction remain present for hours, days or even a few weeks after ischemia and may be explained by the presence of edema [26]. Similar results were demonstrated by Engblom et al. in a human population [27]. The significant decrease in EDV in conjunction with unaffected ESV after ischemia suggests diastolic dysfunction as a result of the ischemia. The decreased regional function in ischemic regions indicates regional systolic dysfunction.

In this study we found that there was a slight, but statistically significant, increase in regional myocardial function in remote areas measured both by wall thickness and radial strain. There was, however, no change in function seen by longitudinal strain. Increased function in remote areas has been described previously [6,7,28] but most other studies have found a decreased function in both animals [29,30] and humans [6,27,31,32]. Reasons for the lack of consensus between studies are unknown but may be related to duration of ischemia, reperfusion and timing of imaging. An advantage of our study is the analysis of strain and wall thickening measurements in the same animal both prior to and after infarction. The presented method for measuring regional left ventricular function in ischemic, adjacent and remote areas may be used in controlled experimental settings to investigate the effect of cardioprotective treatments, such as cooling [33].

In a direct comparison between strain tagging and wall thickening, a previous study by Götte et al. [34] using CMR has shown that the former was more accurate in discriminating infarcted from remote myocardium. In our study, however, we found that wall thickening and radial VE strain were similar in discriminating between

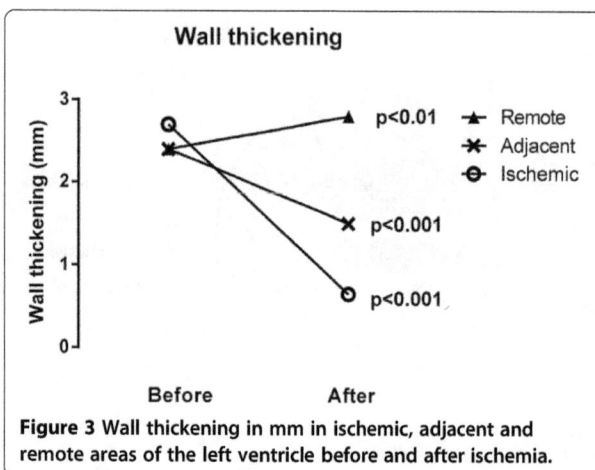

Figure 3 Wall thickening in mm in ischemic, adjacent and remote areas of the left ventricle before and after ischemia.

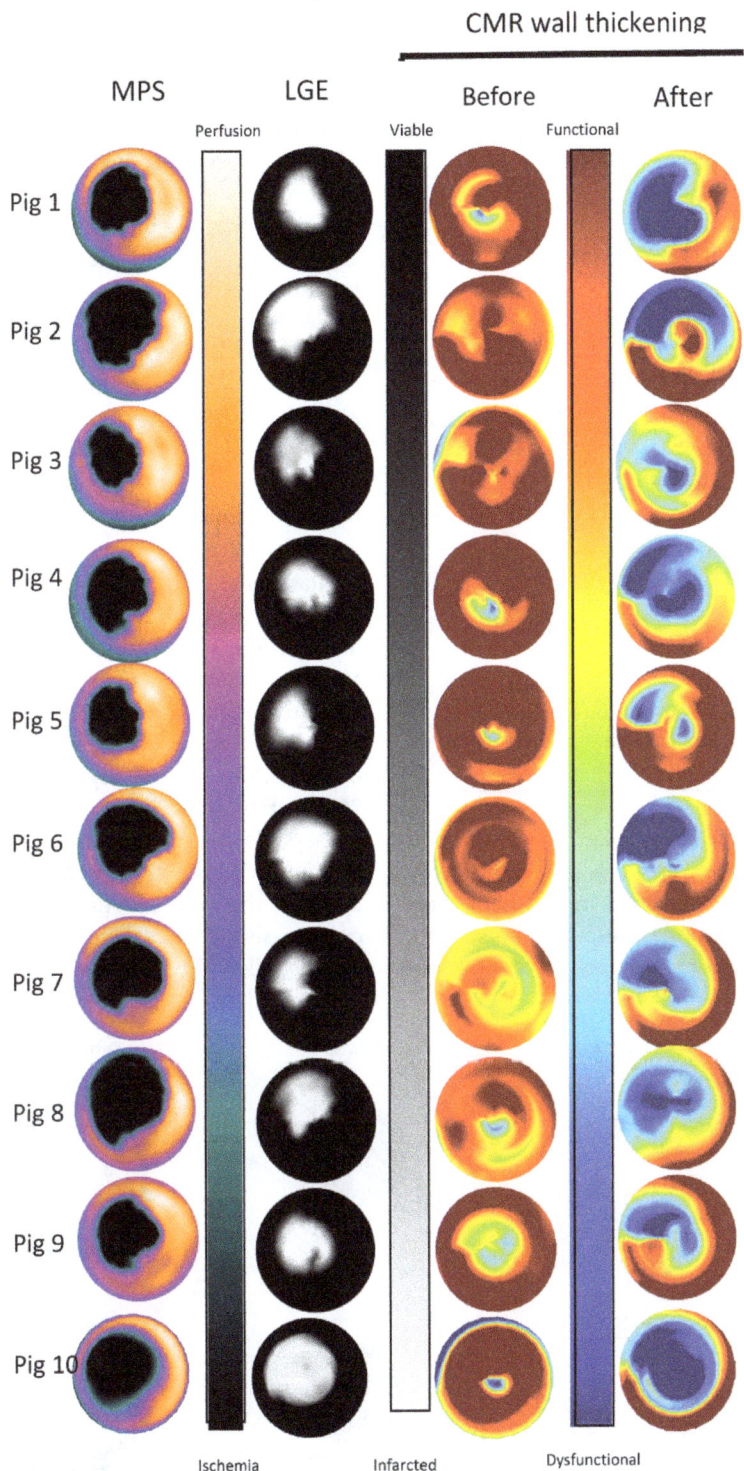

Figure 4 Polar plots of MPS, LGE and CMR absolute wall thickening for each subject. The first column shows the ischemic area by MPS. The second column shows infarct transmurality assessed by LGE. The third column shows cardiac function by CMR absolute wall thickening before ischemia and the fourth column cardiac function by CMR absolute wall thickening after ischemia. The color bars next to the respective polar plots denote the scale.

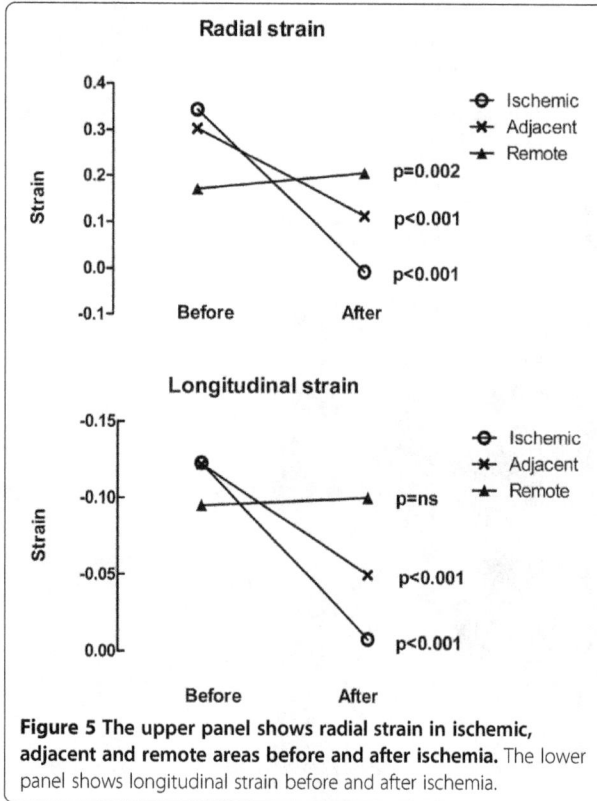

Figure 5 The upper panel shows radial strain in ischemic, adjacent and remote areas before and after ischemia. The lower panel shows longitudinal strain before and after ischemia.

thickening and 15% for strain. The thresholds have limited applicability due to the low sensitivity and specificity. This has implications on trying to differentiate between remote, adjacent and ischemic regions based on regional function regardless of modality. The detection of adjacent sectors alone may be of limited clinical value, however the rational for including adjacent sectors in this study was to differentiate between sectors with high grade ischemia (ischemic sectors) and low grade ischemia (adjacent sectors).

We also found an increase of left ventricular mass of 9% following ischemia that is likely caused by edema. The increase was impressive in the ischemic area, measuring $37\% \pm 3\%$ ($p < 0.01$) compared to $6\% \pm 2$ ($p = ns$) in the combined remote and adjacent areas. This was also supported by end diastolic thickness that was significantly higher in ischemic compared to remote sectors ($p < 0.01$).

Limitations

The study was conducted on 10 pigs, all with occlusion of the LAD. How results for CMR wall thickening and VE-strain would be affected by right coronary artery or left circumflex occlusion remains to be studied. In wall thickening, the most basal slices in end-diastole are often excluded since myocardium cannot be found in 360° of the left ventricular myocardial circumference in end-systole due to long-axis AV-plane motion [35]. No standard definition of ischemic, adjacent and remote areas of the ventricle have been established, therefore caution should be taken when comparing results with other studies.

ischemic and non-ischemic areas. We found that both wall thickening and strain are able to differentiate between ischemic and non-ischemic, remote and non-remote myocardium, respectively. However, the sensitivity to detect adjacent regions was poor, 33% for wall

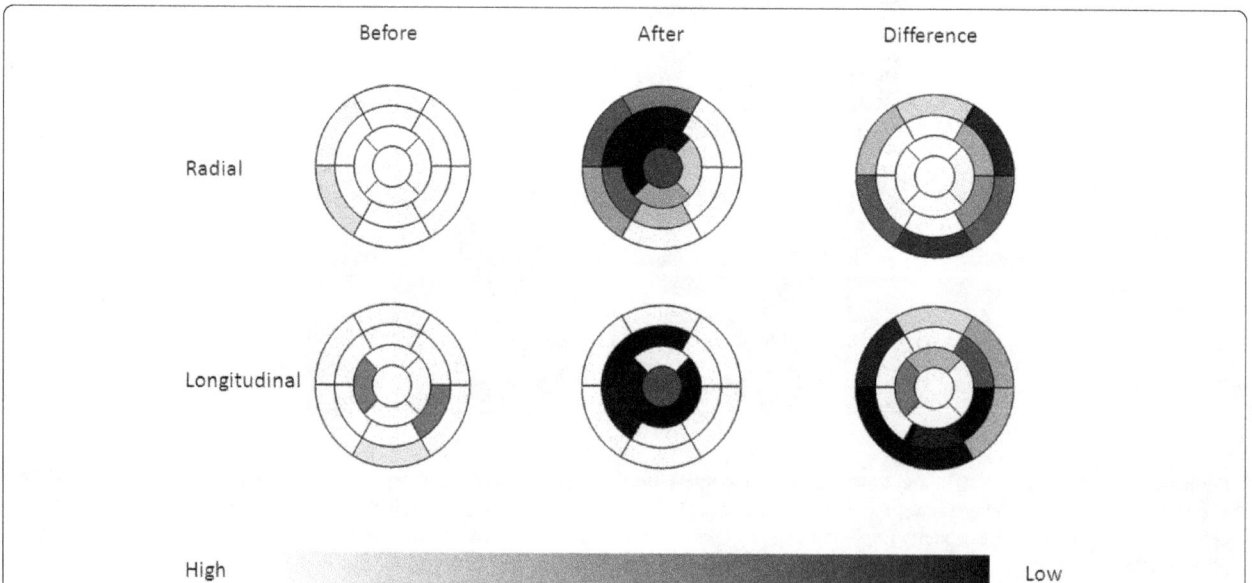

Figure 6 Mean regional function for all subjects expressed as radial strain (top row) and longitudinal strain (bottom row). Left column shows high regional function before ischemia. Middle column shows decreased regional function in segments supplied by left anterior descending artery. Right column shows difference in regional function before and after ischemia. White means high strain and black low strain.

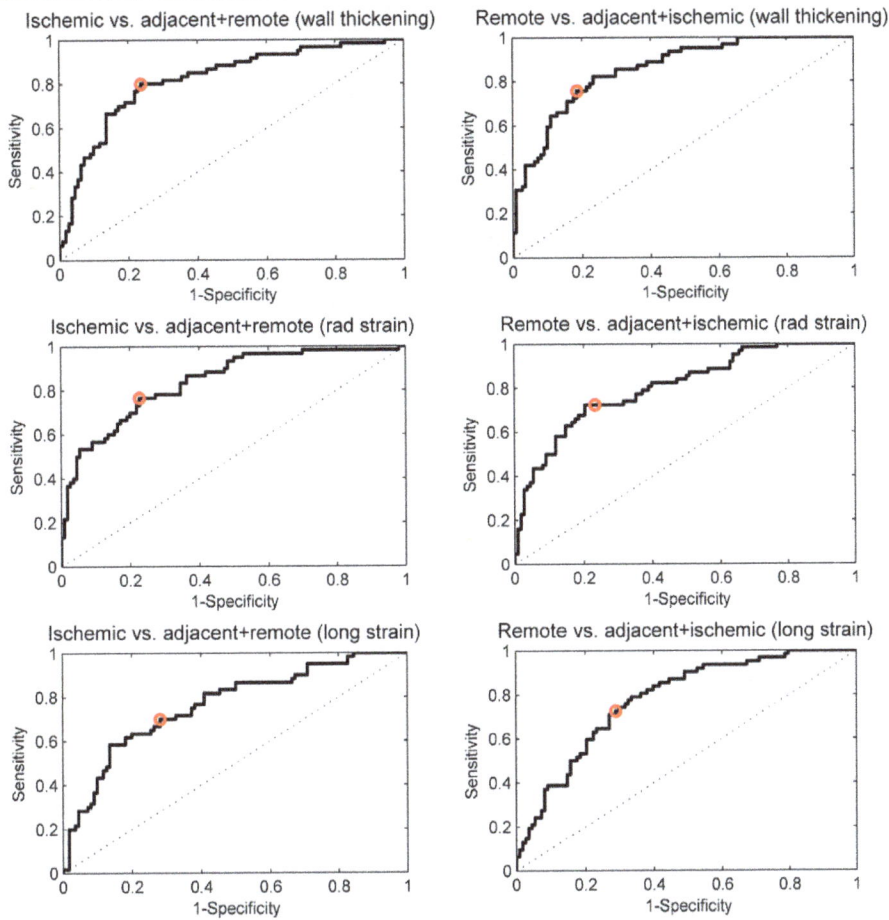

Figure 7 ROC analysis determining threshold. Upper panel shows results for wall thickening. Middle panel shows results for radial strain. Lower panel shows results for longitudinal stain. Left column shows differentiation between ischemic and non-ischemic areas. Right column shows differentiation between remote and non-remote areas. Red marker shows sensitivity and specificity for optimal thresholds.

Table 2 Thresholds for wall thickening, radial strain and longitudinal strain determined by ROC analysis for differentiations between ischemic, adjacent and remote areas

	Threshold	Sensitivity%	Specificity%
Wall thickening ischemic	< 1.4 mm	80	76
Wall thickening adjacent	1.4 - 2.1 mm	35	90
Wall thickening remote	>2.1 mm	76	81
Radial strain ischemic	< 0.06	77	77
Radial strain adjacent	0.06-0.15	33	89
Radial strain remote	>0.15	73	77
Long. strain ischemic	> −0.04	70	72
Long. strain adjacent	−0.04 - −0.07	15	88
Long. strain remote	<−0.07	73	71

Conclusions

Thresholds for wall thickening and strain could be established for differentiation between ischemic, adjacent and remote areas. These thresholds, however will have limited clinical applicability due to the low sensitivity and specificity. Regional left ventricular function is reduced in the ischemic and areas adjacent to the ischemia after reperfused anterior myocardial infarction, while there is a slight increase in radial function in remote areas of the left ventricle. Edema was present mainly in the ischemic region but also to a slighter degree in the combined adjacent and remote areas.

Competing interests

Einar Heiberg is the founder of Medviso AB that produce software for cardiac image processing. All other authors declare that they have no competing interests.

Authors' contribution

UP: Have made substantial contributions to the conception and design of the study, analysis and interpretation of the data and drafted the manuscript.

JU: Have made substantial contributions to the conception and design of the study, the analysis and interpretation, and revised the manuscript for important intellectual content. EH: Have made substantial contributions to the conception and design of the study, analysis and interpretation of the data, and revised the manuscript for important intellectual content. HE: Have made substantial contributions to the analysis and interpretation of the data, and revised the manuscript for important intellectual content. DE: Have made substantial contributions in the acquisition of data, and revised the manuscript for important intellectual content. MG Have made substantial contributions in the acquisition of data, and revised the manuscript for important intellectual content. HA: Have made substantial contributions to the conception and design of the study, and revised the manuscript for important intellectual content. All authors have approved final version of the manuscript.

Acknowledgements
This study was funded by the Swedish Heart Lung Foundation, the Swedish Research Council (VR-2011-3916,VR- 2012–4944), and Region of Scania, Sweden.

Author details
[1]Department of Clinical Physiology, Clinical Sciences, Lund University Hospital, SE-22185 Lund, Sweden. [2]Department of Cardiology, Catharina Hospital Eindhoven, Eindhoven, The Netherlands. [3]Centre for Mathematical Sciences, Lund University, Lund, Sweden. [4]Department of Biomedical Engineering, Faculty of Engineering, Lund University, Lund, Sweden. [5]Department of Cardiology, Clinical Sciences, Lund University, Lund, Sweden.

References
1. Go AS, Mozaffarian D, Roger VL, Benjamin EJ, Berry JD, Borden WB, Bravata DM, Dai S, Ford ES, Fox CS, Franco S, Fullerton HJ, Gillespie C, Hailpern SM, Heit JA, Howard VJ, Huffman MD, Kissels BM, Kittner SJ, Lackland DT, Lichtman JH, Lisabeth JH, Magid D, Marcus GM, Marelli A, Matchar DB, McGuire DK, Mohler ER, Moy CS, Mussolino ME: Heart disease and stroke statistics–2013 update: a report from the American Heart Association. Circulation 2013, 127(1):e6–e245.
2. Shimkunas R, Zhang Z, Wenk JF, Soleimani M, Khazalpour M, Acevedo-Bolton G, Wang G, Saloner D, Mishra R, Wallace AW, Ge L, Baker AJ, Guccione JM, Ratcliffe MB: Left ventricular myocardial contractility is depressed in the borderzone after posterolateral myocardial infarction. Ann Thorac Surg 2013, 95(5):1619–1625.
3. Braunwald E, Kloner RA: The stunned myocardium: prolonged, postischemic ventricular dysfunction. Circulation 1982, 66(6):1146–1149.
4. Kloner RA, Bolli R, Marban E, Reinlib L, Braunwald E: Medical and cellular implications of stunning, hibernation, and preconditioning: an NHLBI workshop. Circulation 1998, 97(18):1848–1867.
5. Rademakers F, Van de Werf F, Mortelmans L, Marchal G, Bogaert J: Evolution of regional performance after an acute anterior myocardial infarction in humans using magnetic resonance tagging. J Physiol 2003, 546(Pt 3):777–787.
6. Kramer CM, Rogers WJ, Theobald TM, Power TP, Petruolo S, Reichek N: Remote noninfarcted region dysfunction soon after first anterior myocardial infarction. A magnetic resonance tagging study. Circulation 1996, 94(4):660–666.
7. Ito S, Suzuki T, Hosokawa H, Inada T, Takeda Y, Suzumura H, Tomimoto S, Yamada Y, Goto A, Horio T, Suzuki S, Fukutomi T, Itho M: Increased hyperkinesis in noninfarcted areas during short-term follow-up in patients with first anterior acute myocardial infarction treated by direct percutaneous transluminal coronary angioplasty. Jpn Heart J 1999, 40(5):549–560.
8. Pennell DJ: Ventricular volume and mass by CMR. J Cardiovasc Magn Reson 2002, 4(4):507–513.
9. Maceira AM, Prasad SK, Khan M, Pennell DJ: Normalized left ventricular systolic and diastolic function by steady state free precession cardiovascular magnetic resonance. J Cardiovasc Magn Reson 2006, 8(3):417–426.
10. Messroghli DR, Bainbridge GJ, Alfakih K, Jones TR, Plein S, Ridgway JP, Sivananthan MU: Assessment of regional left ventricular function: accuracy and reproducibility of positioning standard short-axis sections in cardiac MR imaging. Radiology 2005, 235(1):229–236.
11. Simonetti OP, Kim RJ, Fieno DS, Hillenbrand HB, Wu E, Bundy JM, Finn JP, Judd RM: An improved MR imaging technique for the visualization of myocardial infarction. Radiology 2001, 218(1):215–223.
12. Pennell DJ, Sechtem UP, Higgins CB, Manning WJ, Pohost GM, Rademakers FE, van Rossum AC, Shaw LJ, Yucel EK, European Society of cardiology, Society of Cardiovascular Magnetic Resonance: Clinical indications for cardiovascular magnetic resonance (CMR): Consensus Panel report. J Cardiovasc Magn Reson 2004, 6(4):727–765.
13. Zerhouni EA, Parish DM, Rogers WJ, Yang A, Shapiro EP: Human heart: tagging with MR imaging–a method for noninvasive assessment of myocardial motion. Radiology 1988, 169(1):59–63.
14. Heiberg E, Pahlm-Webb U, Agarwal S, Bergvall E, Fransson H, Steding-Ehrenborg K, Carlsson M, Arheden H: Longitudinal strain from velocity encoded cardiovascular magnetic resonance: a validation study. J Cardiovasc Magn Reson 2013, 15:15.
15. Petitjean C, Rougon N, Cluzel P: Assessment of myocardial function: a review of quantification methods and results using tagged MRI. J Cardiovasc Magn Reson 2005, 7(2):501–516.
16. Aletras AH, Ding S, Balaban RS, Wen H: DENSE: displacement encoding with stimulated echoes in cardiac functional MRI. J Magn Reson 1999, 137(1):247–252.
17. Wedeen VJ: Magnetic resonance imaging of myocardial kinematics. Technique to detect, localize, and quantify the strain rates of the active human myocardium. Magn Reson Med 1992, 27(1):52–67.
18. Kwong RY, Schussheim AE, Rekhraj S, Aletras AH, Geller N, Davis J, Christian TF, Balaban RS, Arai AE: Detecting acute coronary syndrome in the emergency department with cardiac magnetic resonance imaging. Circulation 2003, 107(4):531–537.
19. Cerqueira MD, Weissman NJ, Dilsizian V, Jacobs AK, Kaul S, Laskey WK, Pennell DJ, Rumberger JA, Ryan T, Verani MS: Standardized myocardial segmentation and nomenclature for tomographic imaging of the heart. A statement for healthcare professionals from the Cardiac Imaging Committee of the Council on Clinical Cardiology of the American Heart Association. Circulation 2002, 105(4):539–542.
20. Heiberg E, Engblom H, Engvall J, Hedstrom E, Ugander M, Arheden H: Semi-automatic quantification of myocardial infarction from delayed contrast enhanced magnetic resonance imaging. Scand Cardiovasc J 2005, 39(5):267–275.
21. Cain PA, Ugander M, Palmer J, Carlsson M, Heiberg E, Arheden H: Quantitative polar representation of left ventricular myocardial perfusion, function and viability using SPECT and cardiac magnetic resonance: initial results. Clin Physiol Funct Imaging 2005, 25(4):215–222.
22. Soneson H, Ubachs JF, Ugander M, Arheden H, Heiberg E: An Improved Method for Automatic Segmentation of the Left Ventricle in Myocardial Perfusion SPECT. J Nucl Med 2009, 50(2):205–213.
23. Ugander M, Soneson H, Engblom H, van der Pals J, Erlinge D, Heiberg E, Arheden H: Quantification of myocardium at risk in myocardial perfusion SPECT by co-registration and fusion with delayed contrast-enhanced magnetic resonance imaging–an experimental ex vivo study. Clin Physiol Funct Imaging 2012, 32(1):33–38.
24. Heiberg E, Sjogren J, Ugander M, Carlsson M, Engblom H, Arheden H: Design and validation of Segment–freely available software for cardiovascular image analysis. BMC Med Imaging 2010, 10:1.
25. Hedstrom E, Engblom H, Frogner F, Astrom-Olsson K, Ohlin H, Jovinge S, Arheden H: Infarct evolution in man studied in patients with first-time coronary occlusion in comparison to different species - implications for assessment of myocardial salvage. J Cardiovasc Magn Reson 2009, 11(1):38.
26. Kidambi A, Mather AN, Swoboda P, Motwani M, Fairbairn TA, Greenwood JP, Plein S: Relationship between myocardial edema and regional myocardial function after reperfused acute myocardial infarction: an MR imaging study. Radiology 2013, 267(3):701–708.
27. Engblom H, Hedstrom E, Heiberg E, Wagner GS, Pahlm O, Arheden H: Rapid initial reduction of hyperenhanced myocardium after reperfused first myocardial infarction suggests recovery of the peri-infarction zone: one-year follow-up by MRI. Circ Cardiovasc Imaging 2009, 2(1):47–55.
28. Rechavia E, de Silva R, Nihoyannopoulos P, Lammertsma AA, Jones T, Maseri A: Hyperdynamic performance of remote myocardium in acute infarction. Correlation between regional contractile function and myocardial perfusion. Eur Heart J 1995, 16(12):1845–1850.

29. Epstein FH, Yang Z, Gilson WD, Berr SS, Kramer CM, French BA: **MR tagging early after myocardial infarction in mice demonstrates contractile dysfunction in adjacent and remote regions.** *Magn Reson Med* 2002, **48**(2):399–403.

30. Kramer CM, Lima JA, Reichek N, Ferrari VA, Llaneras MR, Palmon LC, Yeh IT, Tallant B, Axel L: **Regional differences in function within noninfarcted myocardium during left ventricular remodeling.** *Circulation* 1993, **88**(3):1279–1288.

31. Bogaert J, Bosmans H, Maes A, Suetens P, Marchal G, Rademakers FE: **Remote myocardial dysfunction after acute anterior myocardial infarction: impact of left ventricular shape on regional function: a magnetic resonance myocardial tagging study.** *J Am Coll Cardiol* 2000, **35**(6):1525–1534.

32. Kramer CM, Rogers WJ, Theobald TM, Power TP, Geskin G, Reichek N: **Dissociation between changes in intramyocardial function and left ventricular volumes in the eight weeks after first anterior myocardial infarction.** *J Am Coll Cardiol* 1997, **30**(7):1625–1632.

33. Gotberg M, Olivecrona GK, Engblom H, Ugander M, van der Pals J, Heiberg E, Arheden H, Erlinge D: **Rapid short-duration hypothermia with cold saline and endovascular cooling before reperfusion reduces microvascular obstruction and myocardial infarct size.** *BMC Cardiovasc Disord* 2008, **8**:7.

34. Gotte MJ, van Rossum AC, Twisk JWR, Kuijer JPA, Marcus JT, Visser CA: **Quantification of regional contractile function after infarction: strain analysis superior to wall thickening analysis in discriminating infarct from remote myocardium.** *J Am Coll Cardiol* 2001, **37**(3):808–817.

35. Carlsson M, Ugander M, Mosen H, Buhre T, Arheden H: **Atrioventricular plane displacement is the major contributor to left ventricular pumping in healthy adults, athletes, and patients with dilated cardiomyopathy.** *Am J Physiol* 2007, **292**(3):H1452–H1459.

11

Atrial fibrillation in patients hospitalized with acute myocardial infarction: analysis of the china acute myocardial infarction (CAMI) registry

Yan Dai, Jingang Yang, Zhan Gao, Haiyan Xu, Yi Sun, Yuan Wu, Xiaojin Gao, Wei Li, Yang Wang, Runlin Gao, Yuejin Yang[*] on behalf of the CAMI Registry study group

Abstract

Background: The incidence, clinical outcomes and antithrombotic treatment spectrum of atrial fibrillation (AF) in patients hospitalized with acute myocardial infarction (AMI) have not been well studied in Chinese population.

Methods: Twenty-six thousand five hundred ninety-two consecutive patients diagnosed with AMI were enrolled in CAMI registry from January 2013 to September 2014. After excluding 343 patients with uncertain AF status and 1,591 patients transferred out during hospitalization, 24,658 patients were finally included in this study and involved in analysis.

Results: In the CAMI registry, 740 (3.0%) patients were recorded with AF prevalence during hospitalization. Higher-risk baseline clinical profile was observed in patients with AF. These patients were less likely to receive reperfusion/revascularization than those without AF. The in-hospital mortality (including death and treatment withdrawal) was significantly higher in patients with AF than that of without AF (25.2% vs. 7.2%, respectively; $p < 0.01$). The case of composite of adverse events was similar, which included death, treatment withdrawal, re-infarction, heart failure or stroke (42.1% vs. 16.0%, $p < 0.01$). In multivariate logistic regression analysis, AF was an independent predictor for in-hospital mortality (odds ratio, 1.88; 95% confidence interval: 1.27–2.78) and the composite of adverse events (odds ratio, 2.11; 95% CI: 1.63–2.72). Only 5.1% of patients with AF were treated with warfarin, and 1.7% were treated with both warfarin and dual antiplatelet therapy.

Conclusions: The analysis was based on the CAMI registry in China. The patients hospitalized for AMI who developed AF were at significantly higher risk for in-hospital mortality and other adverse events. However, the anticoagulants including warfarin have been largely underused post hospital discharge.

Keywords: Atrial fibrillation, Acute myocardial infarction, Hospital mortality, Anticoagulation treatment

* Correspondence: yangyj_fw@126.com
Department of Cardiology, Fuwai Hospital, National Center for Cardiovascular Diseases, Chinese Academy of Medical Science and Peking Union Medical College, 167 Beilishi Road, Beijing 100037, People's Republic of China

Background

Atrial fibrillation (AF) is a common complication of acute myocardial infarction (AMI). The reported incidence of AF was widely ranged from 2.3 to 21.0%, with an inconsistent relation to high mortality [1–12]. Although guidelines and consensus recommend a combination of warfarin and dual antiplatelet therapy (DAPT) and the duration was determined by hemorrhagic risk [13, 14], it was still complex to select an optimal antithrombotic regimen for patients with AF and AMI. Until now, this triple therapy has been largely underused in real-world clinical practice [15–17].

In China, AMI has become a major cause of emergency medical care, hospitalization and death over the past a few decades [18, 19]. The incidence, impact, and antithrombotic therapy of AF in AMI have not been correspondingly defined and demonstrated. Present analysis was aimed to study this subject with the data from China Acute Myocardial Infarction (CAMI) registry [20]. The data of patients with AMI were applied during January 2013 to September 2014. The baseline characteristics, treatment strategy, clinical data and outcomes were statistically analyzed and explored.

Methods

Study population

The design of the CAMI registry has been demonstrated in previous studies [20]. Briefly, this registry involved three levels of hospitals (representing typical Chinese governmental and administrative models) from all provinces and municipalities throughout mainland China (except for Hong Kong and Macau). Patients diagnosed with AMI were eligible for inclusion in CAMI registry, and were enrolled consecutively. Clinical data, treatments and outcomes were collected by local investigators and captured electronically with a fixed table, including a standardized set of variables and definitions, under a rigorous data quality control. A total of 108 hospitals have participated in the registry after its launch in January 2013 up to September 2014. This project was approved by the institutional review board central committee at Fuwai Hospital, National Center for Cardiovascular Diseases of China of China.

Inclusion and exclusion rules: the patients diagnosed with AMI in involved hospitals during January 2013 up to September 2014 were included. The patients were excluded if AF status was missing or they were transferred out during hospitalization. For the main analysis of in-hospital outcomes, the patients with truncated hospital stay because of outside transfer were also excluded. The presence of AF was documented by a standard 12-lead electrocardiogram or electrocardiogram monitoring during hospitalization.

In-hospital outcomes

The primary outcome of this study was in-hospital mortality, which included death and treatment withdrawal (withdrawal from all medical therapy or premature hospital discharge). In China, many patients withdraw from treatment at terminal status, which could be attributed to the culture or financial affordability. Therefore, single in-hospital mortality without accounting for these patients could lead to an underestimate of actual in-hospital mortality rates. Other recorded in-hospital clinical events included: re-infarction, stroke, heart failure, a composite of adverse events (the combination of death, treatment withdrawal, re-infarction, heart failure or stroke), major bleeding (including an absolute hemoglobin decrease of 3 g/dL, intracranial hemorrhage, any red blood cell transfusion or a bleeding event requiring surgical repairing), and any reported bleeding. Detailed definitions of clinical events were previously demonstrated [20].

Statistical analyses

The patient baseline characteristics, medical history, treatments, and complications were evaluated. Continuous variables are presented as median (interquartile range) and compared with Kruskal Wallis H test. Categorical variables were presented as counts and percentages, and were compared with chi-square or Fisher's exact tests.

Logistic regression analysis was applied to evaluate the association between AF and in-hospital mortality or the composite of adverse events. The variables included in the multivariable model were either statistically significant on univariate analysis ($p < 0.05$) or clinically critical, which were chosen by a stepwise method to minimize colincarity. Included covariates were: sex, age (>75 years), diabetes, hypertension, previous stroke, previous myocardial infarction, prior percutaneous coronary intervention (PCI)/coronary artery bypass graft (CABG), ST-segment elevation myocardial infarction (STEMI), serum creatinine, Global Registry of Acute Coronary Events (GRACE) score >140, CHA2DS2-VASc score >2, and reperfusion therapy. Crude and adjusted odds ratios (ORs) and corresponding 95% confidence intervals (CIs) were reported.

All comparisons were two-sided, with statistical significance defined as p less than 0.05. Statistical analysis was completed with SAS software, version 9.4.

Results

Twenty-six thousand five hundred ninety-two patients diagnosed with AMI were consecutively enrolled in CAMI registry from January 2013 to September 2014. After excluding 343 patients with uncertain AF status and 1,591 patients who were transferred out during hospitalization, 24,658 patients were finally included in this analysis.

Among them, 740 (3.0%) patients were recorded with AF prevalence during hospitalization (Fig. 1).

Baseline characteristics of patients were shown (Table 1). Compared with patients without AF, the age of patients with AF were higher (mean age: 73 vs. 63 years, $p <0.01$), more likely to be women (35.1% vs. 25.5%, $p <0.01$) and with more comorbidities such as hypertension (59.3% vs. 51.2%, $p <0.01$), heart failure (7.7% vs. 2.4%, $p < 0.01$) and stroke (17.8% vs. 9.2%, $p < 0.01$).Patients with AF were less frequently presented with STEMI than those without AF (65.7% vs. 76.0%, $p <0.01$), and had worse left ventricular function. The proportions of CHA2DS2-VASc ≥2 (66.1% vs.45.5%, $p <0.01$) and HAS-BLED ≥3 scores (21.4% vs.10.8%, $p <0.01$) were significantly higher in patients with AF, as well as the GRACE (161 vs.129,$p <0.01$) and Thrombolysis in Myocardial Infarction (TIMI) scores (6 vs.4,$p <0.01$). Patients with AF received reperfusion/revascularization during hospitalization at a lower rate than those without AF (35.9% vs. 48.3%, respectively, $p < 0.01$), as the case for PCI(29.7% vs. 40.5%, respectively, $p <0.01$).

The antithrombotic treatment regimens in AMI patients with and without AF were summarized (Table 2). During hospitalization, 78.0% of patients with AF received DAPT, less than the rate of 86.3% in patients without AF ($p <0.01$). However, the rates of anticoagulants treatment including unfractionated heparin (UFH), low molecular weight heparin (LMWH) and fondaparinux both groups were similar. A majority of patients received DAPT (86.1%) and LMWH (84.2%). Only 3.5% of patients with AF received warfarin, which was nonetheless higher than the rate of 1.4% in patients without AF ($p <0.01$).

At hospital discharge, 76.2% of patients with AF received DAPT, which was lower than the rate of 86.1% in patients without AF ($p <0.01$). However, only 5.1% of patients with AF were discharged on warfarin, and the proportion of warfarin in combination with DAPT was as low as 1.7%. In addition, no new direct oral anticoagulants (dabigatran, rivaroxaban, and apixaban) were applied in any patient.

The in-hospital outcomes were summarized (Table 3). Rate of in-hospital mortality (death or treatment withdrawal) was significantly higher in patients with AF (25.2%) than that of without AF (7.2%) ($p <0.01$). The rate of composite of adverse events (death, treatment withdrawal, re-infarction, heart failure or stroke) was also significantly higher in AF group (42.1% vs. 16.0%, $p <0.01$), which was also the case for individual component of the composite. In multivariate logistic regression analysis, AF was an independent predictor for both in-hospital mortality (odds ratio: 1.88, 95%CI: 1.27–2.78) and the composite of adverse events (2.11, 95% CI: 1.63–2.72, respectively) (Figs. 2 and 3). The rate of major bleeding was 1.7% in patients with AF, numerically higher than the rate of 0.9% for patients without AF ($p =0.65$).

Discussion

CAMI registry was the largest nationwide observational study to date for hospitalized patients with AMI throughout China. The major findings of present analysis were: 1) the overall incidence of AF was 3.0% in Chinese patients with AMI during hospitalization; 2) the risk of baseline profile was higher in patients with AF than patients without AF; 3) patients who developed AF were at a 1.88-fold higher risk of in-hospital mortality than patients without AF; and 4) although the majority of AMI patients complicated with AF received anticoagulation and antiplatelet

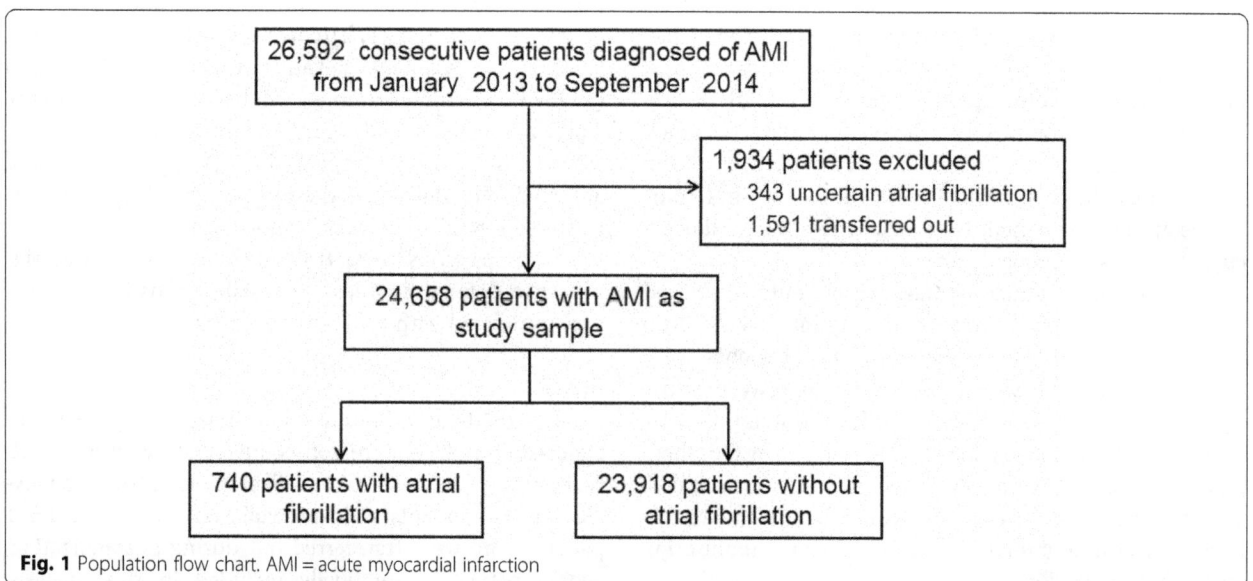

Fig. 1 Population flow chart. AMI = acute myocardial infarction

Table 1 Baseline characteristics

	Overall population (n = 24658)	AF (n = 740)	No AF (n = 23918)	P value
Demographics				
Age(years)	63 (53–72)	73 (65–79)	63 (53–72)	<0.01
Men	74.2	64.9	74.5	<0.01
Medical history				
Previous angina pectoris	28.2	32.0	28.0	0.02
PreviousMI	7.7	7.9	7.6	0.81
PreviousPCI/CABG	5.2	4.5	5.2	0.37
Previous heart failure	2.6	7.7	2.4	<0.01
Previous stroke	9.5	17.8	9.2	<0.01
Previous peripheral arterial disease	0.6	1.1	0.6	0.15
Chronic renal failure	1.4	1.7	1.4	0.60
Cardiovascular risk factors				
Hypertension	51.5	59.3	51.2	<0.01
Hyperlipidemia	8.0	6.3	8.1	0.10
Diabetes mellitus	20.0	18.8	20.0	0.44
Family history of premature CAD	4.0	3.0	4.0	0.12
Current smoker	54.7	44.7	55.0	<0.01
Clinical characteristics				
STEMI	75.7	65.7	76.0	<0.01
LVEF(%)	55(47–60)	50(41–59)	55(47–60)	<0.01
Killip classification III-IV	9.2	24.2	8.7	<0.01
CHA2DS2-VASc ≥ 2	46.1	66.1	45.5	<0.01
HAS-BLED ≥ 3	11.1	21.4	10.8	<0.01
GRACE Score	129 (112–149)	161 (133–182)	129 (112–146)	<0.01
TIMI Score				
STEMI	4 (2–6)	6 (4–8.5)	4 (2–6)	<0.01
NSTEMI	2(2–3)	2(2–3)	2(1–3)	<0.01
Treatments				
Reperfusion Therapy	48.0	35.9	48.3	<0.01
PCI	40.2	29.7	40.5	<0.01
Fibrinolysis	7.8	6.2	7.8	<0.01
ACE/ARB	59.7	54.8	59.9	0.02
β-blockers	69.9	59.9	70.2	<0.01
Anti-arrhythmia drugs	9.8	45.4	8,7	<0.001

Data are presented as median (IQR) or %
AF atrial fibrillation, MI myocardial infarction, PCI percutaneous coronary intervention, CABG coronary artery bypass graft, CAD coronary artery disease, LVEF left ventricular ejection fraction, GRACE global registry of acute coronary events, TIMI thrombolysis in myocardial infarction, STEMI ST-segment elevation myocardial infarction, NSTEMI non-ST-elevation myocardial infarction, ACEI angiotensin-converting enzyme, ARB angiotensin receptor blocker

Table 2 Antithrombotic treatment strategy in-hospital and at hospital discharge

	Overall population (n = 24658)	AF (n = 740)	No AF (n = 23918)	P value
In-hospital[a]				
DAPT	86.1	78.0	86.3	<0.01
UFH	5.9	5.2	5.9	0.43
LMWH	84.2	84.9	84.1	0.59
Fondaparinux	3.8	2.9	3.9	0.16
Warfarin	1.4	3.5	1.4	<0.01
At hospital discharge				
DATP	85.9	76.2	86.1	<0.01
Warfarin	1.9	5.1	1.4	<0.01
Warfarin alone	0.3	1.0	0.3	0.02
Warfarin + single antiplatelet drug	0.9	2.4	0.7	<0.01
Warfarin + DAPT	0.7	1.7	0.5	<0.01

AF atrial fibrillation, DAPT dual antiplatelet therapy, UFH unfractionated heparin, LMWH low molecular weight heparin
[a]Not including anticoagulants administered in catheterization laboratory

therapy during hospitalization, only 5.1% of them were discharged on warfarin, and 1.7% were discharged on both warfarin and DAPT.

In this nationally representative study, it firstly defined an AF incidence of 3.0% in contemporarily treated AMI patients in China. It was much lower compared to the reported data in other countries, ranging from 2.3 to 21% [1–12]. It may be resulted from some possible

Table 3 In-hospital events

	Overall population (n – 24658)	AF (n – 740)	No AF (n – 23918)	P value
Death	4.4	14.0	4.1	<0.01
Treatment withdrawal	3.3	11.2	3.1	<0.01
Death + Treatment withdrawal	7.7	25.2	7.2	<0.01
Re-infarction	0.6	1.4	0.6	0.02
Stroke	0.8	1.9	0.7	<0.01
Ischemic	0.6	1.4	0.5	
Hemorrhagic	0.08	0.13	0.07	
Unknown	0.11	0.4	0.09	
Heart failure	16.7	42.1	16.0	<0.01
Composite of adverse events[a]	19.2	47.5	18.4	<0.01
Major bleeding[b]	0.9	1.7	0.9	0.65
Any bleeding	1.8	2.7	1.8	0.09

[a]Composite of adverse events: death, treatment withdrawal, re-infarction, heart failure or stroke
[b]Major bleeding was defined as an absolute hemoglobin decrease of 3 g/dL, intracranial hemorrhage, any red blood cell transfusion or a bleeding event requiring surgical repair

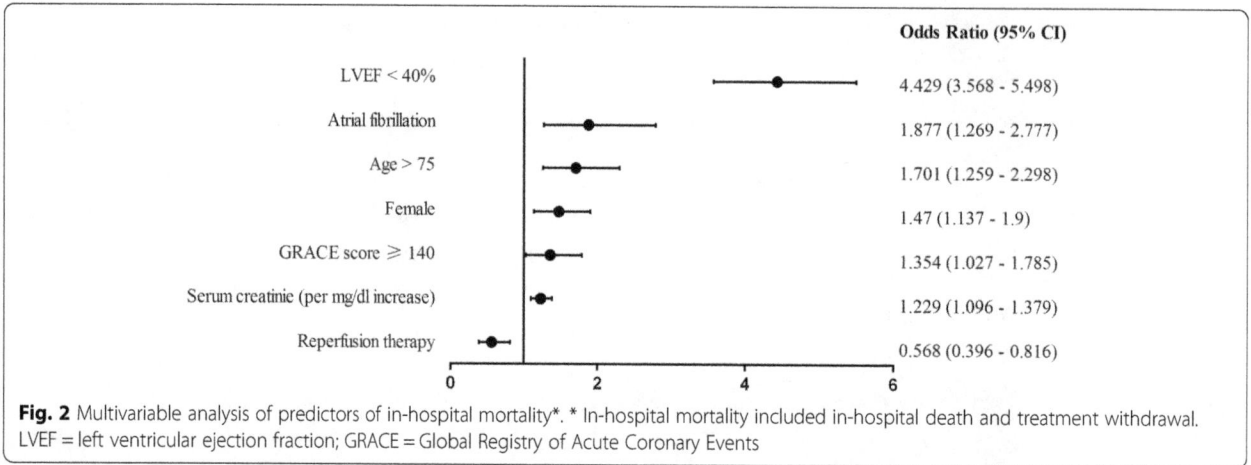

Fig. 2 Multivariable analysis of predictors of in-hospital mortality*. * In-hospital mortality included in-hospital death and treatment withdrawal. LVEF = left ventricular ejection fraction; GRACE = Global Registry of Acute Coronary Events

explanations. First, age was the most commonly reported risk factor for AMI complicated with AF [21, 22], and the low rate of AF in CAMI patients may be associated with an overall lower mean age of 63 years in samples. Second, 48.0% of overall patients in CAMI received reperfusion therapy (42.2% PCI). In previous studies, widespread use of reperfusion therapy, especially PCI, was associated with a notable decline of AF incidence [11, 23]. Third, the majority of patients in CAMI were treated with angiotensin-converting enzymes/angiotensin receptor inhibitors or β-blockers, and trials evaluating the effects of these drugs in patients with AMI have reported lower incidence rates of AF, although mainly making effects on late developing AF [24, 25]. Fourth, ethnic differences may also account for the wide incidence range of AMI complicated AF among different countries. A recently published study reported a low AF incidence of 2.7% in Arabian Gulf patients with acute coronary syndrome (ACS) [4].

Consistent with previous studies [1–12], in CAMI registry, higher-risk baseline clinical characteristics could be observed in AMI patients complicated with AF during hospitalization, including older age, a greater cardiovascular risk factor burden, more comorbidities, poorer left ventricular function, and higher clinical risk scores. The present study also documented that AMI patients with AF were less likely to receive reperfusion/revascularization than those without AF. For the patients with older age and more comorbidities, more conservative management approach would be selected by the physicians [26].

It indicated that AF increased the risk of morbidity and mortality in patients with ACS, and that this association would be mediated to a greater or lesser extent by various comorbidities [1]. However, because of differences in study design and data availability, including study population, AF classification, sample size, and follow-up duration, the association between AF development in ACS and increased in-hospital mortality

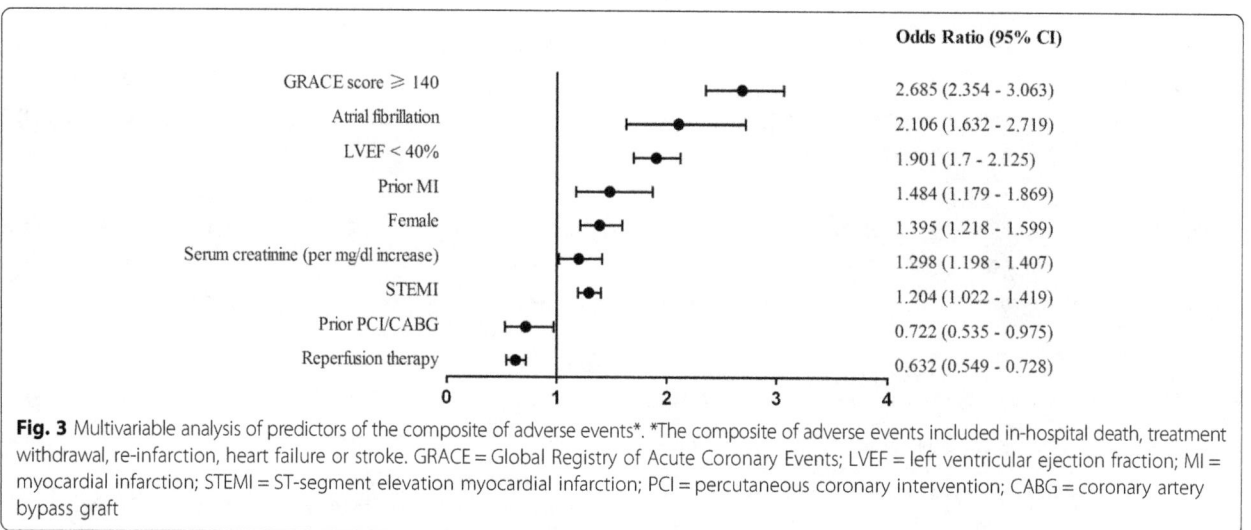

Fig. 3 Multivariable analysis of predictors of the composite of adverse events*. *The composite of adverse events included in-hospital death, treatment withdrawal, re-infarction, heart failure or stroke. GRACE = Global Registry of Acute Coronary Events; LVEF = left ventricular ejection fraction; MI = myocardial infarction; STEMI = ST-segment elevation myocardial infarction; PCI = percutaneous coronary intervention; CABG = coronary artery bypass graft

remained to be controversial. Some variables were reported to be independently associated with AF [2–9], while others reported no association [10–12]. In present analysis, the data was obtained from the CAMI registry, which was a large-scale, national and contemporary registry project for AMI patients in China [20]. The in-hospital mortality was significantly higher in patients with AF in unadjusted analysis. In addition, AF was also an independent multivariate risk factor of mortality after adjusting for possible confounders, although to an attenuated extent. With the consistency of findings, the association was further underscored in unadjusted and adjusted analyses.

The risk of bleeding may be increased by the anticoagulants treatment combined with DAPT therapy for stroke prevention in ACS patients with AF [27, 28]. However, current guidelines and consensus recommend a combination of warfarin and DAPT (triple therapy), with adjustment of duration according to hemorrhagic risk [13, 14]. Nonetheless, in previous studies, it documented that this triple therapy was largely underused, with a frequency ranged from 5.7 to 15.6% [15–17]. In the CAMI national registry, only 5.1% of AMI patients with AF were discharged on warfarin, and the proportion of warfarin in combination with DAPT was even as low as 1.7%. The latter striking gap in China might be secondary to many factors: the uncertainty about the benefits of intense anticoagulation in these high risk patients, inadequate provider knowledge, structural inadequacies of healthcare delivery systems, and/or concern about potential violence and litigation from patients or their families due to complications associated with treatment [29–31]. In addition, although new direct oral anticoagulants (dabigatran, rivaroxaban, and apixaban) have been approved for stroke prevention in non valvular AF patients [13], the CAMI registry indicated that these new anticoagulants have not been applied yet in AMI patients with AF in China.

CAMI registry was compared with REAL (REgistro regionale AngiopLastiche dell'Emilia-Romagna) registry. REAL registry was a multi-center, large scale, prospective study [32–35]. It aimed to collect the clinical data of coronary interventional cases from 4 million residents in Emilia- Romagna. 13 hospitals participated in this registry. The data could be retrieved in database. Many studies were performed based on this database [36]. Similar to REAL registry, CAMI has collected information of patients with acute myocardial infarction (AMI), including the clinical data, treatment, efficacy and prognosis. It aimed to improve the overall treatment efficacy of AMI in China. However, CAMI has only focused the patients from China. Different from REAL registry, CAMI has involved 108 hospitals in Chinese mainland and the hospitals differed in levels in CAMI registry. In addition, the population base was larger in CAMI registry in China.

Finally, the involved cases were updated (since 2013). The study based on CAMI would be promising in improving the treatment efficacy of AMI in China.

Strengths and limitations

CAMI is the largest national registry of patients with AMI. The population in the registry was representative of different regions, economic strata and access to medical resources in China. Therefore, the CAMI registry can adequately reflect the current performance and status of healthcare system in China. The data was valuable, specific and updated, which was based on a larger population base. Nevertheless, our study has several limitations. First, CAMI was subject to inherent limitations and potential biases, including the collection of nonrandomized data, missing or incomplete information, and potential confounding by drug indications or other unmeasured covariates which must be considered in results interpretation. Second, our database did not allow the identification of timing, type and duration of AF (paroxysmal, persistent or permanent), as well as the AF history, which may make effects on the prognosis prediction of the patients. Third, we do not include the follow-up data after hospital discharge, including both the mortality and other clinical events.

Conclusions

In China, AF development in patients with AMI was associated with significantly higher in-hospital mortality, and the anticoagulants including warfarin were largely underused during hospitalization and after hospital discharge. The conclusion on prediction and treatment may be instructional towards both clinical practice and further relevant studies.

Abbreviations

AF: Atrial fibrillation; AMI: Acute myocardial infarction; DAPT: Dual antiplatelet therapy; CAMI: China acute myocardial infarction; PCI: Percutaneous coronary intervention; CABG: Coronary artery bypass graft; STEMI: ST-segment elevation myocardial infarction; GRACE: Global registry of acute coronary events; OR: Odds ratio; CI: Confidence interval; TIMI: Thrombolysis in myocardial infarction; UFH: Unfractionated heparin; LMWH: Low molecular weight heparin; ACS: Acute coronary syndrome

Acknowledgments

The authors expressed their gratitude to all investigators and coordinators who participated in CAMI registry. Further information about the CAMI project, along with a list of participants, is available at http://www.CAMIRegistry.org.

Funding

The project was financial supported by one of the National Twelfth Five-year Science and Technology Support Projects by the Ministry of Science and Technology of China (Grant No. 2011BAI11B02).

Authors' contributions
In this study, YD, JY, ZG, RG and YY were involved in the design and analysis of data, drafting and revising of the manuscript and final approval of the submitted manuscript; HX, YS, YW, XG, WL, and YW were involved in the analysis of data, revising of the manuscript critically for important intellectual content and final approval of the manuscript submitted. All authors read and approved the final manuscript.

Competing interests
The authors declare that they have no competing interests.

References

1. Schmitt J, Duray G, Gersh BJ, Hohnloser SH. Atrial fibrillation in acute myocardial infarction: a systematic review of the incidence, clinical features and prognostic implications. Eur Heart J. 2009;30(9):1038–45.
2. Lopes RD, Pieper KS, Horton JR, Al-Khatib SM, Newby LK, Mehta RH, et al. Short- and long-term outcomes following atrial fibrillation in patients with acute coronary syndromes with or without ST-segment elevation. Heart. 2008;94(7):867–73.
3. Gonzalez-Pacheco H, Marquez MF, Arias-Mendoza A, Alvarez-Sangabriel A, Eid-Lidt G, Gonzalez-Hermosillo A, et al. Clinical features and in-hospital mortality associated with different types of atrial fibrillation in patients with acute coronary syndrome with and without ST elevation. J Cardiol. 2015; 66(2):148–54.
4. Hersi A, Alhabib KF, Alsheikh-Ali AA, Sulaiman K, Alfaleh HF, Alsaif S, et al. Prognostic significance of prevalent and incident atrial fibrillation among patients hospitalized with acute coronary syndrome: findings from the Gulf RACE-2 Registry. Angiology. 2012;63(6):466–71.
5. Lau DH, Huynh LT, Chew DP, Astley CM, Soman A, Sanders P. Prognostic impact of types of atrial fibrillation in acute coronary syndromes. Am J Cardiol. 2009;104(10):1317–23.
6. Jabre P, Roger VL, Murad MH, Chamberlain AM, Prokop L, Adnet F, et al. Mortality associated with atrial fibrillation in patients with myocardial infarction: a systematic review and meta-analysis. Circulation. 2011;123(15): 1587–93.
7. Podolecki T, Lenarczyk R, Kowalczyk J, Kurek T, Boidol J, Chodor P, et al. Effect of type of atrial fibrillation on prognosis in acute myocardial infarction treated invasively. Am J Cardiol. 2012;109(12):1689–93.
8. Rene AG, Genereux P, Ezekowitz M, Kirtane AJ, Xu K, Mehran R, et al. Impact of atrial fibrillation in patients with ST-elevation myocardial infarction treated with percutaneous coronary intervention (from the HORIZONS-AMI [Harmonizing Outcomes With Revascularization and Stents in Acute Myocardial Infarction] trial). Am J Cardiol. 2014;113(2):236–42.
9. McManus DD, Huang W, Domakonda KV, Ward J, Saczysnki JS, Gore JM, et al. Trends in atrial fibrillation in patients hospitalized with an acute coronary syndrome. Am J Med. 2012;125(11):1076–84.
10. Eldar M, Canetti M, Rotstein Z, Boyko V, Gottlieb S, Kaplinsky E, et al. Significance of paroxysmal atrial fibrillation complicating acute myocardial infarction in the thrombolytic era. SPRINT Thrombolytic Surv Groups Circ. 1998;97(10):965–70.
11. Kinjo K, Sato H, Ohnishi Y, Hishida E, Nakatani D, Mizuno H, et al. Prognostic significance of atrial fibrillation/atrial flutter in patients with acute myocardial infarction treated with percutaneous coronary intervention. Am J Cardiol. 2003;92(10):1150–4.
12. Asanin M, Perunicic J, Mrdovic I, Matic M, Vujisic-Tesic B, Arandjelovic A, et al. Prognostic significance of new atrial fibrillation and its relation to heart failure following acute myocardial infarction. Eur J Heart Fail. 2005;7(4): 671–6.
13. Camm AJ, Lip GY, De Caterina R, Savelieva I, Atar D, Hohnloser SH, et al. 2012 focused update of the ESC guidelines for the management of atrial fibrillation: an update of the 2010 ESC guidelines for the management of atrial fibrillation. Developed with the special contribution of the european heart rhythm association. Eur Heart J. 2012;33(21):2719–47.
14. Faxon DP, Eikelboom JW, Berger PB, Holmes DR, Bhatt DL, Moliterno DJ, et al. Consensus document: antithrombotic therapy in patients with atrial fibrillation undergoing coronary stenting. North-American perspect Thromb Haemost. 2011;106(4):572–84.
15. Chamberlain AM, Gersh BJ, Mills RM, Klaskala W, Alonso A, Weston SA, et al. Antithrombotic strategies and outcomes in acute coronary syndrome with atrial fibrillation. Am J Cardiol. 2015;115(8):1042–8.

16. Maier B, Hegenbarth C, Theres H, Schoeller R, Schuehlen H, Behrens S. Antithrombotic therapy in patients with atrial fibrillation and acute coronary syndrome in the real world: data from the berlin AFibACS registry. Cardiol J. 2014;21(5):465–73.
17. Lopes RD, Li L, Granger CB, Wang TY, Foody JM, Funk M, et al. Atrial fibrillation and acute myocardial infarction: antithrombotic therapy and outcomes. Am J Med. 2012;125(9):897–905.
18. Chen ZM, Jiang LX, Chen YP, Xie JX, Pan HC, Peto R, et al. Addition of clopidogrel to aspirin in 45,852 patients with acute myocardial infarction: randomised placebo-controlled trial. Lancet. 2005;366(9497):1607–21.
19. Gao R, Patel A, Gao W, Hu D, Huang D, Kong L, et al. Prospective observational study of acute coronary syndromes in China: practice patterns and outcomes. Heart. 2008;94(5):554–60.
20. Xu H, Li W, Yang J, Wiviott SD, Sabatine MS, Peterson ED, et al. The China Acute Myocardial Infarction (CAMI) Registry: A national long-term registry-research-education integrated platform for exploring acute myocardial infarction in China. Am Heart J. 2016;175(5):193-201.e3
21. Rathore SS, Berger AK, Weinfurt KP, Schulman KA, Oetgen WJ, Gersh BJ, et al. Acute myocardial infarction complicated by atrial fibrillation in the elderly: prevalence and outcomes. Circulation. 2000;101(9):969–74.
22. Fang MC, Chen J, Rich MW. Atrial fibrillation in the elderly. Am J Med. 2007; 120(6):481–7.
23. Goldberg RJ, Yarzebski J, Lessard D, Wu J, Gore JM. Recent trends in the incidence rates of and death rates from atrial fibrillation complicating initial acute myocardial infarction: a community-wide perspective. Am Heart J. 2002;143(3):519–27.
24. Anand K, Mooss AN, Hee TT, Mohiuddin SM. Meta-analysis inhibition of renin-angiotensin system prevents new-onset atrial fibrillation. Am Heart J. 2006;152(2):217–22.
25. Ehrlich JR, Hohnloser SH, Nattel S. Role of angiotensin system and effects of its inhibition in atrial fibrillation: clinical and experimental evidence. Eur Heart J. 2006;27(5):512–8.
26. Fox KA, Anderson Jr FA, Dabbous OH, Steg PG, Lopez-Sendon J, Van de Werf F, et al. Intervention in acute coronary syndromes: do patients undergo intervention on the basis of their risk characteristics? The Global Registry of Acute Coronary Events (GRACE). Heart. 2007;93(2): 177–82.
27. Lamberts M, Gislason GH, Olesen JB, Kristensen SL, Schjerning Olsen AM, Mikkelsen A, et al. Oral anticoagulation and antiplatelets in atrial fibrillation patients after myocardial infarction and coronary intervention. J Am Coll Cardiol. 2013;62(11):981–9.
28. Lamberts M, Olesen JB, Ruwald MH, Hansen CM, Karasoy D, Kristensen SL, et al. Bleeding after initiation of multiple antithrombotic drugs, including triple therapy, in atrial fibrillation patients following myocardial infarction and coronary intervention: a nationwide cohort study. Circulation. 2012; 126(10):1185–93.
29. Du X, Gao R, Turnbull F, Wu Y, Rong Y, Lo S, et al. Hospital quality improvement initiative for patients with acute coronary syndromes in China: a cluster randomized, controlled trial. Circ Cardiovasc Qual Outcomes. 2014;7(2):217–26.
30. Ranasinghe I, Rong Y, Du X, Wang Y, Gao R, Patel A, et al. System barriers to the evidence-based care of acute coronary syndrome patients in China: qualitative analysis. Circ Cardiovasc Qual Outcomes. 2014;7(2):209–16.
31. Lancet T. Chinese doctors are under threat. Lancet. 2010;376(9742):657.
32. Campo G, Guastaroba P, Marzocchi A, Santarelli A, Varani E, Vignali L, et al. Impact of copd on long-term outcome after st-segment elevation myocardial infarction receiving primary percutaneous coronary intervention. Chest. 2013;144(3):750–7.
33. Campo G, Saia F, Guastaroba P, Marchesini J, Varani E, Manari A, et al. Prognostic impact of hospital readmissions after primary percutaneous coronary intervention. Arch Intern Med. 2011;171(21):1948–9.
34. Campo G, Saia F, Percoco G, et al. Long-term outcome after drug eluting stenting in patients with ST-segment elevation myocardial infarction: data from the REAL registry. Int J Cardiol. 2010;140(2):154–60.
35. Percoco G, Manari A, Guastaroba P, et al. Safety and long-term efficacy of sirolimus eluting stent in ST-elevation acute myocardial infarction: the REAL (Registro REgionale AngiopLastiche Emilia-Romagna) registry. Cardiovasc Drugs Ther. 2006;20(1):63–8.

12

Improved treatment and prognosis after acute myocardial infarction in Estonia

Aet Saar[1*], Toomas Marandi[1,2], Tiia Ainla[1,2], Krista Fischer[3], Mai Blöndal[1] and Jaan Eha[1,4]

Abstract

Background: The aim of the study was to explore trends in short- and long-term mortality after hospitalization for acute myocardial infarction (AMI) over the period 2001—2011 in Estonian secondary and tertiary care hospitals while adjusting for changes in baseline characteristics.

Methods: In this nationwide cross-sectional study random samples of patients hospitalized due to AMI in years 2001, 2007 and 2011 were identified and followed for 1 year. Trends in 30-day and 1-year all-cause mortality were analysed using Cox proportional hazards regression model.

Results: The final analysis included 423, 687 and 665 patients in years 2001, 2007 and 2011 respectively. During the study period, the prevalence of most comorbidities remained unchanged while the in-hospital and outpatient treatment improved significantly. For example, the proportion of tertiary care hospital AMI patients who underwent revascularization was almost three times higher in 2011 compared to 2001. The proportion of secondary care patients who were referred to a tertiary care centre for more advanced care increased from 5.8 to 40.1 % (p for trend <0.001). Meanwhile, the 1-year mortality rates decreased from 29.5 to 20.2 % (adjusted $p = 0.004$) in the tertiary and from 32.4 to 23.1 % (adjusted $p = 0.006$) in the secondary care. The decrease in the 30-day mortality rates was statistically significant only in the secondary care hospitals.

Conclusions: The use of evidence-based treatments in Estonian AMI patients improved between 2001 and 2011. At the same time, we observed a significant reduction in the long-term mortality rates, both for patients primarily hospitalized into secondary as well as into tertiary care hospitals.

Keywords: Acute myocardial infarction, Treatment, Mortality rates, Estonia

Background

Coronary artery disease (CAD) is currently the number one cause of death in Europe [1]. Even though the fatality rates for acute myocardial infarction (AMI) have markedly decreased during the last few decades, Estonian death rates from CAD are still among the highest in Europe [2]. Modelling studies from different European countries have attributed declining trends in cardiovascular mortality to improved treatment and changes in cardiovascular risk factors [3, 4].

Important components of AMI treatment are early diagnosis, timely reperfusion and use of evidence-based medications [5, 6]. Earlier studies [7–9] from Estonia show improvement in AMI treatment, emphasizing better access to invasive diagnostics and treatment and wider use of evidence-based medications over time. However, no significant improvement in short- and long-term mortality in Estonian AMI population was seen [8, 9]. A recent overview about quality of care and mortality following AMI from Central and Eastern European countries describes lack of comparable data and wide variation in acute cardiac care, in both between and within European countries [10].

* Correspondence: aetsaar@gmail.com
[1]Department of Cardiology, University of Tartu, Tartu, Estonia
Full list of author information is available at the end of the article

The aim of the present study is to explore trends in short- and long-term mortality rates after hospitalization for AMI over the period 2001—2011 in Estonian secondary and tertiary care hospitals while considering changes in baseline characteristics and treatment.

Methods

We conducted a nationwide cross-sectional study based on hospital records. The formation of the study sample is described in Fig. 1.

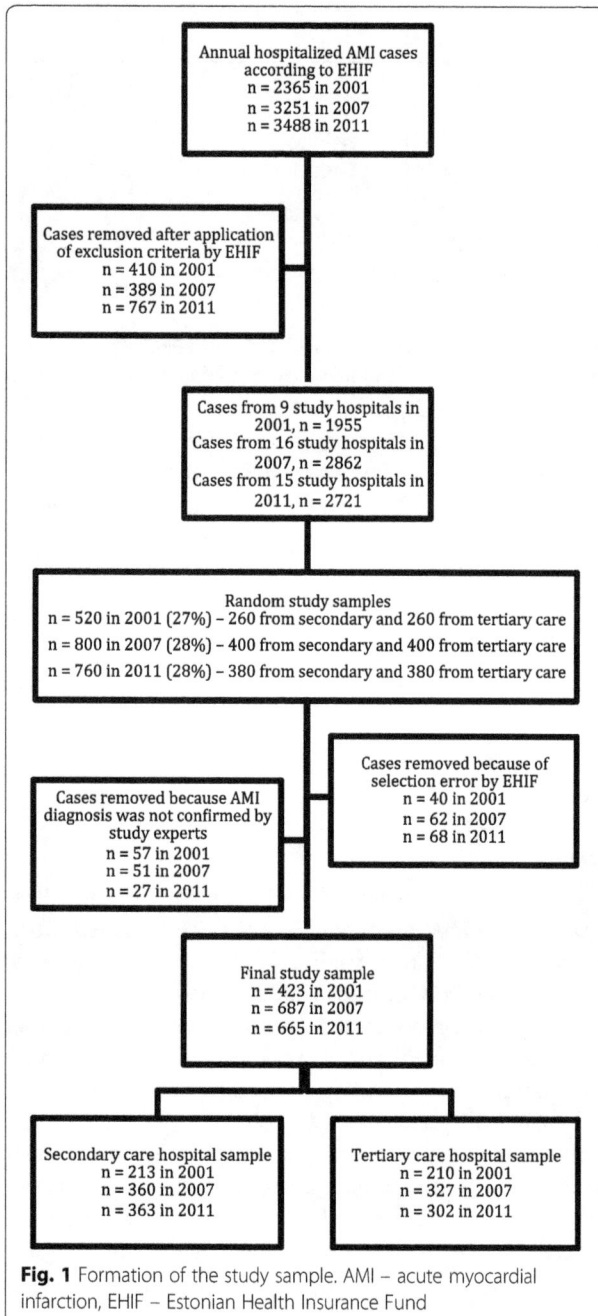

Fig. 1 Formation of the study sample. AMI – acute myocardial infarction, EHIF – Estonian Health Insurance Fund

The list of all the AMI cases for each year was obtained from the Estonian Health Insurance Fund (EHIF) database. During the time period studied, approximately 95 % of the Estonian population was covered with the health insurance. The validity of AMI diagnoses in EHIF database has been established previously [11]. According to the EHIF database, the total number of AMI cases hospitalized (main diagnosis code I21—I22 according to the International Statistical Classification of Diseases [ICD] and Related Health Problems 10th revision) was as 2365 in 2001, 3251 in 2007 and 3488 in 2011. All Estonian hospitals are using ICD codes I21—I22 (acute and subsequent myocardial infarction) with extension to diagnose AMI. As we intended to evaluate treatment of AMI in the hospital where the patient was primarily hospitalized, the following exclusion criteria were applied: (1) patients who were not primarily hospitalized into one of the study hospitals; (2) patients who were re-admitted with AMI diagnosis within 28 days after the first admission (only the second admission was excluded); (3) patients whose length of hospital stay was less than 3 days if they were discharged alive and were not transferred, which made the diagnosis of AMI very unlikely considering the local clinical practice.

From the remaining cases a study sample was formed by the use of random selection. The sampling was performed in clusters in order to get cross-sectional overview from all cases admitted into different types of hospitals. To ensure data comparability across years, the formation of the study sample was similar in all years studied.

In order to have a representative sample of all Estonian AMI patients, we included hospitals that treat the major proportion of annual AMI cases. In 2001, there were two tertiary and seven secondary care hospitals responsible for the treatment of most AMI cases in Estonia. The tertiary care hospitals had percutaneous coronary intervention (PCI) availability during working hours, while the secondary care hospitals did not have PCI availability. In 2007, the study included sixteen hospitals, two of tertiary and fourteen of secondary care. By the year 2007, both tertiary care hospitals had 24/7 PCI availability and one secondary care hospital had PCI available during working hours. In 2011, the study included thirteen secondary and two tertiary care hospitals. The tertiary care hospitals and one secondary care hospital had 24/7 PCI availability and two secondary care hospitals had PCI availability once a week. Thus, ten out of thirteen secondary care hospitals did not have PCI availability.

In Estonia there are two tertiary care hospitals, which did not change during the study period. The number of secondary care hospitals varied in the years studied due to the restructuring of the hospital network of Estonia. Also, it should be noted, that the recommendations of the

Estonian Society of Cardiology to admit patients with ST-segment elevation myocardial infarction (STEMI) for primary PCI to two tertiary care hospitals remained consistent during the study period.

The criteria applied for AMI diagnosis on 2001 and 2007 study populations were based on the consensus document published by the European Society of Cardiology in 2000 [12]. For 2011 cohort, the criteria were based on the redefinition of myocardial infarction published in 2007 [13]. In the data abstraction process, the medical records from study hospitals were obtained and data were collected retrospectively by experts according to the acute coronary syndromes data standards that were later presented in the CARDS Project [14]. The experts were certified cardiologists or cardiologists in training and all had received additional training on the data collection for this study. Every AMI case was reviewed by one expert, which was followed by random re-abstraction by another expert for data quality monitoring purposes. If discrepancies were determined, the experts were additionally trained. Data on mortality were obtained from the Estonian Population Registry. As the aim of the study was to evaluate the quality of care of the first hospital where the patient was admitted, data collection stopped after the patient was referred from a secondary care to a tertiary care hospital. Data on discharge medications were available only for those secondary care patients who were not referred to a tertiary care hospital.

The study was approved by the Research Ethics Committee of the University of Tartu.

Statistical analysis

For all patient characteristics and outcome variables of interest, comparisons between three years (2001, 2007, 2011) and two types of hospital (tertiary vs secondary care) of primary hospitalization were made.

Categorical variables were summarized by percentages and continuous variables by means and standard deviations. Differences in continuous variables were examined by classical linear regression and differences in binary variables by logistic regression. Categorical variables with more than two categories were analysed using the Chi-Square test.

As main outcome variables in this study, 30-day and 1-year all-cause mortality was analysed. In addition to crude mortality rates, baseline adjusted (age, sex, AMI subtype, diabetes, hypertension, previous heart failure, previous myocardial infarction) rates were compared using the Cox proportional hazards regression model. Patients initially hospitalized into a secondary care hospital but transferred and treated in tertiary care hospital, were included in the mortality analysis as secondary care patients. Two sided P values <0.05 were considered statistically significant.

For all statistical analyses, R software (ver. 3.1.1) was used [15].

Results

Final study sample included 423, 687 and 665 cases from years 2001, 2007 and 2011 respectively.

Baseline characteristics

Baseline characteristics are presented in Tables 1 and 2. Although the mean age of the study sample increased in both hospital types during the period, there were no significant changes in the frequency of most comorbidities. The results show increased proportion of patients with non-ST-segment-elevation acute myocardial infarction (NSTEMI) compared to that of patients with STEMI in both hospital types over time.

Treatment

Guideline-recommended treatments were more likely to be used for patients hospitalized in 2011 than in the earlier years in both hospital types (Tables 3 and 4). Cardiac catheterization and percutaneous revascularization became a dominant strategy in the tertiary care setting. The reperfusion rates for STEMI increased from 42.3 to 63.1 % ($p < 0.001$) in the tertiary care hospitals, while there was no statistically significant change in the secondary care hospitals. Meanwhile, there was an important increase in the proportion of patients who were referred from a secondary to a tertiary care hospital for further diagnostics and treatment (from 5.8 to

Table 1 Baseline characteristics of acute myocardial infarction patients hospitalized primarily into tertiary care hospitals

	Year 2001 n = 210	Year 2007 n = 327	Year 2011 n = 302	P value for trend
Hospital days, mean, (SD)	11.4 (9.1)	10.0 (8.4)	9.2 (6.5)	0.002
Mean age (SD), years	68.3 (12.7)	69.7 (12.0)	71.0 (12.0)	0.015
≥75 years, %	31.0	37.0	41.4	0.017
Men, %	66.7	58.1	62.3	0.3
STEMI, %	61.9	49.5	53.0	0.043
Diabetes, %	19.0	27.2	26.2	0.065
Arterial hypertension, %	70.0	70.0	75.2	0.206
Previous MI, %	29.5	29.4	29.1	0.925
Previous heart failure, %	27.1	28.1	25.2	0.626
Time to presentation, %				
≤3 h	47.6	41.9	44.7	0.723
3–12 h	23.8	24.8	23.2	
>12 h	28.6	33.3	32.1	

MI myocardial infarction, *STEMI* ST-segment elevation myocardial infarction, *SD* standard deviation

Table 2 Baseline characteristics of AMI patients hospitalized primarily into secondary care hospitals

	Year 2001 $n = 213$	Year 2007 $n = 360$	Year 2011 $n = 363$	P value for trend
Hospital days, mean, (SD)	11.4 (6.8)	9.4 (7.6)	6.5 (6.3)	<0.001
Mean age (SD), years	68.4 (12.4)	71.8 (11.4)	72.8 (12.2)	<0.001
≥75 years, %	34.3	45.3	47.4	0.002
Men, %	52.1	51.9	48.5	0.4
STEMI, %	59.6	51.4	44.4	<0.001
Diabetes, %	16.4	31.1	21.5	0.225
Arterial hypertension, %	57.3	75.8	74.7	<0.001
Previous MI, %	23.9	27.2	30.9	0.073
Previous heart failure, %	26.8	31.7	32.2	0.176
Time to presentation, %				
≤3 h	31.0	30.6	30.0	0.993
3–12 h	25.8	25.0	26.4	
>12 h	43.2	44.4	43.5	

MI myocardial infarction, *STEMI* ST- segment elevation myocardial infarction, *SD* standard deviation

40.1 %, $p < 0.001$). The prescription rates of cardiovascular medications recommended by guidelines at discharge increased in all five drug groups in both hospital types (Table 5).

Mortality

There was a statistically significant decrease from 20.2 to 12.4 % (adjusted $p = 0.003$) in 30-day mortality rate in the secondary care setting during the period studied (Table 6). 30-day mortality reduction was not statistically significant in the tertiary care hospitals. Results from long-term mortality analysis show decrease from 29.5 to 20.2 % (adjusted $p = 0.004$) in the tertiary care and from 32.4 to 23.1 % (adjusted $p = 0.006$) in the secondary care hospitals in 1-year mortality rates.

From the results of mortality analysis comparing different years and hospital types we found marked decline in mortality rates in both types of hospitals, which took place first in the tertiary and then in the secondary care. Mortality rates were similarly high in 2001. 30-day and 1-year mortality had decreased by year 2007 only in the tertiary care. By 2011, mortality rates had declined in both hospital types; mortality gap between the secondary and the tertiary care had disappeared (Fig. 2).

Discussion

In this countrywide analysis covering period 2001—2011, we demonstrated a decrease in short- and long-term mortality of AMI patients. The mortality reduction is consistent with reports from other countries and is generally attributed to many factors, including improved risk factor management, more frequent use of pharmacological

Table 3 In-hospital management in tertiary care hospitals

	Year 2001 $n = 210$ %	Year 2007 $n = 327$ %	Year 2011 $n = 302$ %	P value for trend
Medications				
Aspirin	87.1	94.2	94.4	0.003
P2Y$_{12}$-receptor inhibitors	17.1	61.5	70.5	<0.001
Anticoagulants	89.0	93.0	92.7	0.133
Glycoprotein IIb/IIIa inh.	12.4	38.8	29.1	<0.001
Betablockers	79.5	82.6	82.1	0.452
Nitrates	92.4	78.9	76.2	<0.001
ACEi/ARB	70.5	74.9	81.1	0.006
Statins	26.7	67.9	77.2	<0.001
Cardiac catheterization	35.7	78.6	80.8	<0.001
Revascularization	27.6	64.2	73.5	<0.001
PCI	22.4	61.5	67.9	<0.001
CABG	5.2	3.7	6.0	0.722
Echocardiography	81.9	85.3	88.4	0.044
Treatment for STEMI	$n = 130$	$n = 162$	$n = 160$	
Reperfusion for STEMI	42.3	64.2	63.1	<0.001
Thrombolysis	35.4	7.4	0.6	<0.001
Primary PCI	6.9	56.8	62.5	<0.001
Treatment for NSTEMI	$n = 80$	$n = 165$	$n = 142$	
PCI	18.8	47.9	53.5	<0.001
CABG	7.5	3.6	9.2	0.56

Anticoagulants – low molecular weight heparins/unfractionated heparin/fondaparinux, *ACEi* angiotensin-converting enzyme inhibitors, *ARB* angiotensin II receptor blockers, P2Y$_{12}$-receptor inhibitors – ticlopidine/clopidogrel/ticagrelol, *CABG* coronary artery bypass grafting, *PCI* percutaneous coronary intervention, *STEMI* ST- segment elevation myocardial infarction, *NSTEMI* non-ST-segment elevation myocardial infarction

agents and more widespread availability of revascularization methods, especially primary PCI [3, 4, 16, 17]. Also, developments in efficacy and safety of coronary artery stents may have improved the outcome [18].

The prevalence of STEMI has decreased in both hospital types, which is counter-balanced by higher proportion of NSTEMI. Improved coronary risk factor management and treatment after first coronary event may have contributed to the observed trend [19]. Another plausible explanation is the rising mean age, which is consistent with earlier studies describing higher prevalence of NSTEMI among the elderly [20]. Third and probably the most important explanation for the growing ratio of NSTEMI to STEMI is the more widespread use of high-sensitivity troponin assays, which has resulted in more sensitive diagnostics [21].

During last decades, led by the Estonian Society of Cardiology, much effort has been offered to improve diagnostics and treatment of AMI. Quality improvement measures have targeted different aspects of the AMI management, including prehospital triage and

Table 4 In-hospital management in secondary care hospitals

	Year 2001	Year 2007	Year 2011	P value for trend
	$n = 213$	$n = 360$	$n = 363$	
	%	%	%	
Medications				
Aspirin	88.3	86.4	85.7	0.383
P2Y$_{12}$-receptor inhibitors	0	10.6	26.4	<0.001
Anticoagulants	85.4	92.8	95.0	<0.001
Glycoprotein IIb/IIIa inh.	0.5	3.1	5.2	0.003
Betablockers	76.1	77.8	73.0	0.384
Nitrates	96.7	85.6	78.8	<0.001
ACEi/ARB	37.1	62.2	55.9	<0.001
Statins	5.6	30.8	49.0	<0.001
Cardiac catheterization	0	6.7	18.5	<0.001
Revascularization	0	4.2	14.3	<0.001
PCI	0	4.2	14.3	<0.001
CABG	0	0	0	-
Echocardiography	52.1	51.9	50.7	0.735
Referred to a tertiary care hospital	5.8	24.8	40.1	<0.001
Treatment for STEMI	$n = 127$	$n = 185$	$n = 161$	
Reperfusion for STEMI	44.1	34.1	37.9	0.251
Thrombolysis	44.1	34.1	29.2	0.008
Primary PCI	0	0	8.7	-
Treatment for NSTEMI	$n = 86$	$n = 175$	$n = 202$	
PCI	0	4.6	10.4	0.002
CABG	0	0	0	-
Referred to a tertiary care hospital	5.8	10.3	28.2	<0.001

Anticoagulants – low molecular weight heparins/unfractionated heparin, fondaparinux, *ACEi* angiotensin-converting enzyme inhibitors, *ARB* angiotensin II receptor blockers, P2Y$_{12}$-receptor inhibitors – ticlopidine/clopidogrel/ticagrelol, *CABG* coronary artery bypass grafting, *PCI* percutaneous coronary intervention, *STEMI* ST-segment elevation myocardial infarction, *NSTEMI* non-ST-segment elevation myocardial infarction

Table 5 Medications prescribed for outpatient use in tertiary and secondary care hospitals

	Year 2001 %	Year 2007 %	Year 2011 %	P value for trend
Tertiary care hospitals	$n = 181$	$n = 290$	$n = 261$	
Aspirin	85.1	93.1	95.4	<0.001
P2Y$_{12}$-receptor inhibitors	18.2	64.8	72.8	<0.001
Betablockers	71.3	80.0	85.4	<0.001
ACEi/ARB	66.3	77.2	84.7	<0.001
Statins	31.5	73.4	80.8	<0.001
Nitrates	61.9	22.1	15.8	<0.001
Secondary care hospitals	$n = 163$	$n = 224$	$n = 184$	
Aspirin	79.8	82.6	91.3	0.004
P2Y$_{12}$-receptor inhibitors	0.6	10.7	32.8	<0.001
Betablockers	68.7	80.9	82.8	0.001
ACEi/ARB	37.4	68.9	68.3	<0.001
Statins	14.7	37.3	65.6	<0.001
Nitrates	85.3	58.2	41.4	<0.001

ACEi angiotensin-converting enzyme inhibitors, *ARB* angiotensin II receptor blockers, P2Y$_{12}$-receptor inhibitors – ticlopidine/clopidogrel/ticagrelol

establishing STEMI network, therapies during hospitalization, at discharge and outpatient care. For example, local STEMI guideline was published [22], European AMI definitions and guidelines were translated into Estonian and several educational events throughout Estonia were organized. At the same time, access to cardiac catheterization facilities has improved.

Reperfusion rates for STEMI are used as performance measures of AMI treatment. Findings indicate that reperfusion rates in the tertiary care hospitals are now comparable with respective rates form North, West, and Central Europe [23, 24]. Results are different for the secondary care – only approximately 40 % of STEMI patients are being offered reperfusion, with no increase during the period studied. However, low reperfusion rates should be interpreted with caution – in 2011 more than 40 % of secondary care patients were referred to a tertiary care centre for further management. We can hypothesize that patients were transferred before receiving reperfusion. Nevertheless, such trend is alarming, because transfer increases the delays and timely PCI is impossible. Data from international EPICOR registry suggest that recommended times are often not met when AMI patients are transferred for primary PCI [25]. Primary PCI is recommended as first line therapy for STEMI but it should be emphasized that thrombolysis is also an appropriate and proven reperfusion strategy [26]. However, more frequent referral to the tertiary care hospitals is in agreement with guidelines that recommend an invasive management for STEMI or high-risk NSTEMI patients [7, 8]. Also, local quality improvement initiatives have stressed the importance of timely referral of STEMI patients without contraindications and most NSTEMI patients to tertiary care centres with catheterization laboratories.

In addition to the reperfusion therapy, the recommended concomitant pharmacological therapy and the discharge medications play a major role in determining prognosis. Lower prescription rates of secondary prevention drugs in the secondary care can be partly explained by differences in the baseline characteristics. Patients in the secondary care hospitals were older and it has been shown that elderly patients are less likely to receive medications recommended by guidelines [27]. Previously described lower adherence to guidelines in smaller non-

Table 6 Mortality of acute myocardial infarction patients primarily hospitalized into tertiary and secondary care hospitals

Mortality	2001 %	2007 %	2011 %	P value for trend, unadjusted	HR (95 % CI) change per year, unadjusted	P value for trend, adjusted[a]	HR (95 % CI) change per year, adjusted[a]
30-day							
Tertiary care hospitals	17.6	13.1	13.2	0.181	0.97 (0.926–1.015)	0.061	0.96 (0.913–1.002)
Secondary care hospitals	20.2	22.5	12.4	0.022	0.96 (0.920–0.994)	0.003	0.94 (0.904–0.980)
1-year							
Tertiary care hospitals	29.5	24.5	20.2	0.026	0.96 (0.928–0.995)	0.004	0.95 (0.917–0.984)
Secondary care hospitals	32.4	35.0	23.1	0.026	0.97 (0.938–0.996)	0.006	0.95 (0.918–0.977)

[a]adjusted for age, sex, AMI subtype (STEMI vs NSTEMI), previous myocardial infarction, previous heart failure, diabetes, hypertension
STEMI ST-segment elevation myocardial infarction, *NSTEMI* Non-ST-segment elevation myocardial infarction, *HR* hazard ratio, *CI* confidence interval

academic hospitals, staffed less frequently with certified cardiologists, is another plausible explanation [28, 29]. However, utilization rates of recommended drugs in the tertiary care hospitals are similar with corresponding rates from the UK, Sweden, and the US [30]. Also, patient compliance with suggested medications plays an important role in determining the prognosis. Failure to adhere to suggested therapies leads to more frequent hospital readmissions and has a negative impact on mortality [31, 32]. Similar problems related to the compliance with suggested drugs after AMI have been previously described in Estonia [33].

Another noteworthy finding from the study is the big proportion of patients who present late after symptom onset. Longer ischaemic times are associated with more myocardial damage and have adverse impact on outcome [34, 35]. Approximately 43 % of patients who present later than 12 h after symptom onset explain why reperfusion rates have remained low in the secondary care hospitals. Unfortunately, presentation delays did not show decrease over time.

Treatment of AMI patients improved mainly in the tertiary care hospitals with the main changes occurring during the first part of the study period. Inconsistency in

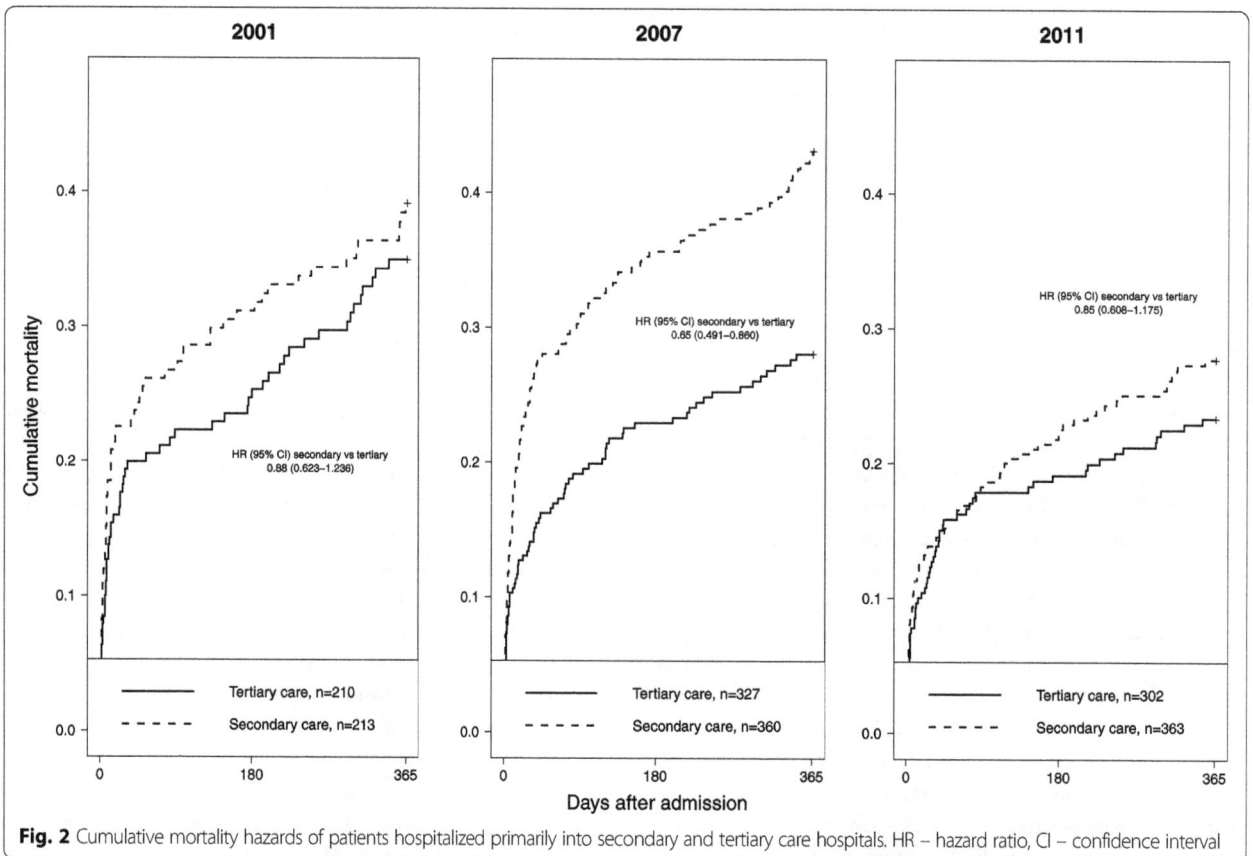

Fig. 2 Cumulative mortality hazards of patients hospitalized primarily into secondary and tertiary care hospitals. HR – hazard ratio, CI – confidence interval

the speed of implementation of new treatment strategies was reflected as a marked mortality gap in 2007 between the secondary and the tertiary care hospitals. By the 2011, the differences in treatment persisted, but a significant proportion of patients were transferred for further management to the tertiary care hospitals. Consequently, the noticeable mortality gap between the secondary and the tertiary care hospitals was no longer present in 2011. A similar initial large variation in treatments between different hospitals and gradual lowering of short- and long-term mortality are previously described in Sweden for period 1996—2007 [36] and in the US between 1995 and 2006 [37].

The present study has several limitations. The first limitation is that it cannot prove clear causality of observed decrease in the mortality rates. Through adjusting for baseline characteristics, we can reduce the possibility that differences in the patient population accounted for the change, but causality between practice patterns and outcomes should not be inferred. Secondly, the present study describes three random patient samples from studied years, thus not describing the complete AMI population for the period. Consequently, the treatment regimens in the present study may not be exactly as of the whole AMI population. Thirdly, we did not collect information about contraindications to certain treatments; therefore, we were not able to evaluate how big proportion of eligible patients received recommended treatment. Fourthly, we did not collect data about drug compliance and utilization of other secondary prevention methods including smoking cessation etc. The importance of compliance with recommended antiplatelet therapy after coronary stent implementation is highlighted in recent study, which describes almost 5-fold increase in cardiac mortality rates for patients who discontinued clopidogrel within 3-months after the PCI procedure [38]. Thus, we were unable to account for the effect of these or any other unmeasured confounders, which might have influence to the long-term outcome.

Conclusions

In this country-wide analysis covering period 2001—2011, we reported a decrease in 1-year mortality of AMI patients. During the study period, prevalence of most comorbidities remained unchanged while AMI management improved significantly. Guideline-recommended acute phase treatments were increasingly used in the tertiary care setting. Secondary care hospitals are still lagging behind, but substantial amount of patients are now referred to a tertiary care centre for more advanced care. In conclusion, we were able to demonstrate improved prognosis for Estonian AMI patients during the decade from 2001 to 2011. Furthermore, we determined that the prognosis

does not depend on the hospital type where patient is hospitalized primarily – by the end of the study period, Estonian hospitals were functioning as an efficient network, delivering quite equal care to AMI patients as it was aimed by the Estonian Society of Cardiology.

Competing interests
The authors declare that they have no competing interests.

Authors' contributions
AS, MB, TA, TM and JE participated in the design of the study and in writing the manuscript. KF and AS performed the statistical analysis. All authors read and approved the final manuscript.

Acknowledgements
We thank Estonian Health Insurance Fund for the list of hospitalized AMI cases. We also thank the experts, Marit Aasaru, Märt Elmet, Viktoria Krjukova, Leili Kütt, Julia Reinmets, Gudrun Veldre and Jaanus Laanoja who participated in abstraction of the data.
This work was supported by Estonian Ministry of Education and Research [SF0180001s07, IUT-2-7] and by the Estonian Science Foundation [Grant no ETF8903, ETF8273].

Author details
[1]Department of Cardiology, University of Tartu, Tartu, Estonia. [2]Centre of Cardiology, North Estonia Medical Centre, Tallinn, Estonia. [3]Estonian Genome Centre, University of Tartu, Tartu, Estonia. [4]Heart Clinic, Tartu University Hospital, Tartu, Estonia.

References
1. Causes of death statistics, Eurostat 5/2014. http://ec.europa.eu/eurostat/statistics-explained/index.php/Causes_of_death_statistics#. Accessed 5 Mar 2015.
2. Nichols M, Townsend N, Scarborough P, Rayner M. Trends in age-specific coronary heart disease mortality in the European Union over three decades: 1980–2009. Eur Heart J. 2013;34:3017–27.
3. Smolina K, Wright L, Rayner M, Goldcare M. Determinants of the decline in mortality from acute myocardial infarction in England between 2002 and 2012: linked national database study. Br Med J. 2012; doi:10.1136/bmj.d8059.
4. Björck L, Rosengren A, Bennett K, Lappas G, Capewell S. Modelling the decreasing coronary heart disease mortality in Sweden between 1986 and 2002. Eur Heart J. 2009;30:1046–56.
5. Steg PG, James SK, Atar D, Badano LP, Blömstrom-Lundqvist C, Borger MA, et al. ESC Guidelines for the management of acute myocardial infarction in patients presenting with ST-segment elevation: The Task Force on the management of ST-segment elevation acute myocardial infarction of the European Society of Cardiology. Eur Heart J. 2012;33:2569–619.
6. Hamm CW, Bassand JP, Agewall S, Bax J, Boersma E, Bueno H, et al. ESC Guidelines for the management of acute coronary syndromes in patients presenting without persistent ST-segment elevation: The Task Force for the management of acute coronary syndromes (ACS) in patients presenting without persistent ST-segment elevation of the European Society of Cardiology (ESC). Eur Heart J. 2011;32:2999–3054.
7. Ainla T, Marandi T, Teesalu R, Baburin A, Elmet M, Liiver A, et al. Diagnosis and treatment of acute myocardial infarction in tertiary and secondary care hospitals in Estonia. Scand J Public Health. 2006;34:327–31.
8. Blöndal M, Ainla T, Marandi T, Baburin A, Eha J. Changes in treatment and mortality of acute myocardial infarction in Estonian tertiary and secondary care hospitals in 2001 and 2007. BMC Res Notes. 2012;5:71.
9. Blöndal M, Ainla T, Marandi T, Baburin A, Rahu M, Eha J. Better outcomes for acute myocardial infarction patients first admitted to PCI hospitals in Estonia. Acta Cardiol. 2010;65:541–8.
10. Smith FG, Brogan RA, Alabas O, Laut KG, Quinn T, Bugiardini R, Gale CP. Comparative care and outcomes for acute coronary syndromes in Central and Eastern European Transitional countries: A review of the literature. Eur Heart J Acute Cardiovasc Care. 2014. [Epub ahead of print]

11. Thetloff M, Palo E. Comparative analysis of morbidity information on the basis of annual statistical reports and the database of Estonian Health Insurance Fund 1994. http://ee.euro.who.int/Haigestumusinfo_vordlus%20SoM_HK.pdf. Accessed 19 May 2015.

12. Alpert JS, Thygesen K, Antman E, Bassand JP. Myocardial infarction redefined – a consensus document of The Joint European Society of Cardiology/American College of Cardiology Committee for the redefinition of myocardial infarction. J Am Coll Cardiol. 2000;36:959–69.

13. Thygesen K, Alpert JS. White HD; Joint ESC/ACCF/ AHA/WHF Task Force for the Redefinition of Myocardial Infarction. Universal Definition of Myocardial Infarction. Eur Heart J. 2007;28:2525–38.

14. Flynn MR, Barrett C, Cosío FG, Gitt AK, Wallentin L, Kearney P, et al. The Cardiology Audit and Registration Data Standards (CARDS), European data standards for clinical cardiology practice. Eur Heart J. 2005;26:308–13.

15. The R Project for Statistical Computing. http://www.r-project.org. Accessed 5 Mar 2015.

16. Fox KA, Steg PG, Eagle KA, Goodman SG, Anderson Jr FA, Granger CB, et al. Decline in rates of death and heart failure in acute coronary syndromes, 1999–2006. JAMA. 2007;297:1892–900.

17. Nauta ST, Deckers JW, Akkerhuis M, Lenzen M, Simoons ML, van Domburg RT. Changes in clinical profile, treatment, and mortality in patients hospitalised for acute myocardial infarction between 1985 and 2008. PLoS One. 2011; doi:10.1371/journal.pone.0026917.

18. Bangalore S, Toklu B, Amoroso N, Fusaro M, Kumar S, Hannan EL, et al. Bare metal stents, durable polymer drug eluting stents, and biodegradable polymer drug eluting stents for coronary artery disease: mixed treatment comparison meta-analysis. BMJ. 2013; doi:10.1136/bmj.f6625.

19. Rogers WJ, Frederick PD, Stoehr E, Canto JG, Ornato JP, Gibson CM, et al. Trends in presenting characteristics and hospital mortality among patients with ST elevation and non-ST elevation myocardial infarction in the National Registry of Myocardial Infarction from 1990 to 2006. Am Heart J. 2008;156:1026–34.

20. Avezum A, Makdisse M, Spencer F, Gore JM, Fox KA, Montalescot G, et al. Impact of age on management and outcome of acute coronary syndrome: observations from the Global Registry of Acute Coronary Events (GRACE). Am Heart J. 2005;149:67–73.

21. McManus DD, Gore J, Yarzebski J, Spencer F, Lessard D, Goldberg RJ. Recent trends in the incidence, treatment, and outcomes of patients with STEMI and NSTEMI. Am J Med. 2011;124:40–7.

22. Soopõld Ü, Marandi T, Ainla T, Liiver A, Elmet M, Laanoja J, et al. Estonian guidelines for the managament of patients with ST-elevation myocardial infarction. Eesti Arst. 2004;12 Suppl 1:2–48 [in Estonian].

23. Puymirat E, Battler A, Birkhead J, Bueno H, Clemmensen P, Cottin Y, et al. Euro Heart Survey 2009 Snapshot: regional variations in presentation and management of patients with AMI in 47 countries. Eur Heart J Acute Cardiovasc Care. 2013;2:359–70.

24. Kristensen SD, Laut KG, Fajadet J, Kaifoszova Z, Kala P, Di Mario C, et al. Reperfusion therapy for ST elevation acute myocardial infarction 2010/2011: current status in 37 ESC countries. Eur Heart J. 2014;35:1957–70.

25. Sinnaeve PR, Zeymer U, Bueno H, Danchin N, Medina J, Sánchez-Covisa J, et al. Contemporary inter-hospital transfer patterns for the management of acute coronary syndrome patients: Findings from the EPICOR study. Eur Heart J Acute Cardiovasc Care. 2015;4(3):254–62.

26. Huber K, Gersh BJ, Goldstein P, Granger CB, Armstrong PW. The organization, function, and outcomes of ST-elevation myocardial infarction networks worldwide: current state, unmet needs and future directions. Eur Heart J. 2014;35:1526–32.

27. Lee HY, Cooke CE, Robertson TA. Use of Secondary Prevention Drug Therapy in Patients With Acute Coronary Syndrome After Hospital Discharge. J Manag Care Pharm. 2008;14:271–80.

28. O'Brien E, Subherwal S, Roe MT, Holmes DN, Thomas L, Alexander KP, et al. Do patients treated at academic hospitals have better longitudinal outcomes after admission for non-ST-elevation myocardial infarction? Am Heart J. 2014;167:762–9.

29. Dorsch MF, Lawrance RA, Sapsford RJ, Durham N, Das R, Jackson BM, et al. An evaluation of the relationship between specialist training in cardiology and implementation of evidence-based care of patients following acute myocardial infarction. Int J Cardiol. 2004;96:335–40.

30. McNamara RL, Chung SC, Jernberg T, Holmes D, Roe M, Timmis A, et al. International comparisons of the management of patients with non-ST segment elevation acute myocardial infarction in the United Kingdom, Sweden, and the United States: The MINAP/NICOR, SWEDEHEART/RIKS-HIA, and ACTION Registry-GWTG/NCDR registries. Int J Cardiol. 2014;175:240–7.

31. Campo G, Saia F, Guastaroba P, Marchesini J, Varani E, Manari A, et al. Prognostic impact of hospital readmissions after primary percutaneous coronary intervention. Arch Intern Med. 2011;171:1948–9.

32. Moretti C, D'Ascenzo F, Omedè P, Sciuto F, Presutti DG, Di Cuia M, et al. Thirty-day readmission rates after PCI in a metropolitan center in Europe: incidence and impact on prognosis. J Cardiovasc Med (Hagerstown). 2015;16:238–45.

33. Marandi T, Baburin A, Ainla T. Use of evidence-based pharmacotherapy after myocardial infarction in Estonia. BMC Public Health. 2010;10:358.

34. Newby LK, Rutsch WR, Califf RM, Simoons ML, Aylward PE, Armstrong PW, et al. Time from symptom onset to treatment and outcomes after thrombolytic therapy. GUSTO-1 Investigators. J Am Coll Cardiol. 1996;27:1646–55.

35. De Luca G, Suryapranata H, Ottervanger JP, Antman EM. Time delay to treatment and mortality in primary angioplasty for acute myocardial infarction: every minute of delay counts. Circulation. 2004;109:1223–5.

36. Jernberg T, Johanson P, Held C, Svennblad B, Lindback J, Wallentin L. Association between adoption of evidence-based treatment and survival for patients with ST-elevation myocardial infarction. JAMA. 2011;305:1677–84.

37. Krumholz HM, Wang Y, Chen J, Drye EE, Spertus JA, Ross JS, et al. Reduction in acute myocardial infarction mortality in the United States: risk-standardized mortality rates from 1995–2006. JAMA. 2009;302:767–73.

38. Thim T, Johansen MB, Chisholm GE, Schmidt M, Kaltoft A, Sørensen HT, et al. Clopidogrel discontinuation within the first year after coronary drug-eluting stent implantation: an observational study. BMC Cardiovasc Disord. 2014;14:100.

13

Use of diagnostic coronary angiography in women and men presenting with acute myocardial infarction

Louise Hougesen Bjerking[1*], Kim Wadt Hansen[2], Mette Madsen[3], Jan Skov Jensen[1,4], Jan Kyst Madsen[5], Rikke Sørensen[1] and Søren Galatius[2]

Abstract

Background: Based on evident sex-related differences in the invasive management of patients presenting with acute myocardial infarction (AMI), we sought to identify predictors of diagnostic coronary angiography (DCA) and to investigate reasons for opting out an invasive strategy in women and men.

Methods: The study was designed as a matched cohort study. We randomly selected 250 female cases from a source population of 4000 patients hospitalized with a first AMI in a geographically confined region of Denmark from January 2010 to November 2011. Each case was matched to a male control on age and availability of cardiac invasive facilities at the index hospital. We systematically reviewed medical records for risk factors, comorbid conditions, clinical presentation, and receipt of DCA. Clinical justifications, as stated by the treating physician, were noted for the subset of patients who did not receive a DCA.

Results: Overall, 187 women and 198 men received DCA within 60 days (75 % vs. 79 %, hazard ratio: 0.82 [0.67-1.00], $p = 0.047$).In the subset of patients who did not receive a DCA ($n = 114$), clinical justifications for opting out an invasive strategy was not documented for 21 patients (18.4 %). Type 2 myocardial infarction was noted in 11 patients (women versus men; 14.5 % vs. 3.8 %, $p = 0.06$) and identified as a potential confounder of the sex-DCA relationship. Receipt of DCA was predicted by traditional risk factors for ischaemic heart disease (family history of cardiovascular disease, hypercholesterolemia, and smoking) and clinical presentation (chest pain, ST-segment elevations). Although prevalent in both women and men, the presence of relative contraindications did not prohibit the use of DCA.

Conclusion: In this matched cohort of patients with a first AMI, women and men had different clinical presentations despite similar age. However, no differences in the distribution of relative contraindications for DCA were found between the sexes. Type 2 MI posed a potentiel confounder for the sex-related differences in the use of DCA. Importantly,clinical justification for opting out an invasive strategy was not documented in almost one fifth of patients not receiving a DCA.

Keywords: Acute myocardial infarction, Coronary angiography, Cardiac catheterization, Gender

* Correspondence: louise_bjerking@hotmail.com
[1]Department of Cardiology, University Hospital Gentofte, Kildegårdsvej 28, 2900 Hellerup, Denmark
Full list of author information is available at the end of the article

Background

Ischemic heart disease (IHD) constitutes the leading cause of years of life lost worldwide and is one of the leading causes of death in both women and men [1]. Despite recommendations for similar treatment of women and men presenting with acute myocardial infarction (AMI) by the European Society of Cardiology and the Danish Society of Cardiology [2, 3], differences in invasive management of women and men have been widely reported [4–7]. The majority of studies have compared men and women with AMI at different ages prohibiting an appropriate comparison of baseline characteristics and comorbidities. Moreover, it has not been properly investigated whether clinical justifications for opting out an invasive strategy in patients presenting with AMI differ between women and men. The objective of this study was to characterize an age-matched cohort of women and men hospitalized with AMI, and to investigate reasons for opting out an invasive treatment strategy in a real-world setting.

Methods

Design overview

This study was designed as a matched cohort study. Using all patients hospitalized between 1 January 2010 and 2 November 2011 with a first AMI in the Greater metropolitan area surrounding Copenhagen ($n = 4000$) as our source population, we randomly selected 250 female cases and matched them in a 1:1 ratio with 250 male controls based on age and availability of cardiac invasive facilities in the index hospital. This matched cohort of 500 patients constituted our *study population* (Fig. 1) for which we conducted a systematic, retrospective collection of patient data from medical records. Patients were followed for 60 days. We identified predictors of receiving a cardiac catheterization during follow-up, frequencies of relative contraindications

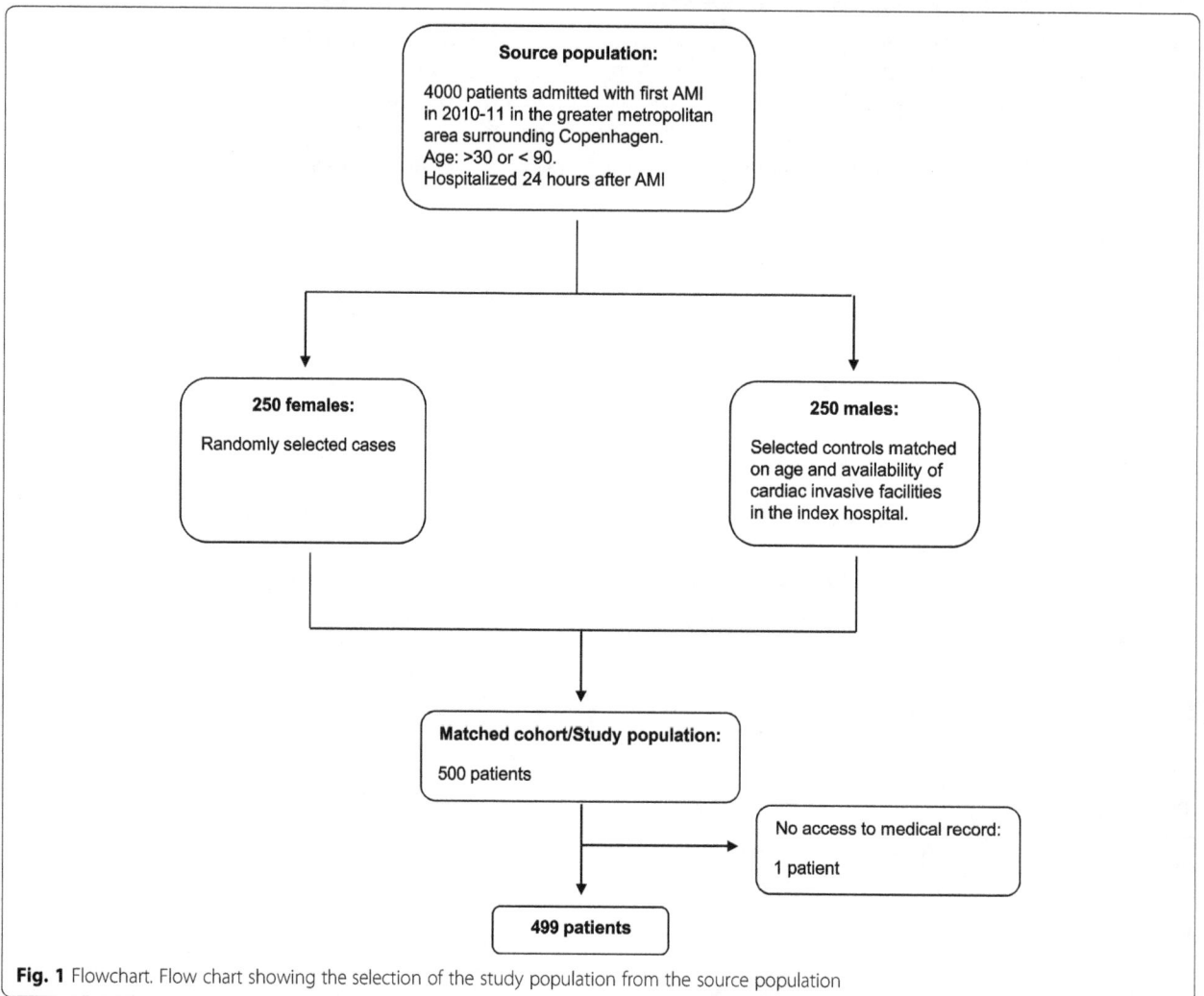

Fig. 1 Flowchart. Flow chart showing the selection of the study population from the source population

for coronary angiography, and documented reasons for opting out an invasive treatment strategy.

Settings

The greater metropolitan area surrounding Copenhagen included 10 hospitals with medical admission wards plus two high-volume hospitals with invasive heart centers performing diagnostic coronary angiography (DCA), percutaneous coronary intervention (PCI) and coronary artery bypass graft surgery (CABG). The hospital catchment areas covered the greater northern capital area and a smaller remote island (Bornholm); a total of 1.68 million inhabitants in 2010 [8]. Pre-hospital triage ensured direct transport of patients presenting with ST-segment elevation myocardial infarction (STEMI) to treatment with primary PCI at an invasive heart center. Non-ST-segment elevation myocardial infarction (NSTEMI) patients were in general initially treated at the nearest hospital and subsequently referred to an invasive heart center for further invasive assessment. The guidelines for treatment of AMI issued by the Danish society of Cardiology follow those of European Society of Cardiology [9] and explicitly state that, unless contraindicated, all patients with AMI irrespective of sex should be offered a DCA.

Patients

We identified a source population of patients hospitalized with a first AMI from 1 January 2010 to 2 November 2011 from the Danish National Patient Register, which contains information on all hospital admissions in Denmark since 1978 [10]. The International Classification of Diseases (ICD) 10th revision codes for AMI (I21-I21.9) in the Danish National Patient Register have previously been validated showing a positive predictive value of 93.5 % [11]. We linked data on dates of index admission, index hospital, and cardiac procedures to information on dates of death from the Danish Register of Causes of Death and demographics from the Danish Civil Registration System using the unique personal civil registration number provided to all Danish citizens at birth or immigration. Further restrictions to the source population were applied; Patients discharged on the day of admission were excluded, as they were unlikely to have experienced an actual myocardial infarction. Similarly, death on the day of admission rendered patients ineligible for invasive treatment and thus were excluded. Finally, we excluded patients younger than 30 years, since AMI in this age group are rarely related to atherosclerosis, and patients older than 90 years, due to frailty in this elderly group [12–14].

From the source population a random draw of 250 female cases matched with 250 male controls of similar age and similar access to invasive cardiac treatment at index hospital constituted the study population. The matching procedure was performed using the *MatchIt* package [15] of statistical software R, version 3.1.0 [16].

Data collection

Patient-level clinical data was collected from electronic medical records. The collection process was standardized using pretested extraction sheets (Additional file 1: Extraction sheet) in order to ensure consistent and comparable data. Each extraction sheet was divided into seven main topics: 1) index admission, 2) risk factors, 3) comorbidities, 4) electrocardiographic (ECG) findings, 5) clinical presentation, 6) in-hospital medications, and 7) blood test results. Only information available to the treating physicians prior to any cardiac catheterization was collected; in patients who did not receive a DCA all information from the hospital stay was collected. Data was entered in an electronic database and compiled with register-based data using the personal civil registration number as described above. Data collection, analysis and interpretation were performed by one specially trained individual (LHB) to ensure consistency and reproducibility. Upon completing the initial data collection process, the process was repeated for the initial 80 medical records and compared the obtained data in order to address potential intra-observer variability.

Contextual variables

For each patient not receiving a coronary angiography we noted the clinical justification, as stated in the medical record by the treating physician, word-for-word and categorized them into 11 arbitrarily defined groups: DCA already performed, death before DCA, DCA declined by patient, DCA not possible to perform or not indicated, comorbidities/bad habitual conditions, lack of symptoms, type 2 MI, high age, DCA not mentioned in the medical record, no AMI, and other. The diagnosis of type 2 MI was assigned when one of two conditions was met: (1) the treating physician documented the qualifying AMI event as a type 2 myocardial infarction directly in the medical records, or (2) the reasons stated by the treating physician for opting out a DCA were consistent with criteria listed in the international definition of type 2 MI [17]. The definitions of relative contraindications for cardiac catheterization were based on guidelines developed by the Danish Society of Cardiology [18]. Uncontrolled hypertension, fever or active infection, malignant or terminal disease, risk of bleeding, ongoing bleeding, moderate to severe heart failure, previous allergy to contrast, digoxin intoxication, and electrolyte disturbances were all considered as individual relative contraindications for DCA. We used data collected from electronic medical records for quantifying the distribution of these relative contraindications in the study population. We defined *uncontrolled hypertension* as an elevated systolic blood pressure (SBP) > [180 mmHg] or diastolic blood pressure (DBP) > [110 mmHg]). *Fever or active infection* was defined as a white blood cell count (WBC) above 8.8 x 10^9/liter or temperature more than 38 degrees Celsius. *Malignant or terminal disease* was defined as severe anemia with hemoglobin below 6 mM or renal failure with serum-creatinine above 250 mM. *Risk of bleeding* was defined as a platelet count below 145 µM or an International Normalized Ratio (INR) above 1.2, and *moderate to severe heart failure* as a history of heart failure, or clinical findings of neck vein distension, dependent edema, or pulmonary edema. *Electrolyte disturbances* were defined as potassium levels above 4.6 or below 3.5 mM.

All collected ECG findings and blood test results were those available to the treating physician as upon hospitalization; but always prior to the time of cardiac catheterization in patients receiving a DCA. The only exception was the second measurement of troponins ("*troponin II*") and the highest troponin value measured during hospitalization ("*peak troponin*") which was sometimes only available subsequent to a coronary angiography. As different troponin assays were used across hospitals we standardized all troponin-levels against the upper reference limit to enable comparisons.

Statistical methods

We present discrete data as counts and percentages, and continuous data as median and interquartile range (IQR). Categorical data were compared using a Chi-squared test or, if the expected number of observations in a group were less than five, using Fisher's exact test. Continuous data were analyzed using the non-parametric Mann-Whitney U-test. In order to identify predictors of DCA we constructed uni- and multivariable logistic regression models with receipt of coronary angiography within 60 days as the dependent variable and patient characteristics as independent variables. The multivariable logistic regression model was build using a backwards stepwise procedure using a p-value of 0.10 as cutoff for inclusion. The final model was tested for collinearity and interactions. Time-to-event analyses of all-cause death and receipt of DCA were conducted using proportional hazards Cox regressions. The assumption of proportional hazards was assessed with log-log curves and by testing the Schoenfeld residuals for time-dependency. Assumptions were found valid. All statistical tests had a two-sided significance level of 0.05. The analyses were conducted using Stata Statistics/Data analysis, MP 14.0 StataCorp, Texas, USA.

Results

The matching procedure successfully balanced the 250 women and 250 men on age and type of index hospital (Additional file 2: Table S1). The study population contained more elderly patients than the source population as expected from the use of female cases. Complete medical records were available for 499 patients (Fig. 1). Table 1 shows baseline characteristics of the study population. A higher proportion of women had heart failure and a family history of cardiovascular diseases (CVD) compared to men. In contrast, more men than women had known ischemic heart disease (IHD), prior PCI, and prior CABG. Numerically, men were more likely to have chest pain than women, whereas more women presented with atypical symptoms such as nausea and vomiting. The only significant difference in ECG patterns was a higher proportion of ST-depressions among men compared to women, although a tendency toward a higher rate of left bundle branch block (LBBB) among women was apparent. Women presented with higher systolic blood pressure, and heart rate but lower serum-creatinine levels than men. Coronary angiography was performed in 385 patients (77.2 %) within 60 days of index hospitalization; 198 men and 187 women. Thus, the cumulative incidence of DCA at 60 days was higher for men than women (79.2 % vs. 75.1 %, HR 0.82 [0.67-1.00], $p = 0.047$). There was no significant difference in all-cause mortality at 60 days between women and men (9.6 % vs. 10.4 %, HR 0.91 [0.52-1.59], $p = 0.74$), even when separated into age-quartiles (Additional file 3: Table S2).

In terms of relative contraindications for DCA women were more likely to have electrolyte-disturbances than men (Table 2). Compared to men, there was a trend towards more cases of uncontrolled hypertension among women, as well as a higher proportion of women with at least one relative contraindication. Among the two most common relative contraindications, uncontrolled hypertension, and risk of bleeding, no sex-related differences were found. The presence of relative contraindications did not preclude the use of DCA.

Table 3 displays univariable predictors of DCA at 60 days. Admission to a hospital with invasive cardiac facilities, known family history of CVD, hypertension, hypercholesterolemia, smoking, and chest pain were all associated with a higher use of DCA. On the other hand, previous CABG, valvular heart disease, atrial fibrillation, COPD, renal failure, stroke, dyspnea, and abdominal pain were associated with less use of DCA. After multivariable analysis arterial hypertension, hypercholesterolemia, smoking, known IHD, chest pain, and ST-elevation persisted as significant positive predictors of DCA. Age, prior CABG, COPD, renal failure, stroke, and Q-wave were negative predictors

Use of diagnostic coronary angiography in women and men presenting with acute myocardial...

99

Table 1 Baseline characteristics and clinical presentations

Number	Study Cohort $n = 499$	Women $n = 249$	Men $n = 250$	p-value $n = 499$
Age *median(IQR)*		74 (62-81)	74 (62-81)	0.96
Admission to invasive heart center		89 (35.6)	92 (36.8)	0.78
Risk factors				
Family history of CVD		80 (32.1)	61 (24.4)	0.06
Arterial hypertension		122 (49.0)	119 (47.6)	0.76
Diabetes mellitus		36 (14.5)	39 (15.6)	0.72
Hypercholesteroleamia		80 (32.1)	85 (34.0)	0.7
Smoking		69 (27.7)	82 (32.8)	0.08
Prior PCI		6 (2.4)	16 (6.4)	0.047
Prior CABG		6 (2.4)	21 (8.4)	0.005
Previous MI		9 (3.6)	9 (3.6)	0.99
Co-morbidities				
Heart-related				
Known IHD		20 (8.0)	46 (18.4)	0.001
Heart failure		35 (14.1)	19 (7.6)	0.020
Valvular heart disease		26 (10.4)	19 (7.6)	0.27
Atrial fibrillation		39 (15.7)	40 (16.0)	0.92
Other				
COPD		23 (9.2)	27 (10.8)	0.56
PAOD		14 (5.6)	20 (8.0)	0.29
Renal failure		11 (4.4)	9 (3.6)	0.66
Neoplasia		4 (1.6)	12 (4.8)	0.07
Liver failure		0 (0.0)	1 (0.4)	1.00
Stroke		25 (10.0)	31 (12.4)	0.40
Symptoms				
Chest pain		189 (75.9)	203 (81.2)	0.15
Dyspnea		96 (38.6)	81 (32.4)	0.15
Neck pain		25 (10.0)	21 (8.4)	0.53
Diaphoresis		30 (12.1)	36 (14.4)	0.44
Nausea/vomiting		47 (18.9)	31 (12.4)	0.046
Fatigue		7 (2.8)	8 (3.2)	0.8
Abdominal pain		14 (5.6)	8 (3.2)	0.19
Back pain		27 (10.8)	21 (8.4)	0.36
Cardiac arrest		15 (6.0)	14 (5.6)	0.84
Other competing acute conditions at admission?[a]		42 (16.9)	34 (13.6)	0.31
ECG				
ST-elevations		104 (41.8)	107 (42.8)	0.82
ST-depressions		59 (23.7)	86 (34.4)	0.008
LBBB		24 (9.6)	16 (6.4)	0.18
Q-wave		37 (14.9)	38 (15.2)	0.92
Systolic blood pressure[e]		140 (126-160)	137 (119.5-155)	0.013
Heart rate[e]		88 (70-105)	81 (66-97)	0.008

Table 1 Baseline characteristics and clinical presentations *(Continued)*

Troponin level I[b,c,e]	3.2 (1.4-9.2)	2.5 (1.0-8.4)	0.25
Troponin level II[b,d,e]	4.5 (2.1-12.5)	6.1 (2.0-35)	0.14
Peak troponin level[b,e]	12.4 (4.7-44.3)	20.3 (4.1-73.6)	0.23
Creatinine level[e]	70 (59-86.5)	87 (74-100)	<0.001

Numbers are counts (%) unless otherwise stated. Numbers of missing values varied from 45 (Systolic blood pressure) to 269 (troponine concentration II). *IQR* interquartile range, *CVD* cardiovascular disease, *PCI* percutaneous coronary intervention, *CABG* coronary artery bypass graft surgery, *AMI* acute myocardial infarction, *IHD* Ischemic heart disease, *COPD* chronic obstructive pulmonary disease, *PAOD* peripheral arterial occlusive Disease, *LBBB* left bundle branch block, *INR* International normalized ratio. [a]Competing acute conditions include infections, dementia, ileus etc. [b]Standardized against upper limit. [c]The first troponin value measured before CAG, [d]the second troponin value measured before CAG. [e]median (IQR)

of DCA (Table 4). In total 114 patients (22.9 %) did not receive a DCA; 52 men and 62 women. Clinical justifications for opting out an invasive treatment strategy, as stated by the treating physician, are summarized in Fig. 2. Most frequent reasons were multiple comorbidities or poor habitual condition (19.3 %), patients who declined invasive examination (16.7 %), or DCA not deemed feasible or indicated (16.7 %). Notably, in 21 (18.4 %) of the cases no reason at all for opting out a coronary angiography was documented in the medical record by the treating physician. There were no significant sex-related differences in any of the 11 groups, but a trend towards more cases of type 2 MI in women compared to men (14.5 % vs. 3.8 %, *p* = 0.06).

Discussion
Key findings
This study used detailed clinical information from 500 medical records of patients hospitalized with a first AMI to investigate the clinical basis for referring men

and women to DCA. Classical risk factors, symptoms and clinical findings predicted the receipt of DCA in this matched cohort. Women had an 18 % lower risk for receipt of DCA at 60 days than men, but a similar risk for all-cause mortality despite accounting for differences in age and type of index hospital. Surprisingly, no clinical justification for refraining from an invasive treatment strategy was documented in almost one fifth of the records of patients who did not receive a DCA.

Interpretations
The matched design of our study was intended to address two issues. First, it has been suggested that differences in patient characteristics, treatments and outcomes can largely be attributed to the differences in age between women and men presenting with ischemic heart disease [6]. Second, the use of cardiac catheterization is strongly associated with hospital-availability of this procedure [19]. By matching on age and hospital, these confounding effects were managed prior to our analyses. Despite the somewhat limited power of our analyses, we identified significant differences in patient characteristics between women and men of similar age; i.e. heart failure was more prevalent in women while more men presented with known IHD and prior revascularizations. Based on these findings a sex-related difference in the etiology of AMI seems more plausible than age in explaining previously observed differences in characteristics between women and men [20].

Our logistic and Cox proportional hazards regression analyses yielded differing results in terms of the association between sex and receipt of DCA. The reason for this lies in the poorer power of the logistic regression which only incorporates counts, as compared to the Cox regression modeling time-to-event data. We relied on the results of the latter, as the logistic regression attributes equal weights to early and late procedures and thus does not address the timing of DCAs, which we deemed of clinical relevance. Thus, despite women having a lower risk for DCA at 60 days than men, we were unable to demonstrate any significant differences in the most common

Table 2 Relative contraindications as defined by national guidelines

	Female	Male	*p*-value
Uncontrolled hypertension	29 (13.1)	18 (8.0)	0.08
Fever or active infection	0 (0.0)	1 (1.47)	0.5
Malignant or terminal disease	11 (5.5)	4 (2.2)	0.12
Risk of bleeding	23 (14.7)	26 (17.3)	0.54
Ongoing bleeding	5 (2.0)	9 (3.6)	0.42
Moderate/severe heart failure	8 (3.2)	5 (2.0)	0.6
Previous allergy to contrast	0(0.0)	0(0.0)	NA
Digoxin intoxication	0 (0.0)	0 (0.0)	NA
Electrolyte-disturbances (4.6 mM < potassium level < 3.5 mM)	49 (24.6)	29 (15.8)	0.031
At least one of the above mentioned relative contraindication (excluding heart failure)	130 (52.0)	120 (48.0)	0.060

Numbers are counts (%) unless otherwise stated
We used clinical data to quantify the distribution of relative contraindications for men and women. The contraindications were not necessarily listed directly by the physicians in the medical records

Use of diagnostic coronary angiography in women and men presenting with acute myocardial...

101

Table 3 Univariable predictors of receipt of DCA at 60 days

	OR	95 % CI	p-value
Female	0.79	0.52-1.20	0.28
Age			
< 60 years	Reference		
60-69 years	1.26	0.33-4.84	0.73
70-79 years	0.26	0.1-0.72	<0.001
≥ 80 years	0.04	0.02-0.10	<0.001
Admission to a hospital with invasive cardiac facilities	4.23	2.43-7.36	<0.001
Risk factors			
Family history of CVD	6.99	3.31-14.79	<0.001
Arterial hypertension	1.67	1.09-2.55	0.019
Diabetes mellitus	0.72	0.42-1.26	0.25
Hypercholesteroleamia	4.21	2.36-7.52	<0.001
Smoking	1.91	1.45-2.52	<0.001
Prior PCI	3.07	0.71-13.33	0.14
Prior CABG	0.41	0.18-0.90	0.027
Previous AMI	1.5	0.43-5.28	0.53
Co-morbidities			
Heart-related			
Known IHD	1.12	0.59-2.10	0.73
Heart failure	0.67	0.36-1.25	0.21
Valvular heart disease	0.40	0.21-0.76	0.005
Atrial Fibrillation	0.36	0.21-0.60	<0.001
Other			
COPD	0.33	0.18-0.60	<0.001
PAOD	0.81	0.37-1.79	0.60
Renal failure	0.11	0.04-0.30	<0.001
Neoplasia	0.88	0.28-2.80	0.84
Liver failure	-	-	-
Stroke	0.19	0.10-0.33	<0.001
Symptoms			
Chest pain	5.64	3.53-9.00	<0.001
Dyspnea	0.47	0.31-0.72	0.001
Neck pain	0.94	0.46-1.91	0.86
Diaphoresis	1.01	0.54-1.87	0.98
Nausea/vomiting	0.71	0.41-1.23	0.22
Fatigue	0.81	0.25-2.59	0.72
Abdominal pain	0.19	0.08-0.45	<0.001
Back pain	1.54	0.70-3.38	0.29
Cardiac arrest	0.76	0.33-1.78	0.53
ECG			
ST-elevations	5.36	3.12-9.21	<0.001
ST-depressions	0.69	0.44-1.08	0.108
LBBB	0.52	0.26-1.03	0.06
Q-wave	0.62	0.36-1.06	0.08

Table 3 Univariable predictors of receipt of DCA at 60 days *(Continued)*

Other			
Systolic BP	1.01	1.00-1.02	0.024
Diastolic BP	1.02	1.01-1.04	0.002
HR	0.99	0.98-1.00	0.010
Troponine 1	0.99	0.99-1.00	0.028
Troponine 2	1.00	1.00-1.00	0.34
Peak troponine	1.00	1.00-1.00	0.59
Creatinine	0.98	0.97-0.99	<0.001

CVD cardiovascular disease, *PCI* percutaneous coronary intervention, *CABG* coronary artery bypass graft surgery, *AMI* acute myocardial infarction, *IHD* Ischemic heart disease, *COPD* Chronic obstructive pulmonary disease, *PAOD* Peripheral Arterial Occlusive Disease, *LBBB* left bundle branch block, *ECG* Electrocardiogram

relative contraindications. Interestingly, non of the defined relative contraindications were listed by the treating physician as reasons for not performing DCA in any patients. Of note, no patients with contrast allergy or pregnancy were found in our cohort; as these contraindications may be considered more severe. Classical risk factors such as family history of CVD, hypercholesterolemia, and smoking; symptoms of chest pain, and clinical findings of ST-segment elevations were significant predictors of an invasive strategy in our cohort. However, women were more likely than men to present with atypical symptoms of nausea and vomiting. Similar findings have been made in other studies [21, 22] and suggest that

Table 4 Multivariable predictors of receipt of DCA at 60 days

	OR	95 % CI	*p*-value
Age	0.90	0.87-0.94	<0.001
Admission to center	2.8	1.27-6.21	0.011
Family history of CVD	2.35	0.92-5.97	0.072
Arteriel hypertension	2.38	1.23-4.62	0.010
Hypercholesteroleamia	3.00	1.38-6.48	0.005
Smoking	2.03	1.39-2.97	<0.001
Prior CABG	0.25	0.06-0.98	0.047
Co-morbidities			
Heart-related			
Known IHD	3.85	1.27-11.63	0.017
Other			
COPD	0.37	0.15-0.87	0.023
Renal failure	0.20	0.05-0.83	0.027
Stroke	0.31	0.13-0.70	0.005
Symptoms			
Chest pain	2.99	1.58-5.67	0.001
ECG			
ST-elevations	4.44	2.05-9.60	0.000
Q-wave	0.35	0.15-0.78	0.011

CABG coronary artery bypass graft surgery, *COPD* Chronic obstructive pulmonary disease, *CVD* cardiovascular disease, *ECG* Electrocardiogram, *IHD* Ischemic heart disease

increased vigilance is required when examining women in the emergency setting. Use of computed coronary tomography might be an option, as some trials suggest this method is effective for identification of patients in need of an invasive strategy [23].

By reviewing medical records containing the treating physicians' reflections and rationale for opting out an invasive treatment strategy in some patients, we got a unique insight into the actual treating process of patients with AMI. Noticeably, we found a trend towards more cases of type 2 MI in women and a potential confounding effect on the sex-DCA relationship. This is in accordance with the findings of Saaby et al. who showed a higher prevalence of type 2 MI in women compared to men, and less cardiac catheterizations in type 2 MI [24]. It is possible that type 2 MI plays a larger role in the sex-related differences in treatment of AMI, than previously known.

Prior studies have proposed several hypotheses as to why sex-related differences in the management of AMI exist. It has been discussed if women were more likely to refuse DCA than men. Golden et al. showed that fewer women preferred DCA in the emergency room and in-hospital [25]. Heidenreich et al. found that elderly women were more likely to refuse DCA than men, but the rate of refusals was low (5.1 %) [26]. In another study, Mumma et al. found that female patients were less likely to receive a cardiac catheterization recommended by the physician, yet this could not explain the gender gap [27]. In our study 17 % of those who were not invasively investigated had refused DCA, without any sex-related differences. Physicians' reasons for not adopting an invasive strategy in women compared to men has previously been investigated [28], but no study examining this issue based on medical records in a real life setting is known by us. Although evidence and guidelines supports that all patients with AMI should undergo DCA, perhaps with the exception of low risk biomarker positive women [29], cases where lack of evidence drives to omitting DCA in patients with AMI exist. According to Poon et al.

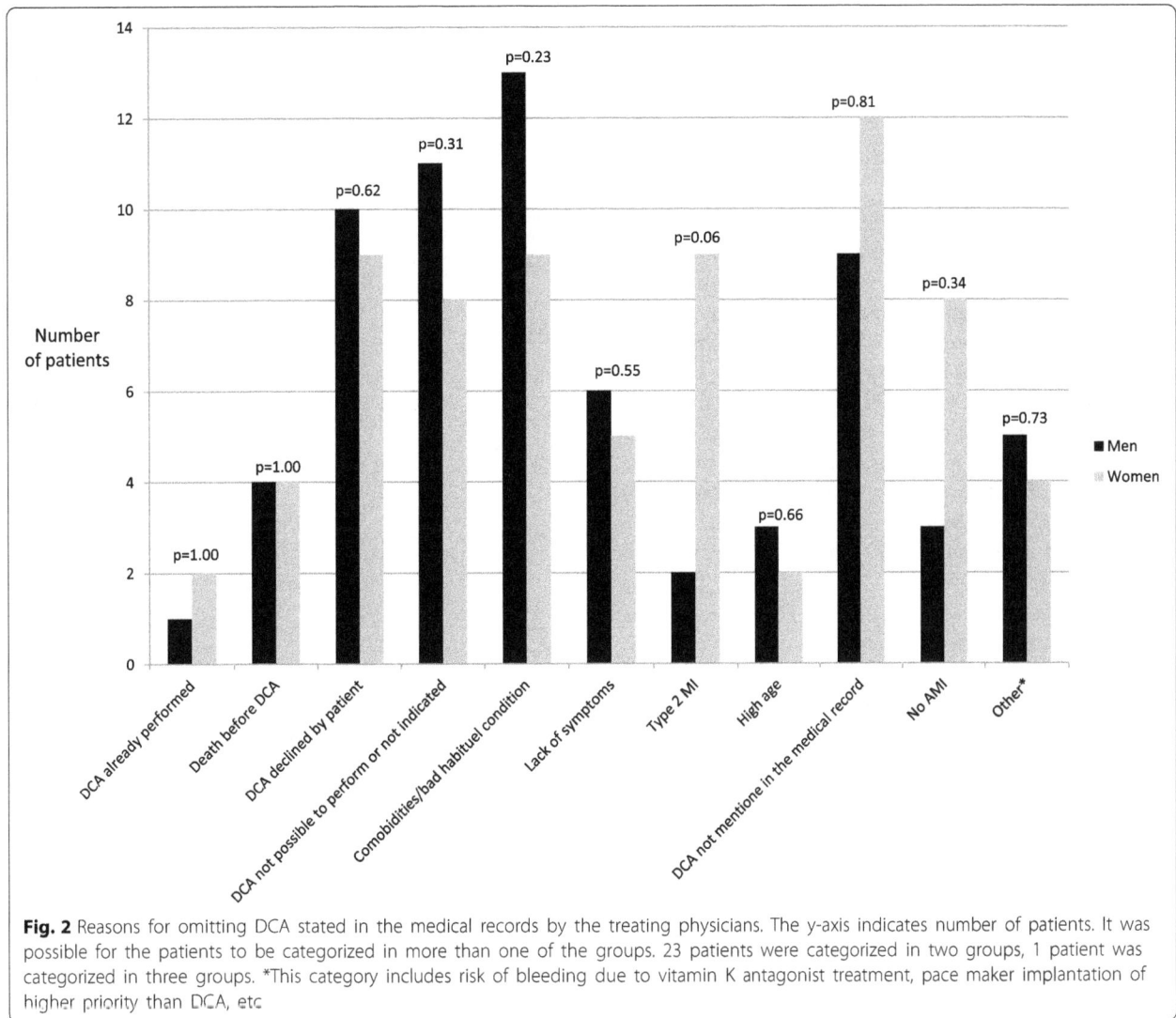

Fig. 2 Reasons for omitting DCA stated in the medical records by the treating physicians. The y-axis indicates number of patients. It was possible for the patients to be categorized in more than one of the groups. 23 patients were categorized in two groups, 1 patient was categorized in three groups. *This category includes risk of bleeding due to vitamin K antagonist treatment, pace maker implantation of higher priority than DCA, etc

significantly more women than men were not referred for DCA because the physician found that it was not supported by evidence [28]. In our study the decision not to refer to a coronary angiography was justified in more than 80 % of the cases, but in the remainder of patients an assessment of indications for cardiac catheterization was not provided. Interestingly, women were more prevalent in this subset of patients. This finding emphasizes the importance of considering and documenting clinical decisions; especially when deviating from guideline-recommended treatments.

Strengths and limitations
Our study included detailed data from medical records representing the actual information available to the treating physicians. This provided unique insights

to the clinical decision underlying referral to cardiac catheterization in a real world-setting.

Our study has some important limitations. First, this was an observational study prohibiting any conclusion regarding causality. Second, given the retrospective data collection process some degree of misclassification cannot be ruled out. Hence, contradictory or inconsistent descriptions in the medical records may have resulted in misinterpretation or missing. We addressed this issue by checking reproducibility through standardized extraction sheets, a specially trained data collector and extensive rereading of the first 80 patients medical records. Third, we did not have information on the level of training or specialization of the treating physicians; particularly the physician who decided whether or not the patient should receive an invasive treatment strategy. Finally, the sample size was small and the study thus underpowered to detect significant differences in the subset analyses of clinical justifications. However, logistic and practical constraints made it impossible to include more than 500 patients.

Conclusion

In this contemporary matched cohort of patients hospitalized with a first AMI we found that patient characteristics differed between women and men despite similar age. Although women had a lower risk for DCA at 60 days than men, we were unable to detect any differences in the distribution of relative contraindications for coronary angiography between the sexes. In patients not referred for DCA, physicians did not document any reasons for opting out this procedure in one fifth of patients. Thus, physicians should focus on managing both women and men in accordance with current guidelines and only refrain from using DCA when evidence-driven. Finally, type 2 MI poses a potential confounder for the sex-DCA relationship and merits further investigations.

Ethics approval and consent to participate

This project was carried out in accordance with current rules of ethics and legislature. It was approved by The Danish Data Protection Agency [record number 2007-58-0015] and the Danish Health and Medicines Authority [record number 3-3013-376/1/]. The approval from the Danish Health and Medicines Authority provided statutory authority for collecting patient information from all 500 medical records without obtaining written informed consent. All personal information was anonymized upon database closure using a positive integer ranging from 1 to 500 as unique patient identifiers and stored on a secure encrypted hard drive. The conversion key was kept on a separate encrypted hard drive. Register-based studies do not require approval from an Ethics Committee in Denmark.

Abbreviations

AMI: acute myocardial infarction; CABG: coronary artery bypass graft; CVD: cardiovascular disease; DBP: diastolic blood pressure; DCA: diagnostic coronary angiography; ECG: electrocardiogram; HR: hazard ratio; ICD: the international classification of diseases; IHD: ischemic heart disease; INR: international ratio; IQR: interquartile range; LBBB: left bundle branch block; NSTEMI: non ST-elevation myocardial infarction; PCI: percutaneous intervention; SBP: systolic blood pressure; STEMI: ST-elevation myocardial infarction; WBC: white blood cell count.

Competing interests

The authors declare that they have no competing interests.

Authors' contributions

LBH, KWH, RS, MM, JKM, JSJ and SG participated in study design. LBH, KWH and SG obtained funding. LBH performed data analysis and wrote the report. All authors interpreted the results, revised the report, and approved the final version. The corresponding author had full access to all of the data in the study and takes responsibility for the integrity of the data and the accuracy of the data analysis.

Acknowledgement

The authors wish to thanks the hospitals in the Greater metropolitan area surrounding Copenhagen for cooperating in the collection of data.

Author details

[1]Department of Cardiology, University Hospital Gentofte, Kildegårdsvej 28, 2900 Hellerup, Denmark. [2]Department of Cardiology, University Hospital Bispebjerg, Copenhagen, Denmark. [3]Department of Public Health, University of Copenhagen, Copenhagen, Denmark. [4]Department of Clinical Medicine, University of Copenhagen, Copenhagen, Denmark. [5]Emergency Department, Holbaek Hospital, University of Copenhagen, Holbaek, Denmark.

References

1. Lozano R, Naghavi M, Foreman K, Lim S, Shibuya K, Aboyans V, Abraham J, Adair T, Aggarwal R, Ahn SY, Alvarado M, Anderson HR, Anderson LM, Andrews KG, Atkinson C, Baddour LM, Barker-Collo S, Bartels DH, Bell ML, Benjamin EJ, Bennett D, Bhalla K, Bikbov B, Bin Abdulhak A, Birbeck G, Blyth F, Bolliger I, Boufous S, Bucello C, Burch M, et al. Global and regional mortality from 235 causes of death for 20 age groups in 1990 and 2010: a systematic analysis for the Global Burden of Disease Study 2010. Lancet. 2012;380:2095–128.
2. Authors/Task Force Members, Hamm CW, Bassand J-P, Agewall S, Bax J, Boersma E, Bueno H, Caso P, Dudek D, Gielen S, Huber K, Ohman M, Petrie MC, Sonntag F, Uva MS, Storey RF, Wijns W, Zahger D, ESC Committee for Practice Guidelines, Bax JJ, Auricchio A, Baumgartner H, Ceconi C, Dean V, Deaton C, Fagard R, Funck-Brentano C, Hasdai D, Hoes A, Knuuti J, et al. ESC Guidelines for the management of acute coronary syndromes in patients presenting without persistent ST-segment elevation: The Task Force for the management of acute coronary syndromes (ACS) in patients presenting without persistent ST-segment elevation of the European Society of Cardiology (ESC). Eur Heart J. 2011;32:2999–3054.
3. Authors/Task Force Members, Steg PG, James SK, Atar D, Badano LP, Lundqvist CB, Borger MA, Di Mario C, Dickstein K, Ducrocq G, Fernandez-Aviles F, Gershlick AH, Giannuzzi P, Halvorsen S, Huber K, Juni P, Kastrati A, Knuuti J, Lenzen MJ, Mahaffey KW, Valgimigli M, van't Hof A, Widimsky P, Zahger D, ESC Committee for Practice Guidelines (CPG), Bax JJ, Baumgartner H, Ceconi C, Dean V, Deaton C, et al. ESC Guidelines for the management of acute myocardial infarction in patients presenting with ST-segment elevation: The Task Force on the management of ST-segment elevation acute myocardial infarction of the European Society of Cardiology (ESC). Eur Heart J. 2012;33:2569–619.
4. Vaccarino V, Rathore SS, Wenger NK, Frederick PD, Abramson JL, Barron HV, Manhapra A, Mallik S, Krumholz HM, National Registry of Myocardial Infarction Investigators. Sex and racial differences in the management of acute myocardial infarction, 1994 through 2002. N Engl J Med. 2005;353:671–82.
5. Nguyen JT, Berger AK, Duval S, Luepker RV. Gender disparity in cardiac procedures and medication use for acute myocardial infarction. Am Heart J. 2008;155:862–8.
6. Hvelplund A, Galatius S, Madsen M, Rasmussen JN, Rasmussen S, Madsen JK, Sand NPR, Tilsted H-H, Thayssen P, Sindby E, Højbjerg S, Abildstrøm SZ. Women with acute coronary syndrome are less invasively examined and subsequently less treated than men. Eur Heart J. 2010;31:684–90.
7. Hansen KW, Soerensen R, Madsen M, Madsen JK, Jensen JS, Kappelgaard LM von, Mortensen PE, Galatius S. Developments in the invasive diagnostic–therapeutic cascade of women and men with acute coronary syndromes from 2005 to 2011: a nationwide cohort study. BMJ Open. 2015;5:e007785.
8. Statistikbanken. http://www.statistikbanken.dk/statbank5a/default.asp?w=1366. Accessed 20 Jan 2016.
9. Guidelines of the Danish society of Cardiology. http://nbv.cardio.dk. Accessed 20 Jan 2016.

10. Andersen TF, Madsen M, Jørgensen J, Mellemkjoer L, Olsen JH. The Danish National Hospital Register: A valuable source of data for modern health sciences. Dan Med Bull. 1999;46:263–8.

11. Madsen M, Davidsen M, Rasmussen S, Abildstrom SZ, Osler M. The validity of the diagnosis of acute myocardial infarction in routine statistics: a comparison of mortality and hospital discharge data with the Danish MONICA registry. J Clin Epidemiol. 2003;56:124–30.

12. Bach RG, Cannon CP, Weintraub WS, DiBattiste PM, Demopoulos LA, Anderson HV, DeLucca PT, Mahoney EM, Murphy SA, Braunwald E. The effect of routine, early invasive management on outcome for elderly patients with non-ST-segment elevation acute coronary syndromes. Ann Intern Med. 2004;141:186–95.

13. Rosengren A, Wallentin L, Simoons M, Gitt AK, Behar S, Battler A, Hasdai D. Age, clinical presentation, and outcome of acute coronary syndromes in the Euroheart acute coronary syndrome survey. Eur Heart J. 2006;27:789–95.

14. Malkin CJ, Prakash R, Chew DP. The impact of increased age on outcome from a strategy of early invasive management and revascularisation in patients with acute coronary syndromes: retrospective analysis study from the ACACIA registry. BMJ Open. 2012;2:e000540.

15. MatchIt: Nonparametric Preprocessing for Parametric Causal Inference. http://gking.harvard.edu/matchit. Accessed 20 Jan 2016.

16. R Core Team. R: A Language and Environment for Statistical Computing. Vienna, Austria: R Foundation for Statistical Computing; 2014.

17. Thygesen K, Alpert JS, Jaffe AS, Simoons ML, Chaitman BR, White HD, et al. Third universal definition of myocardial infarction. J Am Coll Cardiol. 2012;60:1581–98.

18. Rasmussen K, Abildgaard U, Dalsgaard D, Kastrup J, Markenvard J, Pedersen KE, Svendsen TL, Thuesen L. KAG, Hjertekateterisation Og PCI Hos Voksne. Retningslinier Udarbejdet Af En Arbejdsgruppe Nedsat Af Dansk Cardiologisk Selskab. Dansk Cardiologisk Selskab; 2002. http://www.cardio.dk/docman/cat_view/48-rapporter/49-kliniske-rapporter?limit=5&order=name&dir=DESC&start=10. Accessed 21 Apr 2016.

19. Ko DT, Wang Y, Alter DA, Curtis JP, Rathore SS, Stukel TA, Masoudi FA, Ross JS, Foody JM, Krumholz HM. Regional variation in cardiac catheterization appropriateness and baseline risk after acute myocardial infarction. J Am Coll Cardiol. 2008;51:716–23.

20. Shaw LJ, Bugiardini R, Merz CNB. Women and ischemic heart disease: evolving knowledge. J Am Coll Cardiol. 2009;54:1561–75.

21. Dey S, Flather MD, Devlin G, Brieger D, Gurfinkel EP, Steg PG, Fitzgerald G, Jackson EA, Eagle KA, Global Registry of Acute Coronary Events investigators. Sex-related differences in the presentation, treatment and outcomes among patients with acute coronary syndromes: the Global Registry of Acute Coronary Events. Heart Br Card Soc. 2009;95:20–6.

22. Čulić V, Eterović D, Mirić D, Silić N. Symptom presentation of acute myocardial infarction: Influence of sex, age, and risk factors. Am Heart J. 2002;144:1012–7.

23. D'Ascenzo F, Cerrato E, Biondi-Zoccai G, Omedè P, Sciuto F, Presutti DG, et al. Coronary computed tomographic angiography for detection of coronary artery disease in patients presenting to the emergency department with chest pain: a meta-analysis of randomized clinical trials. Eur Heart J Cardiovasc Imaging. 2013;14:782–9.

24. Saaby L, Poulsen TS, Hosbond S, Larsen TB, Pyndt Diederichsen AC, Hallas J, Thygesen K, Mickley H. Classification of myocardial infarction: frequency and features of type 2 myocardial infarction. Am J Med. 2013;126:789–97.

25. Golden KE, Chang AM, Hollander JE. Sex preferences in cardiovascular testing: the contribution of the patient-physician discussion. Acad Emerg Med Off J Soc Acad Emerg Med. 2013;20:680–8.

26. Heidenreich PA, Shlipak MG, Geppert J, McClellan M. Racial and sex differences in refusal of coronary angiography. Am J Med. 2002;113:200–7.

27. Mumma BE, Baumann BM, Diercks DB, Takakuwa KM, Campbell CF, Shofer FS, Chang AM, Jones MK, Hollander JE. Sex bias in cardiovascular testing: the contribution of patient preference. Ann Emerg Med. 2011;57:551–560.e4.

28. Poon S, Goodman SG, Yan RT, Bugiardini R, Bierman AS, Eagle KA, Johnston N, Huynh T, Grondin FR, Schenck-Gustafsson K, Yan AT. Bridging the gender gap: Insights from a contemporary analysis of sex-related differences in the treatment and outcomes of patients with acute coronary syndromes. Am Heart J. 2012;163:66–73.

29. O'Donoghue M, Boden WE, Braunwald E, Cannon CP, Clayton TC, de Winter RJ, Fox KAA, Lagerqvist B, McCullough PA, Murphy SA, Spacek R, Swahn E, Wallentin L, Windhausen F, Sabatine MS. Early invasive vs conservative treatment strategies in women and men with unstable angina and non-ST-segment elevation myocardial infarction: a meta-analysis. JAMA. 2008;300:71–80.

14

Initiation of and long-term adherence to secondary preventive drugs after acute myocardial infarction

Sigrun Halvorsen[1*], Jarle Jortveit[2], Pål Hasvold[3], Marcus Thuresson[4] and Erik Øie[5]

Abstract

Background: Secondary preventive drug therapy following acute myocardial infarction (AMI) is recommended to reduce the risk of new cardiovascular events. The aim of this nationwide cohort study was to examine the initiation and long-term use of secondary preventive drugs after AMI.

Methods: The prescription of drugs in 42,707 patients < 85 years discharged alive from hospital after AMI in 2009–2013 was retrieved by linkage of the Norwegian Patient Register, the Norwegian Prescription Database, and the Norwegian Cause of Death Registry. Patients were followed for up to 24 months.

Results: The majority of patients were discharged on single or dual antiplatelet therapy (91 %), statins (90 %), beta-blockers (82 %), and angiotensin-converting enzyme inhibitors (ACEI)/angiotensin receptor II blockers (ARB) (60 %). Patients not undergoing percutaneous coronary intervention (PCI) (42 %) were less likely to be prescribed secondary preventive drugs compared with patients undergoing PCI. This was particular the case for dual antiplatelet therapy (43 % vs. 87 %). The adherence to prescribed drugs was high: 12 months after index AMI, 84 % of patients were still on aspirin, 84 % on statins, 77 % on beta-blockers and 57 % on ACEI/ARB. Few drug and dose adjustments were made during follow-up.

Conclusion: Guideline-recommended secondary preventive drugs were prescribed to most patients discharged from hospital after AMI, but the percentage receiving such therapy was significantly lower in non-PCI patients. The long-time adherence was high, but few drug adjustments were performed during follow-up. More attention is needed to secondary preventive drug therapy in AMI patients not undergoing PCI.

Keywords: Acute myocardial infarction, Secondary prevention, Medication adherence

Background

Ischemic heart disease is a common cause of death in industrialized countries and accounts for a large proportion of hospital admissions in Norway [1]. Approximately 13,000 men and women are diagnosed annually with acute myocardial infarction (AMI) [2]. Secondary preventive drug therapy, e.g. platelet inhibitors, statins, beta-blockers and angiotensin-converting enzyme inhibitors (ACEI)/angiotensin receptor II blockers (ARB), is recommended following AMI to reduce the risk of new cardiovascular

events and death [3–7]. However, an underuse of secondary preventive drugs has previously been observed following AMI, especially in patients not undergoing percutaneous coronary intervention (PCI) [8]. Despite their elevated cardiovascular risk [9], still many AMI patients are not treated according to guidelines [10]. This may be related to under-prescription, reduced adherence, and/or under-dosing of secondary preventive drug therapy [11, 12]. A potential source for the underuse of recommended secondary preventive drugs could be the shift of treatment responsibility from the hospitals to the general practitioners in the primary care setting. The extent to which the hospital-initiated treatment is continued as initially prescribed, the doses adjusted or drugs switched to another type of drug within the same drug class, is not known. Comprehensive analyses of

* Correspondence: sigrun.h@online.no
[1]Department of Cardiology, Oslo University Hospital Ulleval and University of Oslo, Postboks 4956, Nydalen 0424, Oslo, Norway
Full list of author information is available at the end of the article

initiation and adherence in different patient populations are essential to improve long-term use of secondary preventive drugs and cardiovascular outcomes [13].

The aim of this nationwide cohort study was to examine the initiation and long-term use of secondary preventive drug in patients hospitalized with AMI in Norway during the years 2009 to 2013.

Methods
Data sources
This observational, historical cohort study was based on data from three Norwegian national registries: 1) The Norwegian Patient Register covering all hospital admissions and including diagnoses according to the International Classification of Diseases, 10th revision, Clinical Modification (ICD-10-CM) [14]; 2) the Norwegian Prescription Database registering all pharmacy dispenses [15]; and 3) the Norwegian Cause of Death Registry registering all deaths [16]. The prescription of drugs in patients discharged alive from hospital after AMI in 2009–2013 was retrieved by linkage of the Norwegian Patient Register, the Norwegian Prescription Database, and the Norwegian Cause of Death Registry. Patients were followed for up to 24 months. The Norwegian Institute of Public Health performed the data linkage. Data were anonymised before further analysis. The linked database was managed by The Norwegian University of Science and Technology, Trondheim, Norway.

Study population
All patients below 85 years of age who were admitted to hospital with a primary diagnosis of AMI (index AMI) (ICD-10: I21) between 1 January 2009 and 30 November 2013 and alive 30 days after discharge were included in this study. Patients 85 years or older were excluded for two reasons: 1) their likelihood of long-term use of secondary preventive drugs might be extensively confounded by fragility; 2) older patients have an increased risk of long-term institutional stays where the drug use cannot be captured by the available registries. Patients were classified as PCI and non-PCI patients depending on whether PCI was performed or not up to 30 days after index-AMI. The study population was further stratified into two groups; ≤75 years and 76–84 years.

Index AMI was defined as the first recorded primary diagnosis of AMI for a patient during the specified time-period (not necessarily the patient's first AMI). All residents in Norway are covered by a national health security system with a universal tax-funded access to primary and secondary health care, including secondary preventive drugs recommended after AMI.

Follow-up
Observational data on drug prescriptions were collected up to 24 months following AMI, or until 31 December 2014 or death (whichever occurred first).

Drug treatment and adherence
Drug treatment at discharge for index AMI were calculated from dispensed drugs from pharmacies one year within and until 30 days after the index AMI; either a prior dispensing covering day 0 to day 30 or a new dispensing within day 0 to day 30. Drug adherence was defined as the proportion of patients on the treatment of interest at each day from 12 months prior to the date of hospitalization for AMI until a maximum of 24 months after. The calculation of drug use (days on treatment) was based on the prescribed dose and on the number of pills collected or delivered from the pharmacies. Whether or not the pills were taken by the patients, were not assessed. If a patient had a gap in collection of drugs, the patient was defined as a non-user from last calculated day with available drug. Furthermore, if a patient after a gap, again collected the same drug from the pharmacy, the patient was defined as a user from that actual date, and if a patient was switched to another type of drug within the same drug class after the index AMI episode, the patient was defined as a user.

In the separate analysis of the adherence to the P_2Y_{12}-antagonists clopidogrel, prasugrel or ticagrelor during the first 18 months after AMI, the proportion of all patients still alive continuing on the same P_2Y_{12} antagonist as at discharge was estimated.

In order to describe changes in drug treatment over time, treatment at discharge for index AMI was compared to treatment in the post AMI period (dispensed during 12 18 months after the AMI).

Statistical analyses
Data are presented as mean with standard deviation for continuous variables and absolute and relative frequencies for categorical variables. Patients were stratified by age (≤75 years or 75–84 years) and by PCI status (PCI or no PCI). Statistical analyses were performed using SAS version 9.3 (SAS Institute Inc, Cary, NC, USA) and R version 3.2.2 [17].

Results
A total of 57,106 individuals were admitted to Norwegian hospitals for AMI during the study period, of whom 45,838 (80.3 %) were younger than 85 years. Of these, 42,707 (93.2 %) were alive 30 days after hospital discharge and could be included in the study (Fig. 1). Overall, 70 % of the patients were men and mean age was 65.8 years (standard deviation 11.8) (Table 1). A total of 58 % of the patients underwent PCI, with an increasing proportion

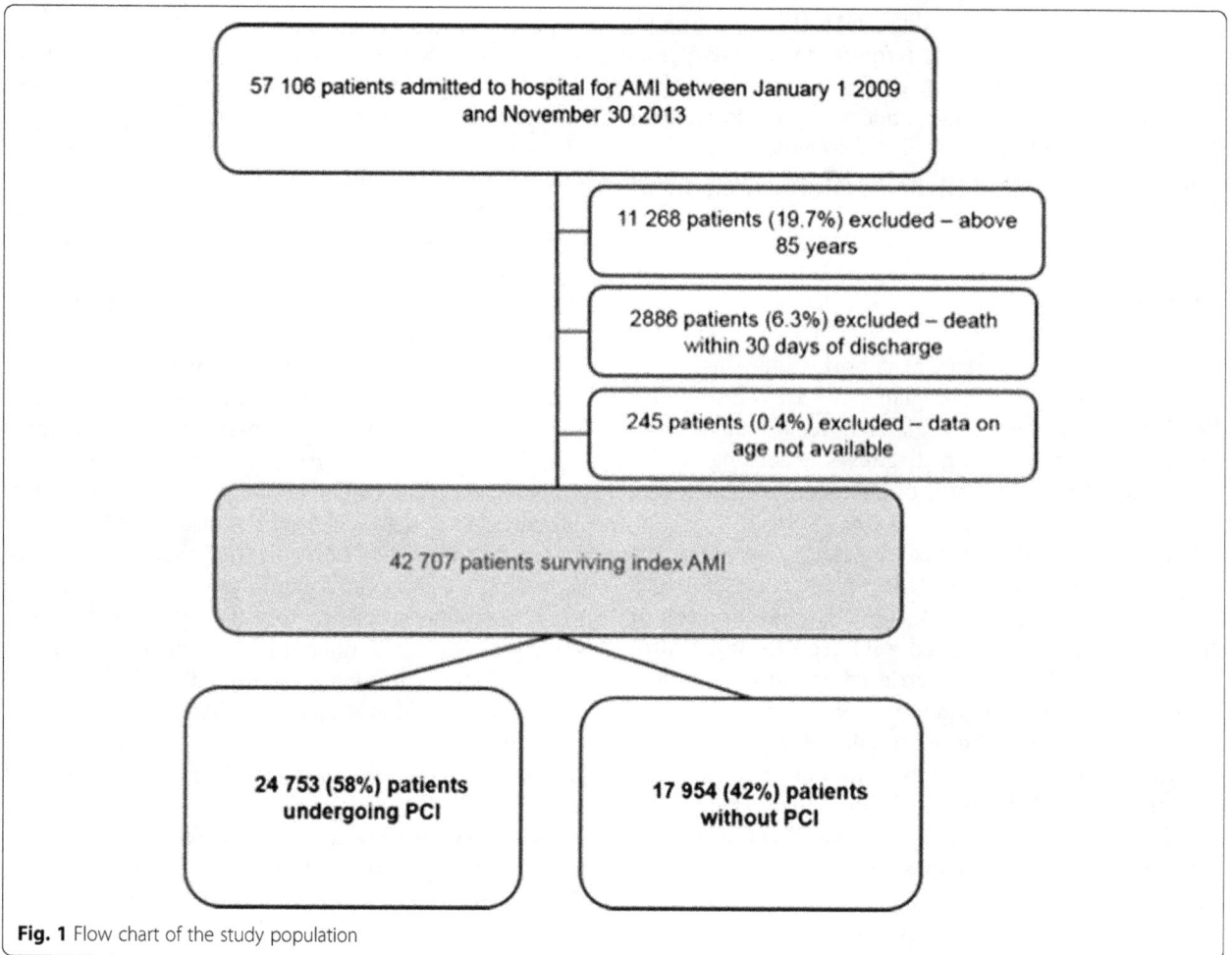

Fig. 1 Flow chart of the study population

during the study period (from 53 % to 63 %) (Additional file 1, Table 1). Patients undergoing PCI were younger and more often male compared with the medically treated patients (Table 1).

Initiation of secondary preventive drugs

The prescription of secondary preventive drugs at discharge is shown in Tables 1 and 2. The majority of patients were discharged on single or dual antiplatelet therapy (DAPT) (19 % and 72 %, respectively), statins (90 %), beta-blockers (82 %), and ACEI/ARB (60 %). The percentage receiving these drugs were slightly lower in patients 75–84 years compared to patients ≤75 years, except for ACEI/ARB which was prescribed slightly more often in the elderly (Table 1).

Patients undergoing PCI were prescribed secondary preventive drug therapy more often than patients not undergoing PCI (Table 1). This was the case both for patients <75 years and patients 75–84 years. The difference in prescriptions was largest with respect to DAPT, which was prescribed in 92 % of the PCI patients vs. 45 % of patients not undergoing PCI (Table 1, Figs. 2 and 3). In

contrast, non-PCI patients were prescribed other kinds of antithrombotic therapy more often than PCI patients: Aspirin monotherapy in 28 % vs. 2 %, oral anticoagulant (OAC) monotherapy in 4 % vs. 0 %, or OAC in combination with single antiplatelet therapy in 6 % vs. 1 %, respectively. However, 14 % of the non-PCI patients were discharged with neither antiplatelet drugs nor OAC, compared to 2 % of the PCI patients. Surprisingly, the differences in prescription pattern between PCI and non-PCI patients were found also with respect to other types of secondary preventive drugs (Table 1).

The mean dose of statins at discharge was 37 mg for simvastatin (55 % of patients) and 57 mg for atorvastatin (40 % of patients). The mean doses of ACEI/ARB and beta-blocker at discharge were 35-60 % and 30-50 % of maximal recommended doses, respectively (Table 2).

Adherence to secondary preventive drugs

The overall long-time adherence was high among all patients initiated on treatment with statins, beta-blockers and ACEI/ARB (Figs. 2 and 3, Table 2). The proportions of patients using statins, ACEI/ARB and beta-blockers

Table 1 Drug treatment at discharge after index AMI. Patients stratified by age (≤75 years or 75–84 years) and by PCI status (PCI or no PCI)

	Age ≤75 years		Age 75–84 years		Total
	n = 30 843		n = 11 864		n = 42 707
	PCI	No PCI	PCI	No PCI	
	n = 19 835	n = 11 008	n = 4918	n = 6946	
	(64.3)	(35.7)	(29.3)	(70.7)	
Women	4065 (20.5)	3478 (31.6)	1819 (37.0)	3357 (48.3)	12 719 (29.8)
Age, mean (SD)	59.8 (9.1)	61.6 (9.6)	79.0 (2.8)	80.0 (2.8)	65.8 (11.8)
DAPT	17 505 (88.3)	5107 (46.4)	3877 (78.8)	2597 (37.4)	29 086 (68.1)
Only P2Y$_{12}$ inhibitor	668 (3.4)	354 (3.2)	202 (4.1)	295 (4.3)	1519 (3.6)
Only ASA	288 (1.5)	3105 (28.2)	151 (3.1)	1860 (26.7)	5404 (12.3)
Only OAC	21 (0.1)	312 (2.8)	15 (0.3)	339 (4.9)	687 (1.6)
OAC + DAPT	925 (4.7)	241 (2.2)	473 (9.6)	165 (2.4)	1804 (4.2)
OAC + P2Y$_{12}$ inhibitor	58 (0.3)	40 (0.4)	28 (0.6)	58 (0.8)	184 (0.4)
OAC + ASA	43 (0.2)	520 (4.7))	32 (0.7)	529 (7.6)	1124 (2.6)
No antiplatelet or OAC	327 (1.7)	1329 (12.1)	140 (2.9)	1103 (15.9)	2899 (6.8)
Statins	19 168 (96.6)	9224 (83.8)	4574 (93.0)	5262 (75.7)	38 228 (89.5)
Beta-blockers	16 763 (84.5)	8529 (77.5)	4238 (86.2)	5456 (78.6)	34 986 (81.9)
ACE inhibitors	7977 (40.3)	3478 (31.7)	2027 (41.2)	2497 (36.0)	15 988 (37.4)
ARB	4822 (24.3)	2945 (26.8)	1597 (32.5)	2072 (29.8)	11 346 (26.8)

Numbers in parentheses are percentages of total number of patients in the group. *SD* denotes standard derivation, *DAPT* dual antiplatelet therapy, *AMI* Acute myocardial infaction, *ASA* Acetylsalicylic acid, *OAC* Oral anticoagulants, *ACE* Angiotensin-converting enzyme, *ARB* Angiotensin II receptor blocker

were reduced by 6 %, 3 % and 4 %, respectively, after one year. No major differences in drug adherence was observed between PCI and non-PCI patients, or between patients ≤75 and 76–84 years. When primary health care physicians took over the prescription responsibility for these patients (approximately 3 months after the AMI), no overall change in adherence was found. Approximately 20 % of patients changed to another drug within the same drug class, or changed the dose of statin, beta-blocker and ACEI/ARB within 12–18 months after the AMI (Table 2).

The adherence to antiplatelet drugs was also high (Figs. 2 and 3). After 12 months, 84 % of patients were still on aspirin; 83 % after 18 months. The adherence to P_2Y_{12} inhibitors are shown in more detail in Fig. 4 and Additional file 1: Table S2. Patients not undergoing PCI had a shorter length of time on treatment with a P_2Y_{12} inhibitor compared with PCI patients, with a substantial proportion of these patients discontinuing treatment already after three months. The majority of the PCI patients treated with ticagrelor and prasugrel maintained the treatment through 12 months. Many PCI patients on clopidogrel discontinued P_2Y_{12} inhibitor after nine months.

Discussion

This nationwide observational cohort study, including all patients younger than 85 years surviving an AMI in Norway during the years 2009 to 2013, showed a generally high long-term adherence to the prescribed treatment with antiplatelet drugs, statins, beta-blockers and ACEI/ARB. The shift of responsibility for prescribing secondary preventive drugs from hospital to primary health care showed a sustained high use of the originally prescribed drugs. Only few patients switched to another type of statin or changed the dose of statin, beta-blocker and ACEI/ARB during the first two years after the AMI. For patients not undergoing PCI, a smaller proportion was discharged with secondary preventive drugs following their AMI compared with patients undergoing PCI, and less than half were prescribed DAPT at discharge.

Contemporary national level data describing long-term adherence to secondary preventive medications, i.e. antiplatelet drugs, statins, beta-blockers, and ACEI/ARB in AMI populations comparing younger vs. older and PCI vs. non-PCI patients are scarce. Furthermore, little is known on the impact of change in drug treatment responsibilities as AMI patients are transferred from hospital care to primary health care.

The initiation of secondary preventive drugs in our study was considerably higher than was found in a previous Danish nationwide study [12]. In patients admitted with a first AMI between 1995 and 2002 in Denmark, only 58 % received beta-blockers, 29 % ACE-inhibitors, and 34 % statins at discharge [12].

Table 2 Secondary preventive drugs at discharge from hospital for index AMI and 12–18 months later; patients <85 years

	Secondary preventive drugs at discharge for index AMI (n = 42 707)		Secondary preventive drugs 12–18 months after index AMI (n = 28 767)		n (%) switched to another drug within same drug class in post-AMI period	n (%) changed dose of actual drug in post-AMI period
	n (%)	Mean dose (mg)	n (%)	Mean dose (mg)		
Statins	38 228 (89.5)		24 062 (83.6)			
Simvastatin	23 528 (55.1)	37.2	12 478 (43.4)	38.4	2571 (15.7)	1415 (8.7)
Atorvastatin	17 084 (40.0)	56.9	10 913 (37.9)	52.1	592 (6)	1755 (17.8)
Rosuvastatin	225 (0.5)	17.7	367 (1.3)	19.6	10 (9.6)	13 (12.5)
Pravastatin	1158 (2.7)	33.5	651 (2.3)	33.5	120 (20.9)	39 (6.8)
ACEI/ARB[a]	25 445 (59.6)		16 274 (56.6)			
Losartan	3658 (8.6)	66.6	2049 (7.1)	66.5	153 (6.9)	238 (10.8)
Candersartan	4157 (9.7)	13.1	2778 (9.7)	13.5	145 (5.4)	467 (17.4)
Valsartan	1503 (3.5)	124.9	865 (3.0)	125.2	68 (7.2)	127 (13.4)
Irbesartan	1530 (3.6)	235.6	770 (2.7)	237.3	72 (7.8)	61 (6.6)
Enalapril	2951 (6.9)	11.8	1657 (5.8)	11.9	170 (8.9)	324 (16.9)
Ramipril	11 492 (26.9)	3.5	6999 (24.3)	4.5	733 (8.8)	2156 (25.8)
Lisinopril	1753 (4.1)	11.3	949 (3.3)	11.3	121 (10.3)	207 (17.5)
Beta-blockers	34 986 (81.9)		22 061 (76.7)			
Metoprolol	30 874 (72.3)	60.6	18 920 (65.8)	62.3	702 (3.2)	4452 (20.3)
Atenolol	1381 (3.2)	52.4	457 (1.6)	51.0	117 (21.6)	54 (10)
Propranolol	305 (0.7)	66.2	82 (0.3)	80.4	26 (26.3)	6 (6.1)
Sotalol	358 (0.8)	80.3	138 (0.5)	75.9	49 (33.3)	14 (9.5)
Bisoprolol	2477 (5.8)	4.1	1856 (6.5)	4.4	64 (4)	310 (19.3)
Carvedilol	1298 (3.0)	15.8	813 (2.8)	15.6	73 (9.1)	123 (15.3)

Numbers in parentheses are percentages of total number of patients in the group
ACEI Angiotensin-converting enzyme inhibitor, *AMI* Aciute myocardial infraction, *ARB* Angiotensin II receptor blocker
[a]some patients were prescribed both ACEI and ARB

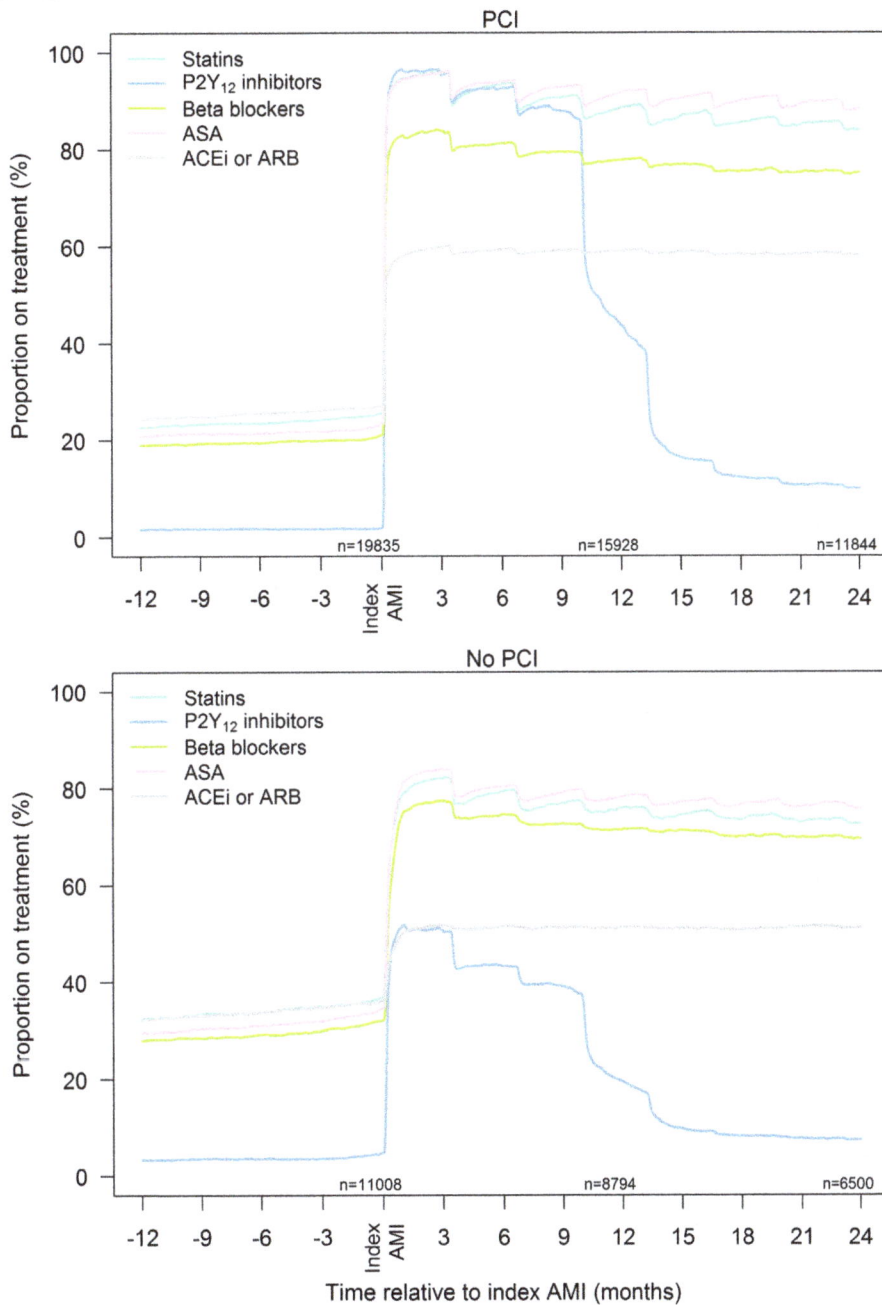

Fig. 2 Adherence to secondary preventive drugs over time in AMI patients ≤75 years with or without PCI. Norway 2009–2013. *Abbreviations:* ASA, acetylsalicylic acid; ACEI, angiotensin-converting enzyme inhibitor; AMI, acute myocardial infarction; ARB, angiotensin II receptor blocker; PCI, percutaneous coronary intervention

Although long-term compliance was reasonably good, patients who did not start treatment shortly after discharge had a low probability of starting treatment later [12]. In a more recent Swedish study, both initiation and long-term adherence to secondary preventive drug therapy was higher and similar to our findings: 82 % of AMI patients were still on aspirin 12 months post AMI, 73 % on statins and 80 % on beta-blockers [18].

A high degree of initiation of secondary preventive drug therapy was also observed in a recent study from the United States [13]. However, when patients were divided into risk groups based on the Global Registry of Acute Coronary Event (GRACE) risk score at hospital discharge, high-risk patients had a lower likelihood of receiving all appropriate therapies at discharge compared with low-risk patients.

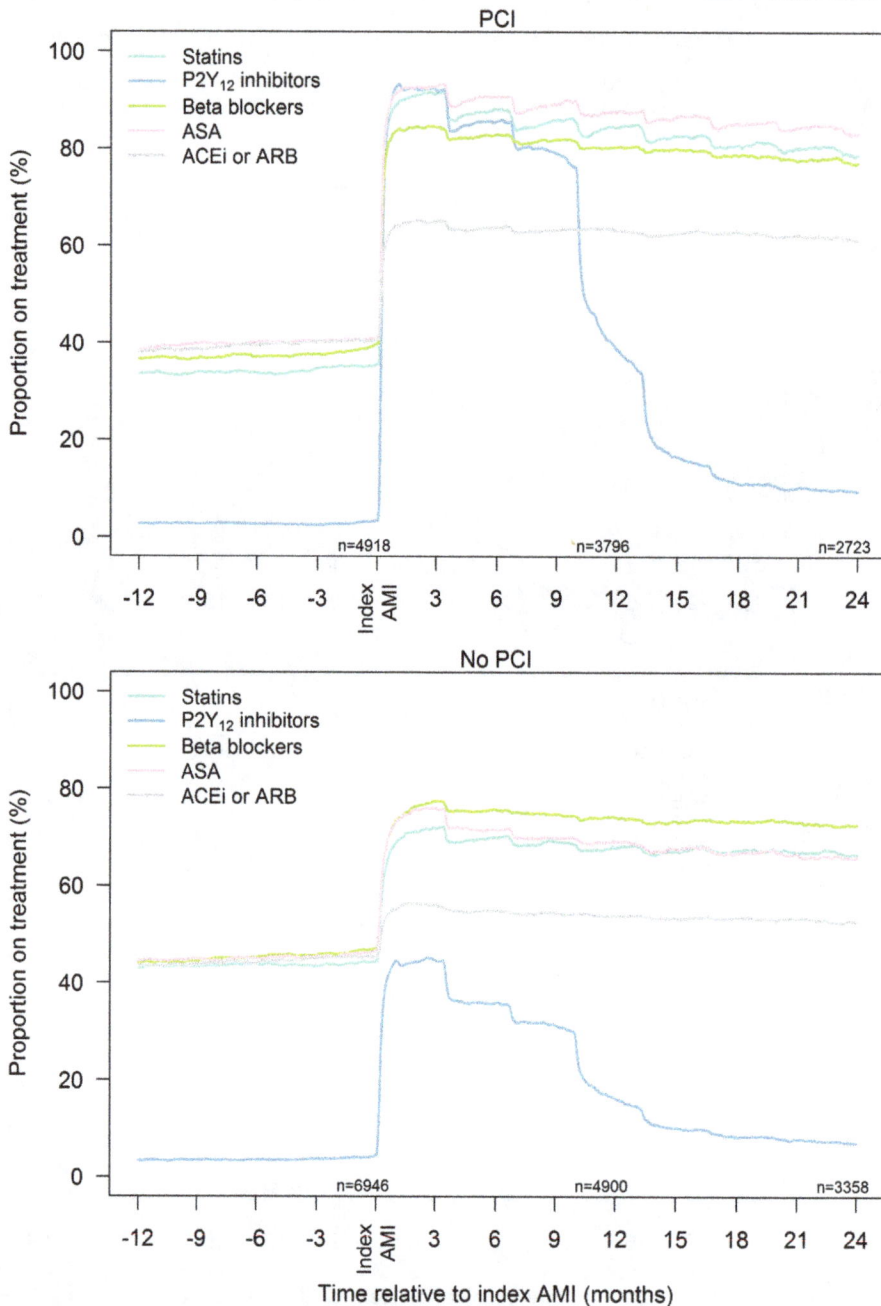

Fig. 3 Adherence to secondary preventive drugs over time in AMI patients 76–84 years with and without PCI. Norway 2009–2013. *Abbreviations*: ASA, acetylsalicylic acid; ACEI, angiotensin-converting enzyme inhibitor; AMI, acute myocardial infarction; ARB, angiotensin II receptor blocker; PCI, percutaneous coronary intervention

Our data may indicate that if secondary preventive drug therapy after AMI is not prescribed at hospital discharge, the likelihood of receiving such treatment is limited. Thus, initiation of guideline-recommended secondary preventive drug therapy after AMI seems to depend on the hospital physicians, in accordance with the previous observations from Denmark [12]. The present study further demonstrates that only minor dose adjustments for drugs prescribed at discharge were performed by the primary care physicians during follow-up. Thus, Norwegian primary care physicians seemed reluctant to changing already prescribed secondary preventive drug therapies after AMI.

This finding further underscores the importance of drug prescription prior to discharge of AMI patients from hospitals. Not only should AMI patients be prescribed guideline-recommended secondary preventive drugs, but the hospital

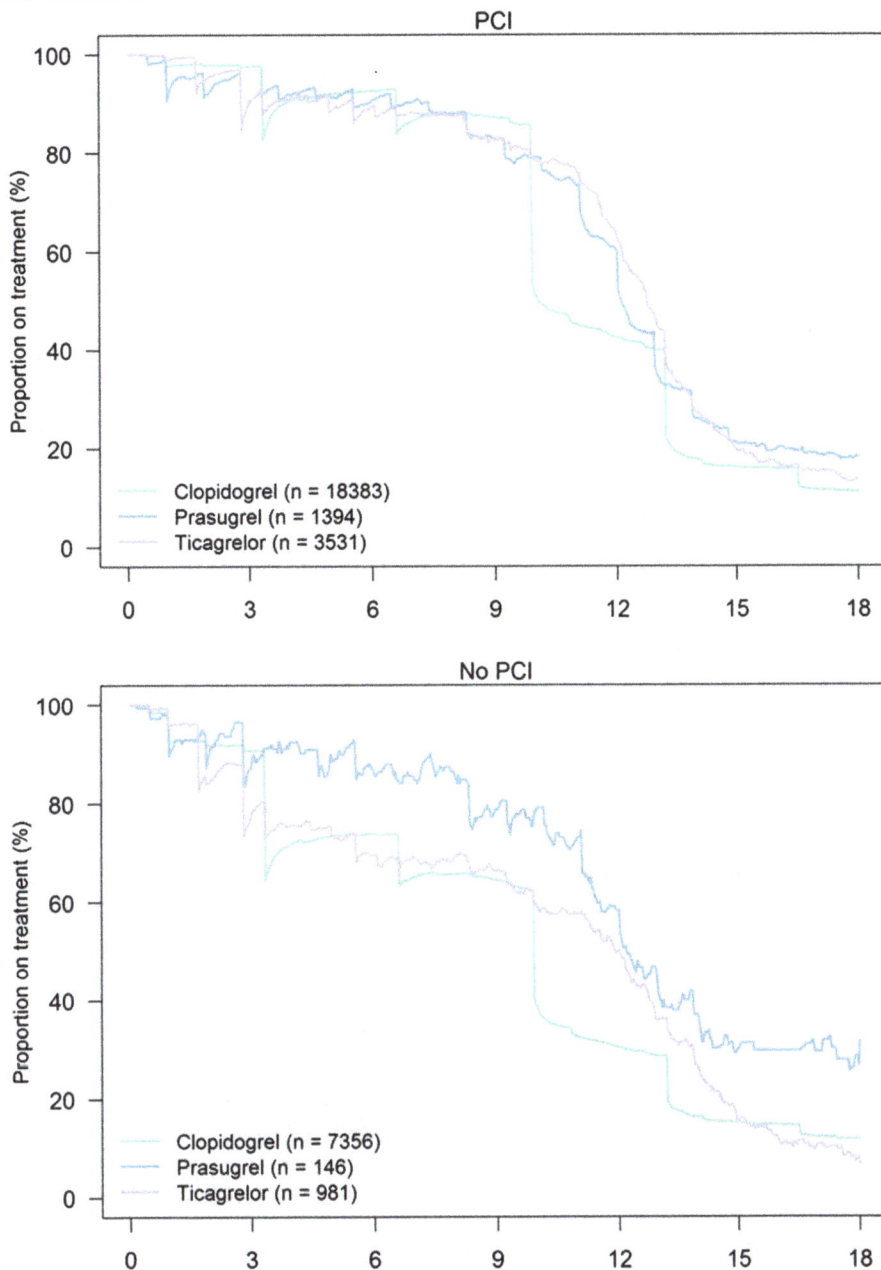

Fig. 4 Adherence to treatment with different P2Y$_{12}$ inhibitors in AMI patients <85 years with and without PCI. Norway 2009–2013. *Abbreviations:* AMI, acute myocardial infarction; PCI, percutaneous coronary intervention

physicians could also advice on further up-titration and the target doses of the prescribed drugs in the discharge summary sent to the patient's general practitioner. It is also important that the general practitioners are updated on current guidelines and take the responsibility for optimizing secondary preventive treatment after AMI. Interestingly, patients not undergoing PCI were less likely to receive guideline-recommended secondary preventive drugs compared with patients undergoing PCI. For example, a 10–20 % higher use of statins and beta-blockers was seen in PCI patients vs. patients not undergoing PCI. Furthermore, a larger portion of patients not undergoing PCI was discharged without a P2Y$_{12}$ inhibitor (48 % and 55 %, respectively, in patients ≤75 or 76–84 years) compared with PCI patients (4 % and 7 %). The reasons for this undertreatment of non-PCI patients are not known. We might speculate that a higher degree of comorbidities might be present in these patients, making the physicians more selective in their prescription of secondary preventive drugs.

The mean doses of both ACEI, ARB and beta-blockers in our study were lower than the target doses in randomized trials studying the efficacy and safety of these drugs. The reasons for the choice of these lower doses, or the lack of up-titration of doses after hospital discharge, are unknown. These drugs are used for a variety of indications, and since we have limited data on weight, blood pressure, heart rate, ejection fraction, comorbidities and on the specific indications for the various drugs (e.g. for ACEI/ARB), we find it difficult to draw any firm conclusions regarding target doses and whether the doses used in our study were too low or not. With respect to statin treatment, it should be noted that during most of our study period, no specific statin dose was recommended and statins were prescribed mainly according to LDL-cholesterol levels.

We observed a generally short duration of P_2Y_{12} inhibitor treatment for patients not undergoing PCI (Fig. 4), with a significant proportion of patients treated for only three months as also observed in a recent study from Sweden [19]. One possible reason for the longer treatment duration after PCI may be that $P2Y_{12}$ inhibition is regarded particularly important after stent implantation to avoid stent thrombosis. However, ESC guidelines recommend P_2Y_{12} inhibition for 12 months in all ACS patients [3–6].

A large proportion of patients discontinued P_2Y_{12} inhibitor after nine months; mainly patients on clopidogrel treatment. One likely explanation to this finding was the nine months' limited reimbursement of clopidogrel in Norway until September 2011 [20]. Prasugrel and ticagrelor have not had such reimbursement limitations. This finding demonstrates the influence the health authorities have on medical treatment by determining the prescription rules for reimbursements of various drugs.

Limitations

Our data set provides a unique possibility to examine adherence to antiplatelet therapy, statins, beta-blockers and ACEI/ARB. It includes nationwide data from all patients hospitalized in Norway for AMI in 2009–2013, allowing analyses of a complete and unselected cohort of patients, and also allowing differentiation between younger and older patients and between patients undergoing PCI or not. This reduces potential problems arising from selection bias due to inclusion of selected hospitals, regions, or health care insurance systems. Furthermore, by restricting the inclusion to patients below 85 years of age, this study focuses on patients who normally would be considered to be treated according to guidelines. However, this register-based analysis also has certain limitations. As our analysis relied on ICD-10 codes, the possibility of coding errors cannot be ruled out, although the primary diagnoses of AMI

previously have been shown to have high sensitivity and specificity [21]. A further subclassification of patients into those presenting with and without persistent ST-segment elevation on the electrocardiogram could not be performed due to non-validated ICD-10 coding specification at this level.

Further, due the study aim describing secondary drug adherence in a nationwide patient population, patients were included based on their first AMI during the observational period, i.e. not necessarily their first time AMI. Thus, the patient population changed during the inclusion period. While patients included early in the inclusion period may have had a recent history of AMI, patients included towards the end of the study period had to be event-free for a longer time. Following from this study design, the yearly numbers of included AMIs in our study decreased during the observational period (Additional file 1, Table 1). Furthermore, how a recent prior AMI episode would affect selection for invasive treatment and secondary prevention drugs is difficult to predict, but it cannot be excluded that these patients would receive a higher attention, and thus a higher likelihood of receiving guideline-recommended treatment.

The registry data were collected for administrative purposes and we did not have any information on smoking patterns, weight, blood pressure, laboratory data or socioeconomic status. Furthermore, the Norwegian Patient Register has only had nationwide coverage since 2009 and medical history from previous hospitalizations was not available.

Conclusions

This nationwide observational study, including all patients in Norway below 85 years of age being alive 30 days after AMI during the years 2009 to 2013, showed a generally high long-term adherence to antiplatelet therapy, as well as treatment with statins, beta-blockers and ACEI/ARB. To a large extent, PCI patients received guideline-recommended treatment with secondary preventive drugs. Patients not undergoing PCI were less likely to be discharged with the recommended drugs. The shift of responsibility for prescribing drug treatment from hospital to primary health care did not to any major extent alter the already prescribed treatments. Thus, the majority of AMI patients remained on the secondary preventive treatment originally prescribed, further underlining the importance of prescribing guideline-recommended drug treatment at hospital discharge, and preferably including specialist guidance on future target doses in the discharge summary. The present study also indicates a need for more careful attention to secondary preventive drug therapy in AMI patients not undergoing PCI.

Abbreviations

ACEI, angiotensin-converting enzyme inhibitor; AMI, acute myocardial infarction; ARB, angiotensin II receptor blocker; ASA, acetylsalicylic acid; DAPT, dual antiplatelet therapy; ICD-10-CM, International Classification of Diseases, 10th revision, Clinical Modification; OAC, oral anticoagulant; PCI, percutaneous coronary intervention.

Funding

This work was supported by AstraZeneca. Project management was provided by AstraZeneca. The statistical analysis was agreed upon by the study steering committee, and data analysis was performed by the study database owner in collaboration with AstraZeneca. AstraZeneca took part as members of the study steering committee in the interpretation of the data and the drafting of the manuscript.

Authors' contributions

S. Halvorsen, J. Jortveit, P. Hasvold, M. Thuresson, and E. Øie, participated equally in the study conception, design, and statistical analysis planning. M. Thuresson was responsible for the statistical analyses and S. Halvorsen for the manuscript draft and finalization. All authors had access to study data, and had authority over manuscript preparation, approval of the final version, and the decision to submit for publication.

Competing interests

All authors have completed the Unified Competing Interest form at http://www.icmje.org/coi_disclosure.pdf (http://www.icmje.org/coi_disclosure.pdf) (available on request from the corresponding author). SH declare support from AstraZeneca for the submitted work, and personal fees from AstraZeneca, Pfizer, BMS, Eli Lilly, Sanofi, Novartis and MSD outside of the submitted work. JJ declare support from AstraZeneca for the submitted work, and personal fees from AstraZeneca, Pfizer and Sanofi outside of the submitted work. PH is employed by AstraZeneca. MT is employed by an independent statistical consultant company, Statisticon, for which AstraZeneca is a client. EØ declare support from Astra Zeneca for the submitted work, and personal fees from AstraZeneca, Pfizer, BMS, Takeda, Novartis, Sanofi and MSD outside of the submitted work.

Author details

[1]Department of Cardiology, Oslo University Hospital Ulleval and University of Oslo, Postboks 4956, Nydalen 0424, Oslo, Norway. [2]Department of Cardiology, Sørlandet Hospital, Arendal, Norway. [3]AstraZeneca NordicBaltic, Södertälje, Sweden. [4]Statisticon, Uppsala, Sweden. [5]Department of Internal Medicine, Diakonhjemmet Hospital, and Center for Heart Failure Research, University of Oslo, Oslo, Norway.

References

1. Patient statistics, 2014. Available at: https://www.ssb.no/en/helse/statistikker/pasient. Accessed 1 Oct 2015.

2. Jortveit J, Govatsmark RE, Digre TA, Risøe C, Hole T, Mannsverk J, Slørdahl SA, Halvorsen S. Myocardial infarction in Norway in 2013. Tidsskr Nor Legeforen. 2014;134:1841–6.

3. Task Force for Diagnosis and Treatment of Non-ST-Segment Elevation Acute Coronary Syndromes of European Society of Cardiology, Bassand JP, Hamm CW, Ardissino D, Boersma E, Budaj A, et al. Guidelines for the diagnosis and treatment of non-ST-segment elevation acute coronary syndromes. Eur Heart J. 2007;28:1598–660.

4. Hamm CW, Bassand JP, Agewall S, Bax J, Boersma E, Bueno H, Caso P, Dudek D, Gielen S, Huber K, Ohman M, Petrie MC, Sonntag F, Uva MS, Storey RF, Wijns W, Zahger D. ESC Committee for Practice Guidelines ESC Guidelines for the management of acute coronary syndromes in patients presenting without persistent ST-segment elevation: The task force for the management of acute coronary syndromes (ACS) in patients presenting without persistent ST-segment elevation of the European Society of Cardiology. Eur Heart J. 2011;32:2999–54.

5. Van de Werf F, Bax J, Betriu A, Blomstrom-Lundqvist C, Crea F, Falk V, Filippatos G, Fox K, Huber K, Kastrati A, Rosengren A, Steg PG, Tubaro M, Verheugt F, Weidinger F, Weis M. ESC Committee for Practice Guidelines (CPG). Management of acute myocardial infarction in patients presenting with persistent ST-segment elevation: the Task Force on the Management of ST-Segment Elevation Acute Myocardial Infarction of the European Society of Cardiology. Eur Heart J. 2008;29:2909–45.

6. Steg PG, James SK, Atar D, Badano LP, Blömstrom-Lundqvist C, Borger MA, Di Mario C, Dickstein K, Ducrocq G, Fernandez-Aviles F, Gershlick AH, Giannuzzi P, Halvorsen S, Huber K, Juni P, Kastrati A, Knuuti J, Lenzen MJ, Mahaffey KW, Valgimigli M, van't Hof A, Widimsky P, Zahger D. ESC Guidelines for the management of acute myocardial infarction in patients presenting with ST-segment elevation. Eur Heart J. 2012;33:2569–19.

7. Jneid H, Anderson JL, Wright RS, Adams CD, Bridges CR, Casey Jr DE, Ettinger SM, Fesmire FM, Ganiats TG, Lincoff AM, Peterson ED, Philippides GJ, Theroux P, Wenger NK, Zidar JP, Anderson JL. American College of Cardiology Foundation; American Heart Association Task Force on Practice Guidelines. 2012 ACCF/AHA focused update of the guideline for the management of patients with unstable angina/Non-ST-elevation myocardial infarction (updating the 2007 guideline and replacing the 2011 focused update): a report of the American College of Cardiology Foundation/American Heart Association Task Force on practice guidelines. Circulation. 2012;126:875–910.

8. Sørensen R, Gislason GH, Fosbøl EL, Rasmussen S, Køber L, Madsen JK, Torp-Pedersen C, Abildstrom SZ. Initiation and persistence with clopidogrel treatment after acute myocardial infarction: a nationwide study. Br J Clin Pharmacol. 2008;66:875–84.

9. Varenhorst C, Jensevik K, Jernberg T, Sundstrom A, Hasvold P, Held C, Lagerqvist B, James S. Duration of dual antiplatelet treatment with clopidogrel and aspirin in patients with acute coronary syndrome. Eur Heart J. 2014;35:969–78.

10. Hambraeus K, Tydén P, Lindahl B. Time trends and gender differences in prevention guideline adherence and outcome after myocardial infarction: Data from the SWEDEHEART registry. Eur J Prev Cardiol. 2015. [Epub ahead of print]

11. Kotseva K, Wood D, De Backer G, De Bacquer D, Pyörälä K, Keil U. EUROASPIRE Study Group EUROASPIRE III: a survey on the lifestyle, risk factors and use of cardioprotective drug therapies in coronary patients from 22 European countries. Eur J Cardiovasc Prev Rehabil. 2009;16:121–37.

12. Gislason GH, Rasmussen JN, Abildstrøm SZ, Gadsbøll N, Buch P, Friberg J, Rasmussen S, Køber L, Stender S, Madsen M, Torp-Pedersen C. Long-term compliance with beta-blockers, angiotensin-converting enzyme inhibitors, and statins after acute myocardial infarction. Eur Heart J. 2006;27:1153–8.

13. Shore S, Jones PG, Maddox TM, Bradley SM, Stolker JM, Arnold SV, Parashar S, Peterson P, Bhatt DL, Spertus J, Ho PM. Longitudinal persistence with secondary prevention therapies relative to patient risk after myocardial infarction. Heart. 2015;101:800–7.

14. Bakken IJ, Nyland K, Halsteinli V, Kvam U, Skjeldestad F. Norsk pasientregister: administrativ database med mange forskningsmuligheter. Nor Epidemiol. 2004;14:65–9.

15. Furu K, Wettermark B, Andersen M, Martikainen JE, Almarsdottir AB, Sørensen HT. The Nordic countries as a cohort for pharmacoepidemiological research. Basic Clin Pharmacol Toxicol. 2010;106:86–94.

16. The Cause of Death Register. https://www.ssb.no/en/helse/statistikker/pasient10. Accessed 1 Oct 2015.

17. Core Team R. R Foundation for Statistical Computing. Vienna: Austria. URL; 2015. R: A language and environment for statistical computing, https://www.r-project.org/.

18. Jernberg T, Hasvold P, Henriksson M, Hjelm H, Thuresson M, Janzon M. Cardiovascular risk in post-myocardial infarction patients: nationwide real world data demonstrate the importance of a long-term perspective. Eur Heart J. 2015;36:1163–70.

19. Angerås O, Hasvold P, Thuresson M, Deleskog A, Braun O. Treatment pattern of contemporary dual antiplatelet therapies after acute coronary syndrome: a Swedish nationwide population-based cohort study. Scand Cardiovasc J. 2016;50:99–107.

20. Nytt om legemidler. http://tidsskriftet.no/Ekstra/Nytt-om-legemidler/Nytt-om-legemidler-2011. Accessed 1 Oct 2015.

21. Hassani S, Lindman AS, Kristoffersen DT, Tomic O, Helgeland J. 30-Day Survival Probabilities as a Quality Indicator for Norwegian Hospitals: Data Management and Analysis. PLoS One. 2015;10, e0136547.

15

Expression of circulating miR-486 and miR-150 in patients with acute myocardial infarction

Rui Zhang, Chao Lan, Hui Pei, Guoyu Duan, Li Huang and Li Li[*]

Abstract

Background: With its high morbidity and mortality, acute myocardial infarction (AMI) places a major burden on society and on individual patients. Correct, early correct diagnosis is crucial to the management of AMI.

Methods: In this study, the expression of circulating miR-486 and miR-150 was investigated in AMI patients and the two miRNAs were evaluated as potential biomarkers for AMI. Plasma samples from 110 patients with AMI (65 patients with ST-segment elevation myocardial infarction (STEMI) and 45 patients with non-ST-segment elevation myocardial infarction (NSTEMI)) and 110 healthy adults were collected. Circulating levels of miR-486 and miR-150 were detected using quantitative real-time PCR in plasma samples.

Results: Results showed that the levels of miR-486 and miR-150 were significantly higher in AMI patients than in healthy controls. Receiver operating characteristic (ROC) curve analyses indicated that the two plasma miRNAs were of significant diagnostic value for AMI, especially NSTEMI. The combined ROC analysis revealed an AUC value of 0.771 in discriminating AMI patients from healthy controls and an AUC value of 0.845 in discriminating NSTEMI patients from healthy controls.

Conclusion: Results indicated that the levels of circulating miR-486 and miR-150 are associated with AMI. They may be novel and powerful biomarkers for AMI, especially for NSTEMI.

Keywords: Acute myocardial infarction, MicroRNAs, Biomarker

Background

Acute myocardial infarction (AMI) is the acute necrosis of myocardial tissue due to persistent and severe ischemia [1]. AMI is one of the most frequently occurring cardiovascular diseases and one of the leading causes of morbidity and mortality in both developed and developing countries [2–4]. With China's aging population and the projected increase in the rate of this disease, it is estimated that 16 million people will suffer from AMI in 2020 and 23 million in 2030 [5]. Because it is the world's largest developing country, China is challenged to provide care for its large and growing population of AMI patients [6]. AMI is separated into two categories based on changes seen in the electrocardiography (ECG): ST-segment elevation myocardial infarction (STEMI) and non-ST-segment elevation myocardial infarction (NSTEMI). In STEMI, the

infarct-related artery is usually totally occluded by fibrin-rich clots, and immediate reperfusion therapy is the initial approach. In contrast, the initial conservative strategy or the initial invasive strategy can be taken in patients with NSTEMI whose infarct-related artery is partially occluded by platelet-rich clots. Prompt diagnosis is critical to controlling the development of AMI and initiating appropriate therapy to reduce the mortality rate and improve prognosis. ECG is significant to differentiate the two AMI types. However, ECG has several limitations. For example, normal findings do not exclude the possibility of AMI. NSTEMI patients are often misdiagnosed because they frequently lack typical symptoms and obvious elevated ST-segment in their ECG. At present, some conventional biomarkers, such as blood troponins, cardiac myoglobin and creatine kinase-MB (CK-MB) are wildly used for clinical diagnosis [7]. However, the search for novel biomarkers for AMI is ongoing.

In recent years, with advances in molecular biology and technology, nucleotide-based biomarkers that may enhance diagnostic or prognostic effectiveness have attracted

* Correspondence: lilieme@126.com
Department of emergency, The First Affiliated Hospital of Zhengzhou University, No.1 Jianshe Road, Zhengzhou, Henan 450052, China

considerable attention. MicroRNAs (miRNAs) are small, non-coding, cellular RNAs 17–27 nucleotides in length. By pairing with the 3' UTR of target mRNAs, they act as sequence-specific regulators of gene expression through translational repression and transcript cleavage [8, 9]. Many studies suggest that miRNAs play crucial roles in a variety of essential biological processes, including proliferation, development, differentiation, and apoptosis [10]. Aberrant expression of miRNAs in tissues contributes to various diseases, such as cancer and cardiovascular disease [11–13]. In addition, many miRNAs are remarkably stable and readily detectable in the peripheral blood or plasma [14, 15]. The levels of circulating miRNAs are different in specific ways under specific pathological conditions [16–18]. This indicates that circulating miRNAs may be excellent candidate diagnostic and prognostic biomarkers of various diseases [19, 20]. Recently, it has been reported that the levels of several miRNAs such as miR-1, miR-133a, miR-208b, miR-499, and miR-328 in the blood and plasma alter during AMI, suggesting the diagnostic value of circulating miRNAs in early AMI [21–26].

It has been reported that miR-486 is a potent modulator in cardiac/skeletal muscle and miR-150 is involved in many cardiovascular diseases [27]. We also performed a preliminary plasma miRNA microassay chip analysis of AMI patients and healthy controls and the results showed significant changes in the levels of miR-486 and miR-150 in AMI patients which was in accordance with a recent study about serum miR-486 and miR-150 [28]. The purpose of the present study was to measure the levels of circulating miR-486 and miR-150 in AMI patients, so as to determine whether miR-486 and miR-150 could serve as novel biomarkers for the early diagnosis of AMI.

Methods

Patient characteristics

This study was approved by the Research Ethics Committee of Zhengzhou University, China, and the samples were collected with each patient's informed consent.

One hundred and ten consecutive AMI patients were enrolled in this study from the First Affiliated Hospital of Zhengzhou University between June 2013 and May 2014. The clinical characteristics of all patients are given in Table 1. AMI patients were diagnosed using the following criteria: 1) acute ischemic chest pain; 2) abnormal electrocardiogram (pathological Q wave, ST-segment elevation, or depression); 3) levels of myocardial necrosis markers (troponins (cTns) and creatine kinase (CK)) more than twice the upper limit of the normal range. These patients were admitted to hospital no more than 24 h after the emergence of symptoms. Patients with previous MI or percutaneous coronary intervention (PCI), any hematological disease, acute or chronic infection, significant hepatic

dysfunction, kidney failure (glomerular filtration rate (GFR) < 15 mL/min/1.73 m^2 or on dialysis), or known or treated malignancies were excluded. In addition, 110 healthy adult volunteers (normal electrocardiograms and no history of cardiovascular diseases) were enrolled in this study. Five milliliter venous blood samples of patients with AMI were collected in EDTA anticoagulant tubes at admission. Samples were centrifuged at 3000 × g for 10 min at 4 °C, then the supernatant was isolated and centrifuged at 12,000 × g for 10 min at 4 °C. Plasma was collected and stored at –80 °C until RNA extraction.

RNA extraction

Total RNA was extracted from plasma using an miRNeasy Serum/Plasm Kit (Qiagen), in accordance with the manufacturer's instructions. The RNA was dissolved in 20 µl of diethylpyrocarbonate-treated (DEPC-treated) water. The concentration and quality of the RNA samples were determined using NanoDrop2000c spectrophotometer (NanoDrop, Thermo Fisher Scientific, U.S.).

Quantitative reverse transcription-polymerase chain reaction (qRT-PCR)

The levels of expression of miR-486 or miR-150 were quantified using quantitative real-time PCR (qRT-PCR) using TaqMan human microRNA assay kits (Applied Biosystems) according to the manufacturer's instructions. The 15 µL RT reaction mix contains 0.3 µL of 100 mM dNTPs, 3 µL of MultiScribe Reverse Transcriptase (50 U/µL), 1.5 µL of 10 × RT buffer, 0.19 µL of RNase inhibitor (20 U/µL), 6 µL of RT primer, 3 µL of RNA sample and 1.01 µL of Nuclease-free water. For RNA from plasma samples, the concentration was diluted to 180 ng/µL. The reagent mixes were incubated at 16 °C for 30 min, 42 °C for 30 min and 85 °C for 5 min, the RT products were stored at – 20 °C until used for qRT-PCR. The 20 µL PCR reaction mix includes 1.0 µL 20 × TaqMan MicroRNA Assays, 0.16 µL RT product, 10 µL TaqMan Universal Master Mix II, No AmpErase UNG (2×), 8.84 µL Nuclease-free water. The PCR cycles consisted of an initial denaturation at 95 °C for 10 min, followed by 40 cycles of 95 °C for 15 s and 60 °C for 60 s. U6 snRNA served as an internal normalized reference. Each specimen was measured in triplicate. The relative expression values of each miRNA were calculated using the $2^{-\Delta Ct}$ method.

Biochemical assays

The concentrations of plasma cardiac troponin T (cTnT) were measured using a Roche high-sensitivity assay performed on a Cobas C8000 system (Roche Diagnostics, Germany) with a detection limit of 0.003 µg/L, a 99th-percentile cutoff of 0.014 µg/L, and a CV of ≤10 % at

Table 1 Clinical features, risk factors, and laboratory data of the cohort

Characteristics	All cohort (n = 220)	AMI cases (n = 110)		Control cases (n = 110)	P
		STEMI (n = 65)	NSTEMI (n = 45)		
Age (years)	57.99 ± 11.63	57.54 ± 12.07	57.93 ± 11.98	58.28 ± 11.32	0.712
Men/women (n/n)	170/50	51/14	36/9	83/27	0.520
Risk factors					
Hypertension (Y/N)	103/117	34/31	17/28	52/58	0.893
Hyperlipidemia (Y/N)	26/119	9/56	3/42	14/96	0.676
Diabetes mellitus (Y/N)	50/170	13/52	10/35	27/83	0.520
Smoking (Y/N)	47/173	15/50	8/37	24/86	0.869
Physical examination					
SBP (mmHg)	124.64 ± 18.89	125.88 ± 21.51	121.76 ± 16.35	124.23 ± 20.26	0.754
DBP (mmHg)	75.95 ± 11.58	76.68 ± 13.70	73.31 ± 9.60	77.30 ± 10.68	0.132
Heart rate (beats/ min)	74.10 ± 12.98	74.20 ± 13.03	75.38 ± 11.54	73.53 ± 13.57	0.511
Lab examination					
TC (mmol/L)	3.9232 ± 0.99	3.91 ± 1.07	3.92 ± 1.09	3.90 ± 0.91	0.998
TG (mmol/L)	1.3727 ± 0.80	1.48 ± 1.17	1.39 ± 0.88	1.30 ± 0.42	0.197
HDL (mmol/L)	1.0470 ± 0.22	0.98 ± 0.23	1.05 ± 0.27	1.09 ± 0.18	0.080
LDL (mmol/L)	2.5300 ± 1.00	2.52 ± 0.97	2.43 ± 0.87	2.58 ± 1.08	0.504
WBC (×10^9/L)	8.589 ± 3.62	9.51 ± 4.13	10.02 ± 4.01	7.46 ± 2.68	<0.001
BUN (mmol/L)	5.9365 ± 2.73	6.25 ± 3.05	6.16 ± 2.64	5.66 ± 2.55	0.135
CK-MB (U/L)	35.68 ± 59.13	58.80 ± 90.75	48.46 ± 58.17	16.79 ± 8.63	<0.001
Cardiac troponin T (ng/mL)	0.68 ± 1.40	1.44 ± 1.89	1.16 ± 1.57	0.05 ± 0.12	<0.001
EF%	58.14 ± 7.83	56.35 ± 7.89	55.80 ± 8.28	60.15 ± 7.13	<0.001

Abbreviations: *AMI* acute myocardial infarction, *STEMI* ST-segment-elevation myocardial infarction, *NSTEMI* non-ST-segment elevation myocardial infarction, *SBP* systolic blood pressure, *DBP* diastolic blood pressure, *TC* total cholesterol, *TG* total triglyceride, *HDL* high-density lipoprotein, *LDL* low-density lipoprotein, *WBC* white blood cell, *BUN* blood urea nitrogen, *CK-MB* creatine kinase-MB, *EF* ejection fractions
Data are expressed as mean ± standard deviation. *P*: comparison between AMI patients with healthy controls

0.013 µg/L. CK-MB was also measured on Cobas C8000 instrument with a Roche IFCC-recommended method.

Statistical analysis

Statistical treatment was performed using SPSS 20.0 software. All data were subjected to a normality test (Kolmogorov-Smirnov). Continuous data are presented as mean ± SD or median with interquartile range. Categorical variables are presented as counts and percentages. Independent sample t-tests and Mann–Whitney U tests were used to compare two groups of continuous variables and the chi-square test was used for categorical variables. Receiver operating characteristic (ROC) curve analysis and comparison of the derived area under the curve (AUC) were performed to assess miRNAs as predictors for distinguishing AMI from healthy controls. Multiple logistic regression analysis was carried out for evaluating the combined diagnostic accuracy of circulating miRNAs. The statistical significance was set at $P < 0.05$.

Results

Clinical characteristics of patients

Among 110 patients with AMI, 65 were diagnosed with STEMI and 45 were diagnosed with NSTEMI. Both the AMI group and control group were predominantly male (87/110 in the AMI group and 83/110 in the control group). The basic clinical characteristics of the patients in this study are shown in Table 1. There were no obvious differences in disease or personal history including hypertension, hyperlipidemia, diabetes, or smoking between AMI patients and control cases. Significant differences were observed between the two groups in white blood cells (WBC), CK-MB, cTnT, and the left ventricular ejection fraction (EF).

Circulating miR-486 or miR-150 levels were significantly higher in AMI patients

The blood samples of AMI patients were immediately collected after admission. We detected the miR-486 and miR-150 levels in plasma of 110 AMI patients (65

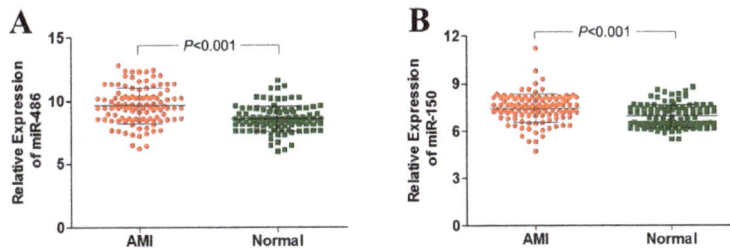

Fig. 1 Expression of circulating miRNAs in AMI patients and control group. Plasma samples were collected upon admission no more than 24 h after AMI onset. **a**: The relative expression levels of miR-486 between AMI group and control group ($P < 0.001$). **b**: The relative expression levels of miR-150 between AMI group and control group ($P < 0.001$). Results were reported as mean ± SD

STEMI patients and 45 NSTEMI patients) and 110 non-AMI controls to assess the value of circulating miRNAs levels for predicting the onset of AMI. As shown in Fig. 1a, the plasma concentrations of miR-486 were markedly higher in AMI patients than in healthy controls ($P < 0.001$). In addition, the expression of miR-150 was markedly higher during the early phase, shortly after the occurrence of AMI in patients, than in controls ($P < 0.001$) (Fig. 1b).

Circulating miR-486 and miR-150 expression levels as predictors of AMI

To further evaluate the predictive power of circulating miR-486 and miR-150 for AMI, ROC curve and areas under ROC curve (AUC) analyses were performed. As shown in Fig. 2a and b, ROC curve analysis of miR-486 or miR-150 exhibited strong differentiation power between AMI patients and healthy controls during the early phase of AMI.

The AUC of miR-486 or miR-150 in AMI patients was 0.731 ($P < 0.001$), 0.678 ($P < 0.001$). Interestingly, the combination of the two miRNAs resulted in a higher AUC value of 0.771 ($P < 0.001$) than the AUC of miR-486 or miR-150 (Fig. 2a, b, c). These data suggested that the combination of circulating miR-486 and miR-150, which both

had both high sensitivity and specificity, might be more suitable than miR-486 or miR-150 alone for diagnosing AMI.

Expression pattern of miR-486 and miR-150 in STEMI and NSTEMI

A follow-up investigation was performed to determine whether the plasma miRNA levels in patients were associated with specific types of AMI. There was distinct difference between the level of plasma miR-486 ($P = 0.015$) and miR-150 ($P = 0.016$) between STEMI patients and NSTEMI patients (Fig. 3a and b). ROC curve analysis of miRNAs showed the AUC of plasma miR-486 and miR-150 in STEMI patients to be 0.695 and 0.639, respectively (Fig. 4a and b), which was lower than in NSTEMI patients (0.782, 0.734) (Fig. 4d and e). There was also a higher AUC value, 0.845, for the combination of miR-486 and miR-150 in the NSTEMI group than in the STEMI group (Fig. 4c and f). These data suggested miR-486 or miR-150 were highly sensitive and specific for the discrimination of NSTEMI cases from controls, and the combination of the two miRNAs was shown to predict NSTEMI with even higher power.

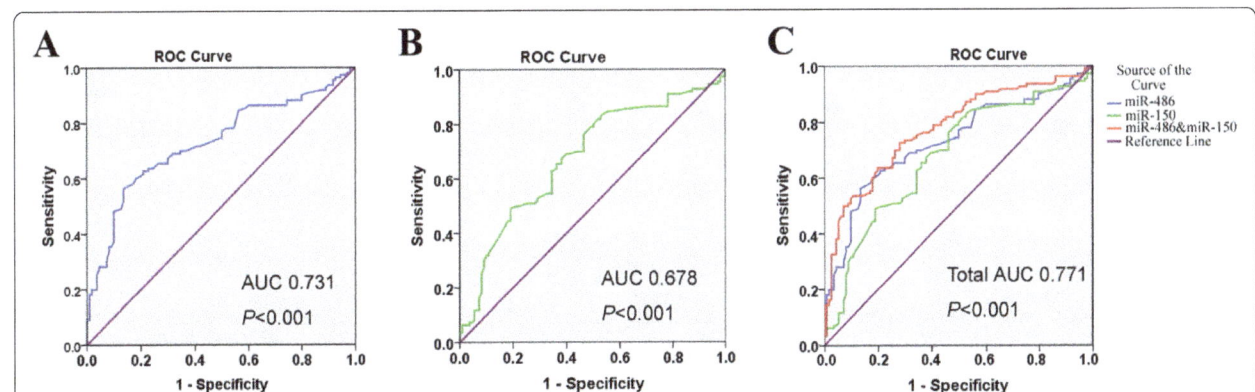

Fig. 2 Receive operating characteristic (ROC) curves analyzed for the diagnostic value of circulating miRNAs. ROC curve for plasma (**a**) miR-486, (**b**) miR-150, and (**c**) the combination of the two miRNAs were able to distinguish AMI from the control group

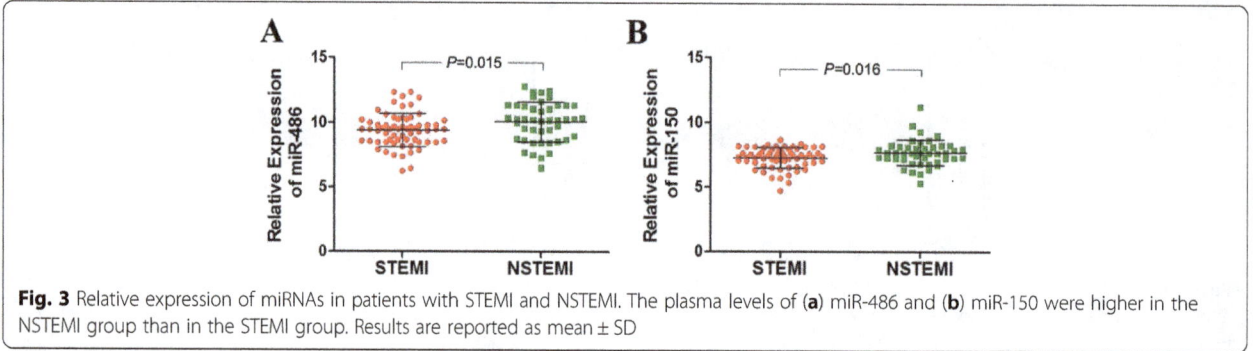

Fig. 3 Relative expression of miRNAs in patients with STEMI and NSTEMI. The plasma levels of (**a**) miR-486 and (**b**) miR-150 were higher in the NSTEMI group than in the STEMI group. Results are reported as mean ± SD

Discussion

AMI remains an important cause of death in the world. Early and reliable diagnosis may prompt patients to undergo reperfusion therapy early and this may improve the survival rate of AMI patients.

Recent studies have revealed that miRNA are important regulators in the pathogenesis of many diseases. Results have demonstrated that miRNAs can be exported or released by cells and circulate in bloodstream; these are called circulating miRNAs [29]. Numerous circulating miRNAs are involved in AMI. These include cardiac-specific miRNAs (miR-208a) and non-cardiac-specific miRNAs (miR-126, miR-328, miR-134) [30–33]. On account of their tissue specificity, rapid release kinetics and stability in plasma, circulating miRNAs are considered promising biomarkers for detecting a large number of diseases, especially cardiovascular diseases. However, studies on the expression of circulating miRNAs in AMI patients are limited.

In this study, qRT-PCR results showed that plasma miR-486 and miR-150 were visibly overexpressed in 110 AMI patients. The ROC analyses showed that the two miRNAs might be suitable diagnostic markers of AMI. Here, the expression of miRNAs was measured in STEMI patients and NSTEMI patients. There was a distinct difference in levels of miR-486 and miR-150 expression between the STEMI and NSTEMI groups. The results of

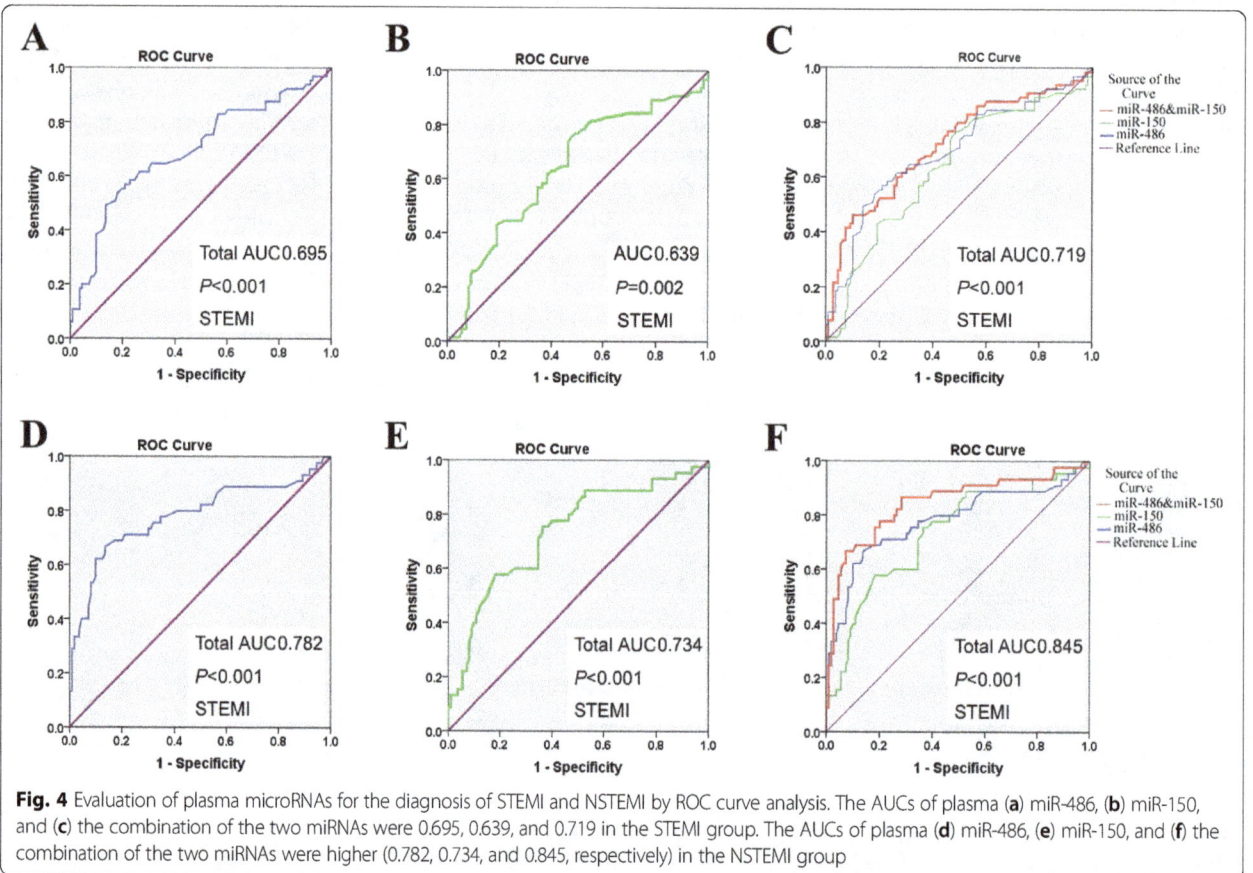

Fig. 4 Evaluation of plasma microRNAs for the diagnosis of STEMI and NSTEMI by ROC curve analysis. The AUCs of plasma (**a**) miR-486, (**b**) miR-150, and (**c**) the combination of the two miRNAs were 0.695, 0.639, and 0.719 in the STEMI group. The AUCs of plasma (**d**) miR-486, (**e**) miR-150, and (**f**) the combination of the two miRNAs were higher (0.782, 0.734, and 0.845, respectively) in the NSTEMI group

ROC analyses indicated that miR-486 and miR-150 are specific and sensitive for the early diagnosis of NSTEMI.

miR-486 is a muscle-enriched miRNA. It was found to be downregulated in several muscular diseases, such as Duchenne's muscular dystrophy and denervation-induced muscle atrophy [34, 35]. Overexpression of miR-486 could lead to muscle hypertrophy. The upregulation of circulating miR-486 in AMI patients may be related to cardiac hypertrophy. miR-150, an miRNA related to inflammation, was reported to be implicated in the pathogenesis of various cardiovascular diseases [36–38]. A microarray screen of plasma samples showed reduced levels of miR-150 in patients with pulmonary arterial hypertension compared to healthy controls. Moreover, plasma miR-150 level in these patients was a significant predictor of survival [39]. miR-150 was also dysregulated in serum of patients with unstable angina pectoris. The diagnostic accuracy for unstable angina pectoris was obviously improved by applying the miRNA panel including miR-132, miR-150, and miR-186 [40]. Furthermore, miR-150 may inhibit cardiac structural and functional remodeling during ischemic injury partly by direct repression of the pro-apoptotic gene egr2 and p2x7r (pro-inflammatory ATP receptor) in cardiomyocytes [41]. In addition, the transcription factor c-Myb, NOTCH3 receptor, and nonmetastatic melanoma protein B were the potential targets of miR-150. Dysregulation of these two miRNAs may be associated with pathological conditions other than cardiac damage.

Conclusion

In conclusion, results demonstrated that miR-486 and miR-150 levels to be significantly high in the plasma of AMI patients, both STEMI and NSTEMI, suggesting that circulating miR-486 and miR-150 might be responsible for the onset of AMI, especially NSTEMI. It is possible that miR-486 and miR-150 could be suitable biomarkers against AMI.

Abbreviations
AMI: Acute myocardial infarction; STEMI: ST-segment elevation myocardial infarction; NSTEMI: Non-ST-segment elevation myocardial infarction.

Competing interests
The authors declare that they have no competing interests.

Authors' contributions
LL, RZ and CL conceived of the study, participated in its design and coordination, and helped to draft the manuscript. HP, GYD and LH collected the samples. CL, RZ, HP, GYD and LH carried out some of the experiments and composed the manuscript. HP, RZ and LL performed the statistical analysis. All authors have read and approved the final manuscript.

Acknowledgements
This research was supported by the innovation foundation of youth in the First Affiliated Hospital of Zhengzhou University.

References
1. White HD, Chew DP. Acute myocardial infarction. Lancet. 2008;372(9638):570–84.
2. Yusuf S, Reddy S, Ounpuu S, Anand S. Global burden of cardiovascular diseases: part I: general considerations, the epidemiologic transition, risk factors, and impact of urbanization. Circulation. 2001;104(22):2746–53.
3. Sodha NR, Clements RT, Feng J, Liu Y, Bianchi C, Horvath EM, et al. Hydrogen sulfide therapy attenuates the inflammatory response in a porcine model of myocardial ischemia/reperfusion injury. J Thorac Cardiovasc Surg. 2009;138(4):977–84.
4. Ueshima H, Sekikawa A, Miura K, Turin TC, Takashima N, Kita Y, et al. Cardiovascular disease and risk factors in Asia: a selected review. Circulation. 2008;118(25):2702–9.
5. Moran A, Gu D, Zhao D, Coxson P, Wang YC, Chen CS, et al. Future cardiovascular disease in china: markov model and risk factor scenario projections from the coronary heart disease policy model-china. Circ Cardiovasc Qual Outcomes. 2010;3(3):243–52.
6. Yang G, Wang Y, Zeng Y, Gao GF, Liang X, Zhou M, et al. Rapid health transition in china, 1990–2010: findings from the global burden of disease study 2010. Lancet. 2013;381(9882):1987–2015.
7. Jaffe AS, Ravkilde J, Roberts R, Naslund U, Apple FS, Galvani M, et al. It's time for a change to a troponin standard. Circulation. 2000;102(11):1216–20.
8. Zamore PD, Haley B. Ribo-genome: the big world of small RNAs. Science. 2005;309(5740):1519–24.
9. Mattick JS, Makunin IV: Non-coding RNA. Hum Mol Genet 2006, 15 Sepc No 1:R17-29.
10. Plasterk RH. Micro RNAs in animal development. Cell. 2006;124(5):877–81.
11. Small EM, Olson EN. Prevasive roles of microRNAs in cardiovascular biology. Nature. 2011;469(7330):336–42.
12. Meltzer PS. Cancer genomics: small RNAs with big impacts. Nature. 2005;435(7043):745–6.
13. Sayed D, Abdellatif M. MicroRNAs in development and disease. Physiol Rev. 2011;91(3):827–87.
14. van Rooij E, Liu N, Olson EN. MicroRNAs flex their muscles. Trends Genet. 2008;24(4):159–66.
15. Lagos-Quintana M, Rauhut R, Yalcin A, Meyer J, Lendeckel W, Tuschl T. Identification of tissue-specific microRNAs from mouse. Curr Biol. 2002;12(9):735–9.
16. van Empel VP, De Windt LJ, da Costa Martins PA. Circulating miRNAs: reflecting or affecting cardiovascular disease? Curr Hypertens Rep. 2012;14(6):498–509.
17. Kloosterman WP, Plasterk RH. The diverse functions of microRNAs in animal development and disease. Dev Cell. 2006;11(4):441–50.
18. Mitchell PS, Parkin RK, Kroh EM, Fritz BR, Wyman SK, Pogosova-Agadjanyan EL, et al. Circulating microRNAs as stable blood-based markers for cancer detection. Proc Natl Acad Sci U S A. 2008;105(30):10513–8.
19. Gilad S, Meiri E, Yogev Y, Benjamin S, Lebanony D, Yerushalmi N, et al. Serum microRNAs are promising novel biomarkers. PLoS One. 2008;3(9), e3148.
20. Chen X, Ba Y, Ma L, Cai X, Yin Y, Wang K, et al. Characterization of microRNAs in serum: a novel class of biomarkers for diagnosis of cancer and other diseases. Cell Res. 2008;18(10):997–1006.
21. Häntzsch M, Tolios A, Beutner F, Nagel D, Thiery J, Teupser D, et al. Comparison of whole blood RNA preservation tubes and novel generation RNA extraction kits for analysis of mRNA and MiRNA profiles. PLoS One. 2014;9(12), e113298.
22. Zhou H, He XY, Zhuang SW, Wang J, Lai Y, Qi WG, et al. Clinical and procedural predictors of no-reflow in patients with acute myocardial infarction after primary percutaneous coronary intervention. World J Emerg Med. 2014;5(2):96–102.
23. Long G, Wang F, Duan Q, Chen F, Yang S, Gong W, et al. Human circulating microRNA-1 and microRNA-126 as potential novel indicators for acute myocardial infarction. Int J Biol Sci. 2012;8(6):811–8.
24. Bostjancic E, Zidar N, Stajer D, Glavac D. MicroRNAs miR-1, miR-133a, miR-133b and miR-208 are dysregulated in human myocardial infarction. Cardiology. 2010;115(3):163–9.
25. Xiao J, Shen B, Li J, Lv D, Zhao Y, Wang F, et al. Serum microRNA-499 and microRNA-208a as biomarkers of acute myocardial infarction. Int J Clin Exp Med. 2014;7(1):136–41.
26. He F, Lv P, Zhao X, Wang X, Ma X, Meng W, et al. Predictive value of circulating miR-328 and miR-134 for acute myocardial infarction. Mol Cell Biochem. 2014;394(1–2):137–44.
27. Chen D, Goswami CP, Burnett RM, Anjanappa M, Bhat-Nakshatri P, Muller W, et al. Cancer affects microRNA expression, release, and function in cardiac and skeletal muscle. Cancer Res. 2014;74(16):4270–81.

28. Hsu A, Chen SJ, Chang YS, Chen HC, Chu PH. Systemic approach to identify serum microRNAs as potential biomarkers for acute myocardial infarction. Biomed Res Int. 2014;2014:418628.

29. Zheng HW, Wang YL, Lin JX, Li N, Zhao XQ, Liu GF, et al. Circulating MicroRNAs as potential risk biomarkers for hematoma enlargement after intracerebral hemorrhage. CNS Neurosci Ther. 2012;18(12):1003–11.

30. Olivieri F, Antonicelli R, Capogrossi MC, Procopio AD. Circulating microRNAs (miRs) for diagnosing acute myocardial infarction: an exciting challenge. Int J Cardiol. 2013;167(6):3028–9.

31. Recchioni R, Marcheselli F, Olivieri F, Ricci S, Procopio AD, Antonicelli R. Conventional and novel diagnostic biomarkers of acute myocardial infarction: a promising role for circulating microRNAs. Biomarkers. 2013;18(7):547–58.

32. Sayed AS, Xia K, Yang TL, Peng J. Circulating microRNAs: a potential role in diagnosis and prognosis of acute myocardial infarction. Dis Markers. 2013;35(5):561–6.

33. Kuwabara Y, Ono K, Horie T, Nishi H, Nagao K, Kinoshita M, et al. Increased microRNA-1 and microRNA-133a levels in serum of patients with cardiovascular disease indicate myocardial damage. Circ Cardiovasc Genet. 2011;4(4):446–54.

34. Small EM, O'Rourke JR, Moresi V, Sutherland LB, McAnally J, Gerard RD, et al. Regulation of PI3-kinase/Akt signaling by muscle-enriched microRNA-486. Proc Natl Acad Sci U S A. 2010;107(9):4218–23.

35. Alexander MS, Casar JC, Motohashi N, Myers JA, Eisenberg I, Gonzalez RT, et al. Regulation of DMD pathology by an ankyrin-encoded miRNA. Skelet Muscle. 2011;1:27.

36. Devaux Y, Vausort M, McCann GP, Zangrando J, Kelly D, Razvi N, et al. MicroRNA-150: a novel marker of left ventricular remodeling after acute myocardial infarction. Circ Cardiovasc Genet. 2013;6(3):290–8.

37. Devaux Y, Vausort M, McCann GP, Kelly D, Collignon O, Ng LL, et al. A panel of 4 microRNAs facilitates the prediction of left ventricular contractility after acute myocardial infarction. PLoS One. 2013;8(8), e70644.

38. Li X, Kong M, Jiang D, Qian J, Duan Q, Dong A. MicroRNA-150 aggravates H2O2-induced cardiac myocyte injury by down-regulating c-myb gene. Acta Biochim Biophys Sin (Shanghai). 2013;45(9):734–41.

39. Rhodes CJ, Wharton J, Boon RA, Roexe T, Tsang H, Wojciak-Stothard B, et al. Reduced microRNA-150 is associated with poor survival in pulmonary arterial hypertension. Am J Respir Crit Care Med. 2013;187(3):294–302.

40. Zeller T, Keller T, Ojeda F, Reichlin T, Twerenbold R, Tzikas S, et al. Assessment of microRNAs in patients with unstable angina pectoris. Eur Heart J. 2014;35(31):2106–14.

41. Tang Y, Wang Y, Park KM, Hu Q, Teoh JP, Broskova Z, Ranganathan P, Jayakumar C, Li J, Su H, Tang Y, Ramesh G, Kim IM: MicroRNA-150 protects the mouse heart from ischemic injury by regulating cell death. Cardiovasc Res 2015 (in press).

16

Is non-HDL-cholesterol a better predictor of long-term outcome in patients after acute myocardial infarction compared to LDL-cholesterol?

Wanwarang Wongcharoen, Satjatham Sutthiwutthichai, Siriluck Gunaparn and Arintaya Phrommintikul*

Abstract

Background: It has recently been shown that non-high density lipoprotein cholesterol (non-HDL-C) may be a better predictor of cardiovascular risk than low density lipoprotein cholesterol (LDL-C). Based on known ethic differences in lipid parameters and cardiovascular risk prediction, we sought to study the predictability of attaining non-HDL-C target and long-term major adverse cardiovascular event (MACE) in Thai patients after acute myocardial infarction (AMI) compared to attaining LDL-C target.

Methods: We retrospectively obtained the data of all patients who were admitted at Maharaj Nakorn Chiang Mai hospital due to AMI during 2006–2013. The mean non-HDL-C and LDL-C during long-term follow-up were used to predict MACE at each time point. The patients were classified as target attainment if non-HDL-C <100 mg/dl and/or LDL-C <70 mg/dl. The MACE was defined as combination of all-cause death, nonfatal coronary event and nonfatal stroke.

Results: During mean follow-up of 2.6 ± 1.6 years among 868 patients after AMI, 34.4% achieved non-HDL-C target, 23.7% achieved LDL-C target and 21.2% experienced MACEs. LDL-C and non-HDL-C were directly compared in Cox regression model. Compared with non-HDL-C <100 mg/dl, patients with non-HDL-C of >130 mg/dl had higher incidence of MACEs (HR 3.15, 95% CI 1.46–6.80, $P = 0.003$). Surprisingly, LDL-C >100 mg/dl was associated with reduced risk of MACE as compared to LDL <70 mg/dl (HR 0.42, 95% CI 0.18–0.98, $p = 0.046$) after direct pairwise comparison with non-HDL-C level.

Conclusions: Non-attaining non-HDL-C goal predicted MACE at long-term follow-up after AMI whereas non-attaining LDL-C goal was not associated with the higher risk. Therefore, non-HDL-C may be a more suitable target of dyslipidemia treatment than LDL-C in patients after AMI.

Keywords: Non-HDL-cholesterol, LDL-cholesterol, Acute myocardial infarction, Major adverse cardiovascular events

Background

It is well-established that low-density lipoprotein cholesterol (LDL-C) is an important risk factor for coronary heart disease. The international guidelines recommend LDL-C as a primary target of therapy in persons with hypercholesterolemia and non-high-density lipoprotein cholesterol (non-HDL-C) as a secondary target of ther-

apy in persons with triglyceride at least 200 mg/dl [1, 2].

Previous epidemiologic studies have shown that non-HDL-C is more strongly associated with coronary heart disease risk than LDL-C [3–5]. In addition, recent post-hoc analyses have demonstrated that the on-treatment level of non-HDL-C is more closely associated with cardiovascular outcome than levels of LDL-C. These findings suggest that the residual risk after lipid-lowering treatment may be better quantified by non-HDL-C than by LDL-C [6].

A number of studies have shown that there are ethnic differences in risk prediction of coronary artery disease.

* Correspondence: arintaya.p@cmu.ac.th
Department of Internal Medicine, Faculty of Medicine, Chiang Mai University, Chiang Mai, Thailand

The Framingham prediction model accurately predicts the coronary artery disease risk among Caucasians and blacks living in the United States, however, it overestimates the risk in South-East Asians [7]. In addition, the data from the Electricity Generating Authority of Thailand (EGAT) cohort study showed that only HDL-C was negatively associated with cardiovascular disease mortality [8]. However, triglyceride and LDL-C were not associated with cardiovascular death in Thai population, which was inconsistent with previous studies in other ethnic populations [9]. Although a growing body of evidence supports that non-HDL-C is superior to LDL-C in predicting long-term cardiovascular risk, there is limited data in South-East Asian population.

Based on known ethic differences in lipid parameters and cardiovascular risk prediction, we sought to study the predictability of attaining non-HDL-C target and long-term cardiovascular outcome in Thai patients after acute myocardial infarction (AMI) compared to attaining LDL-C target.

Methods
Studied population
This is a retrospective cohort study. The 868 patients admitted in Maharaj Nakorn Chiang Mai hospital with a diagnosis of AMI during a period of 2006–2013 were enrolled into the study. The patients who did not have lipid profile data during the treatment and patients who had a follow-up period less than 3 months were excluded from the study.

The primary objective of the study was to assess the predictability of attaining non-HDL-C goal and LDL-C goal on the long-term major adverse cardiovascular events (MACE) occurrence in patients after AMI. The secondary objective of the study was to identify other predictors of long-term MACE occurrence in patients after AMI.

The study protocol was approved by the Medical Ethics Committee of Faculty of Medicine, Chiang Mai University.

Definitions
• Acute myocardial infarction:

  – Typical rise and/or fall of biochemical markers of myocardial necrosis with at least one of the followings:
     a. Ischemic symptoms
     b. Development of pathologic Q waves in the ECG
     c. Electrocardiographic changes indicative of ischemia (ST-segment elevation or depression)
     d. Imaging evidence of new loss of viable myocardium or new regional wall motion abnormality

• Major adverse cardiovascular outcomes

  – Defined as a composite outcome of all-cause death, myocardial infarction, stroke and cardiovascular hospitalization.

• Achieved target of non-HDL-C and LDL-C

  – The patients were classified as achieving target if the mean non-HDL-C was less than 100 mg/dL and/or the mean LDL-C was less than 70 mg/dl.
  – The patients were classified as failure to achieve target if the mean non-HDL-C was more than 130 mg/dL and/or the mean LDL-C was more than 100 mg/dl.

Data collection
The medical records of patients diagnosed with AMI and admitted in the hospital during 2006–2013 were reviewed. Data from medical record included baseline characteristic, cardiovascular risk, diagnostic data of AMI, lipid parameters, and MACE outcomes. Lipid parameters used in the data analysis included LDL-C and non-HDL-C. In this analysis, we examined the relationship between the lipid parameters at admission, the mean lipid parameters during long-term follow-up and cardiovascular outcomes (Additional file 1).

Statistical analysis
Differences between continuous variables were assessed using an unpaired 2-tailed t test for normally distributed continuous variables and the Mann-Whitney test for skewed variables. Proportions were compared by Chi-square test or Fisher exact test when appropriate. The recurrence— free survival curve was plotted via the Kaplan-Meier method with the statistical significance examined by the log-rank test. Multivariate Cox regression analysis was performed for variables with a p value of less than 0.1 in univariate analysis. All statistical significances were set at p value <0.05 and all statistical analyses were carried out by SPSS 17.0 (SPSS Inc. USA).

Results
Between 2006 and 2013, there were 868 patients admitted due to AMI and enrolled into the study. The mean age was 63 ± 11 years. There was higher prevalence of male (62%) in this population. Majority of patients presented with acute ST-segment elevation MI (STEMI). There were 20.9% presented with non-ST-segment elevation MI (non-STEMI) and only 1.5% presented with unstable angina. Among 674 patients who had ST-elevation MI, 399 (59.2%) patients underwent primary PCI, 222 (32.9%) patients received fibrinolytic therapy while 53 (7.9%) did not receive reperfusion therapy. All patients

had been receiving antiplatelets. Beta-blocker, angiotensin converting enzyme inhibitor (ACEI) and angiotensin receptor blocker (ARB) had been prescribed in 79.7%, 64.9% and 28.0% of the patients, respectively.

During a mean follow-up of 2.6 ± 1.6 years, patients had lipid parameter evaluation according to their physicians and the mean interval of lipid parameters follow-up was 6.5 ± 7.5 months. Among 868 patients, 23.7% achieved LDL-C target and 34.4% achieved non-HDL-C target. Table 1 shows the baseline characteristics of the three groups as defined by their LDL-C level: <70 mg/dl, 70–100 mg/dl, and >100 mg/dl. Table 2 shows the baseline characteristics of the three groups as defined by their non-HDL-C level: <100 mg/dl, 100–130 mg/dl, and >130 mg/dl. The patients who attained either LDL-C target or Non-HDL-C target were significantly older and had higher prevalence of chronic kidney disease, compared to those who did not attain the corresponding target. In addition, the baseline LDL-C and baseline non-HDL-C were significantly lower in those with attaining either LDL-C or non-HDL-C target. Statin had been prescribed in 93.0% of the patients, similarly across different LDL-C and non-HDL-C groups. Ezetimibe had been prescribed in addition to statin in 3.9% of the patients. There was a higher proportion of patients with mean LDL-C >100 mg/dl receiving ezetimibe compared to those with lower LDL-C level (Tables 1 and 2).

During follow up, total MACE occurred in 184 (21.2%) patients. There were 25.2, 19.0 and 21.4% of patients developed MACEs in group of LDL-C <70 mg/dl, LDL-C 70–100 mg/dl and LDL >100 mg/dl respectively. There were 20.1, 18.9 and 25.8% of patients developed MACEs in group of non-HDL-C <100 mg/dl, non-HDL-C 100–130 mg/dl and non-HDL-C >130 mg/dl respectively.

We first examined the predictability of LDL-C and long-term MACEs and the predictability of non-HDL-C and long-term MACEs individually. After cox regression analysis adjusted with age, gender, comorbidities, and baseline lipid parameters, patients with LDL70–100 mg/dl and LDL >100 mg/dl had neutral risk of long-term MACEs with the adjusted HR of 0.98 (95% CI 0.57–1.60) and 1.02 (95% CI 0.56–1.84), compared to patients with LDL-C <70 mg/dl. On the contrary, we found that non-attaining non-HDL-C goal could predict the risk of long-term MACEs. Compared to patients with non-HDL-C <100 mg/dl, those with non-HDL-C 100–130 mg/dl had a non-significantly increased risk of MACEs (adjusted HR 1.10; 95% CI 0.65–1.85) and those with non-HDL-C >130 mg/dl had significantly higher risk of long-term MACEs (adjusted HR 1.75; 95% CI 1.02–3.00, $P = 0.04$).

Then, we directly compared the strengths of the association of LDL-C and non-HDL-C with long-term MACEs by including LDL-C and non-HDL-C in the Cox model simultaneously. We demonstrated the stronger association

Table 1 Baseline characteristics of patients among different mean LDL-C groups

Parameter	LDL-C <70 mg/dl (N = 206, 24%)	LDL-C 70–100 mg/dl (N = 405, 46%)	LDL-C >100 mg/dl (N = 257, 30%)	P-value
Age (years)	66.0 ± 11.2	63.3 ± 11.0	60.7 ± 11.1	<0.001
Male	65.6%	62.2%	58.7%	0.312
Body mass index (kg/m^2)	22.5 ± 4.4	22.8 ± 4.5	23.5 ± 5.2	0.122
LVEF (%)	50.0 ± 13.8	50.1 ± 13.8	50.9 ± 14.0	0.772
Creatinine (mg/dl)	2.2 ± 10.2	1.6 ± 2.2	1.7 ± 7.6	0.492
Hemoglobin (g/dl)	12.5 ± 2.8	12.4 ± 2.1	12.7 ± 2.0	0.224
Baseline LDL-C (mg/dl)	97.3 ± 38.5	111.2 ± 39.0	135.3 ± 44.0	<0.001
Baseline non-HDL-C (mg/dl)	121.9 ± 39.5	137.5 ± 43.9	162.7 ± 48.6	<0.001
Baseline HDL-C (mg/dl)	40.4 ± 11.3	39.2 ± 11.6	40.4 ± 9.6	0.322
Smoking	38.0%	35.6%	37.4%	0.714
Hypertension	61.2%	57.3%	53.3%	0.222
Dyslipidemia	29.6%	30.4%	38.1%	0.978
Diabetes mellitus	30.1%	27.4%	24.1%	0.348
Chronic kidney disease	9.7%	7.9%	3.9%	0.039
History of CAD	10.2%	8.9%	12/1%	0.419
History of stroke	4.9%	4.2%	4.7%	0.921
STEMI	78.0%	80.0%	73.7%	0.190
Statin	92.2%	93.8%	92.2%	0.65
Ezetimibe	2.4%	2.5%	7.4%	0.003

CAD coronary artery disease, *LVEF* left ventricular ejection fraction, *STEMI* ST elevation myocardial infarction

Table 2 Baseline characteristics of patients among different mean non-HDL-C groups

Parameter	Non-HDL-C <100 mg/dl (N = 299, 34%)	Non-HDL-C 100–130 mg/dl (N = 333, 38%)	Non-HDL-C >130 mg/dl (N = 236, 27%)	P-value
Age (years)	65.9 ± 11.0	62.5 ± 11.1	60.6 ± 11.0	<0.001
Male	66.2%	60.1%	59.3%	0.173
Body mass index (kg/m²)	22.5 ± 4.5	23.0 ± 5.5	23.4 ± 3.9	0.252
LVEF (%)	49.9 ± 14.4	50.8 ± 13.0	50.0 ± 14.2	0.715
Creatinine (mg/dl)	2.1 ± 8.7	1.7 ± 6.8	1.4 ± 2.2	0.528
Hemoglobin (g/dl)	12.5 ± 2.5	12.5 ± 2.1	12.6 ± 2.0	0.681
Baseline LDL-C (mg/dl)	101.1 ± 38.5	116.1 ± 39.6	131.7 ± 46.1	<0.001
Baseline non-HDL-C (mg/dl)	122.1 ± 38.7	142.1 ± 42.5	164.3 ± 51.4	<0.001
Baseline HDL-C (mg/dl)	39.7 ± 11.3	40.2 ± 11.0	39.8 ± 10.5	0.822
Smoking	37.8%	35.0%	38.6%	0.850
Hypertension	57.9%	59.2%	53.8%	0.477
Dyslipidemia	25.8%	34.2%	38.6%	0.0.05
Diabetes mellitus	27.1%	26.4%	28.0%	0.920
Chronic kidney disease	9.0%	5.4%	7.2%	0.210
History of CAD	8.4%	9.0%	14.0%	0.07
History of stroke	5.0%	3.9%	4.7%	0.788
STEMI	79.3%	79.9%	72.5%	0.181
Statin	93.0%	92.8%	93.2%	0.981
Ezetimibe	3.3%	2.4%	6.8%	0.024

CAD coronary artery disease, *LVEF* left ventricular ejection fraction, *STEMI* ST elevation myocardial infarction

between non-HDL-C and long-term MACEs after the direct comparison with LDL-C. Compared to non-HDL-C <100 mg/dl, patients with non-HDL-C >130 mg/dl tripled the risk of long-term MACEs (adjusted HR 3.15, 95% CI 1.46–6.80, $P = 0.003$). Conversely, LDL-C >100 mg/dl was inversely associated with the long-term MACEs when compared to LDL <70 mg/dl (adjusted HR 0.42, 95% CI 0.18 – 0.98, $p = 0.046$) (Table 3 and Fig. 1). With this regard, we demonstrated that for a given non-HDL-C level, an increase in LDL-C was associated with a reduced risk of long-term MACEs. Due to the possibility of the correlation between LDL-C and non-HDL-C, we performed the collinearity analysis for variance inflation factor (VIF) and demonstrated no collinearity between LDL-C and non-HDL-C.

The association between the incidence of MACEs and the frequency that the patients achieved LDL or Non-HDL targets during the long-term follow-up were also examined. The patients with long-term MACEs had similar percentage of dosage on Non-HDL target compared to those without long-term MACEs (31.0 ± 31.4% vs. 29.1 ± 32.3%, $P = 0.496$). On the contrary, patients

Table 3 Individual relationships and direct pairwise comparison of LDL-C and non-HDL-C and time to the first major adverse cardiovascular events

Variables	Adjusted hazard ratio[a]	95% CI	P-value	Adjusted hazard ratio[b]	95% CI	P-value
LDL-C <70 mg/dl	1.00			1.00		
LDL-C 70–100 mg/dl	0.98	0.57–1.60	0.934	0.74	0.39–1.40	0.350
LDL-C >100 mg/dl	1.02	0.56–1.84	0.956	0.42	0.18–0.98	0.046
Non-HDL-C <100 mg/dl	1.00			1.00		
Non-HDL-C 100–130 mg/dl	1.10	0.65–1.85	0.715	1.40	0.74–2.65	0.304
Non-HDL-C >130 mg/dl	1.75	1.02–3.00	0.04	3.15	1.46–6.80	0.003

[a]Individual relationships of LDL-C, non-HDL-C and time to the first major adverse cardiovascular events calculated by a Cox proportional hazard model with adjustment for age, sex and comorbidities
[b]Direct pairwise comparison of LDL-C, non-HDL-C and time to the first major adverse cardiovascular events calculated by a Cox proportional hazard model with adjustment for age, sex and comorbidities

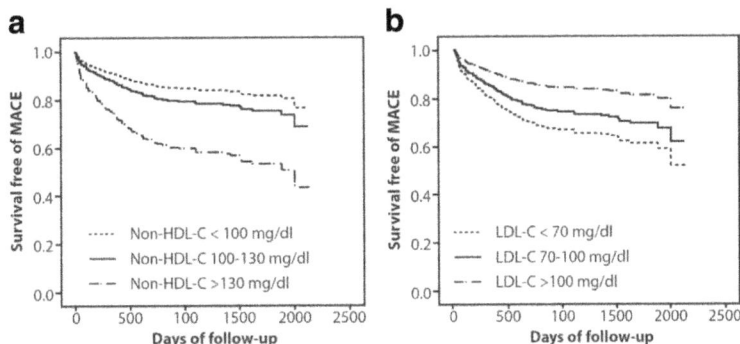

Fig. 1 Time to first major adverse cardiovascular events. Cox regression analysis of time to the first major adverse cardiovascular events after direct pairwise comparison of LDL-C and non-HDL-C. **a** Time to first major adverse cardiovascular events among three different non-HDL-C groups. **b** Time to first major adverse cardiovascular events among three different LDL-C groups

with long-term MACEs had higher percentage of dosage on LDL target than those without long-term MACEs (27.2 ± 28.8% vs. 20.6 ± 28.8%, $P = 0.006$).

Furthermore, the other independent predictors of long-term MACEs were observed. After adjustment with covariates, we found that age, the lower left ventricular ejection fraction (LVEF) and non-STEMI were also the independent predictors of long-term MACE in this population.

Discussion
Main findings
Our study demonstrated that (1) relatively low proportion of patients after AMI achieved lipid treatment goal. Only 24% and 34% of patients after AMI attained LDL-C goal and non-HDL-C goal during long-term follow-up. (2) After cox regression analysis, we demonstrated that non attaining non-HDL-C goal was associated with higher risk of long-term MACE, whereas the non-attaining LDL-C goal was not associated with the increased risk of long-term MACE. (3) The other independent predictors of long-term MACE were age, impaired LVEF and non-STEMI.

Pharmacologic lipid management after AMI is crucial for secondary prevention of cardiovascular events [10–12]. We observed that the low proportion of our studied population could attain lipid target goal during long-term follow-up. Therefore, aggressive lipid-lowering treatment should be reinforced in order to achieve the therapeutic target which may lead to the lower risk of long-term MACE in this high-risk population.

Non-HDL-C composites of all atherogenic apolipoprotein B-containing lipoproteins, including LDL-C, very low-density lipoprotein cholesterol (VLDL-C), intermediate-density lipoprotein cholesterol (IDL-C), lipoprotein(a), chylomicrons, and chylomicron remnants [4]. Therefore, non-HDL-C is a more comprehensive measure of atherogenic particles than LDL-C.

Previous studies have investigated the relationships between LDL-C or non-HDL-C and the risk of coronary heart disease. The Health Professionals Follow-up Study showed that non-HDL-C was more strongly associated with coronary heart disease risk than LDL-C [5]. Similarly, the Framingham Heart Study showed that at every non-HDL-C level, the concentration of LDL-C was not associated with the risk for coronary heart disease. On the contrary, at every LDL-C level, a strong positive and graded association between non-HDL-C and risk of coronary heart disease was observed [13]. In addition, Liu et al. showed that coronary heart disease risk in patients with diabetes was significantly associated with increasing non-HDL-C, but not with increasing LDL-C. They concluded that among patients with diabetes, non-HDL-C was a stronger predictor of coronary heart disease death than LDL-C [3].

A number of studies have shown that there are ethnic differences in risk prediction of coronary artery disease as well as response to treatment [7–9, 14]. In the present study, we demonstrated that Thai patients who did not attain non-HDL-C goal had higher risk of long-term MACE, compared to those who attained non-HDL-C goal. Our findings were in accordance with other studies of western population. Interestingly, we observed that non-attaining LDL-C goal did not correlate with the long-term risk of MACEs. Counter intuitively, patients with mean LDL-C >100 mg/dl had fewer cardiovascular events than those with mean LDL-C <70 mg/dl after direct pairwise comparison with non-HDL-C. This indicated that for a given non-HDL-C level, an increase in LDL-C was associated with a reduced risk of long-term MACEs. It is well-established that the large LDL particle is associated with the lower risk of cardiovascular events than the small dense LDL particle [15]. The inverse association between LDL-C and long-term MACEs observed in the present study may be explained by the fact that patients with higher LDL-C level had larger LDL particle size than those with lower LDL-C level after adjustment with non-HDL-C level. Previous study by Kastelein and colleagues reported similar findings that LDL-C level after statin treatment was inversely associated with adverse cardiovascular outcome after direct pairwise comparison with non-HDL-C level [6].

We demonstrated that non-HDL-C was a more accurate predictor of long-term MACEs than LDL-C in our population after AMI. As the non-HDL-C can be simply calculated by subtracting HDL-C from total cholesterol, therefore, measurement of non-HDL-C incurs no additional cost. With these regards, non-HDL-C should favorably be used as a therapeutic target in the treatment of dyslipidemia in patients after AMI. Our findings support the recommendations from the international atherosclerosis society and national institute of health and care excellence (NICE) which favor the use of non-HDL-C over LDL-C as targets of therapy [16, 17].

Conclusions

Non-attaining non-HDL-C goal was associated with higher risk of long-term MACEs. However, we did not find the correlation between non-attaining LDL-C goal and the increased risk of MACEs. Therefore, non-HDL-C may be a more suitable target of dyslipidemia treatment than LDL-C in patients after AMI. In addition, we demonstrated that only small proportion of patients after AMI could achieve lipid targets during long-term follow-up. More aggressive lipid-lowering strategy should be implemented aiming to reduce the risk of cardiovascular outcome in this high-risk population.

Abbreviations

ACEI: Angiotensin converting enzyme inhibitor; AMI: Acute myocardial infarction; ARB: Angiotensin receptor blocker; CAD: Coronary artery disease; LDL-C: Low-density lipoprotein cholesterol; LVEF: Left ventricular ejection fraction; MACE: Major adverse cardiovascular events; Non-HDL-C: Non-high-density lipoprotein cholesterol; Non-STEMI: Non ST-segment elevation myocardial infarction; STEMI: ST-segment elevation myocardial infarction

Acknowledgment

We would like to thank all staffs in the Northern Cardiac Center and Cardiovascular Division, Department of Internal Medicine, Faculty of Medicine, Chiang Mai University. We also thank Ms. Prapaphan Daoram, a research coordinator.

Funding

This study was supported by the Faculty of Medicine Fund for Medical Research, Faculty of Medicine, Chiang Mai University. A.P. was supported by Thailand Research Fund (RSA5780040). W.W. was supported by Thailand Research Fund (RSA5780039).

Authors' contributions

Study concept and design: WW, AP. Acquisition of the data: WW, SS, SG. Statistical analysis and interpretation of the data: WW, AP. Drafting the manuscript: WW, SS, AP. Critical revision of the manuscript for the important intellectual content: WW, SS, AP. Study supervision: AP. Final approval of the manuscript: WW, SS, SG, AP.

Competing interests

The authors declare that they have no competing interests.

References

1. Expert Panel on Detection, Evaluation, and Treatment of High Blood Cholesterol in Adults. Executive Summary of The Third Report of The National Cholesterol Education Program (NCEP) Expert Panel on Detection, Evaluation, and Treatment of High Blood Cholesterol In Adults (Adult Treatment Panel III). JAMA. 2001;285(19):2486–97.
2. Grundy SM, Cleeman JI, Daniels SR, Donato KA, Eckel RH, Franklin BA, Gordon DJ, Krauss RM, Savage PJ, Smith Jr SC, et al. Diagnosis and management of the metabolic syndrome: an american heart association/national heart, lung, and blood institute scientific statement. Circulation. 2005;112(17):2735–52.
3. Liu J, Sempos C, Donahue RP, Dorn J, Trevisan M, Grundy SM. Joint distribution of non-HDL and LDL cholesterol and coronary heart disease risk prediction among individuals with and without diabetes. Diabetes Care. 2005;28(8):1916–21.
4. Robinson JG. Are you targeting non-high-density lipoprotein cholesterol? J Am Coll Cardiol. 2009;55(1):42–4.
5. Cui Y, Blumenthal RS, Flaws JA, Whiteman MK, Langenberg P, Bachorik PS, Bush TL. Non-high-density lipoprotein cholesterol level as a predictor of cardiovascular disease mortality. Arch Intern Med. 2001;161(11):1413–9.
6. Kastelein JJ, van der Steeg WA, Holme I, Gaffney M, Cater NB, Barter P, Deedwania P, Olsson AG, Boekholdt SM, Demicco DA, et al. Lipids, apolipoproteins, and their ratios in relation to cardiovascular events with statin treatment. Circulation. 2008;117(23):3002–9.
7. Kent DM, Griffith J. The Framingham scores overestimated the risk for coronary heart disease in Japanese, Hispanic, and native american cohorts. ACP J Club. 2002;136(1):36.
8. Sritara P, Patoomanunt P, Woodward M, Narksawat K, Tulyadachanon S, Ratanachaiwong W, Sritara C, Barzi F, Yamwong S, Tanomsup S. Associations between serum lipids and causes of mortality in a cohort of 3,499 urban Thais: the electricity generating authority of Thailand (EGAT) study. Angiology. 2007;58(6):757–63.
9. Sharma SB, Garg S. Small dense LDL: risk factor for coronary artery disease (CAD) and its therapeutic modulation. Indian J Biochem Biophys. 2012; 49(2):77–85.
10. Fruchart JC, Sacks F, Hermans MP, Assmann G, Brown WV, Ceska R, Chapman MJ, Dodson PM, Fioretto P, Ginsberg HN, et al. The residual risk reduction initiative: a call to action to reduce residual vascular risk in patients with dyslipidemia. Am J Cardiol. 2008;102(10 Suppl):1K–34K.
11. Cannon CP, Braunwald E, McCabe CH, Rader DJ, Rouleau JL, Belder R, Joyal SV, Hill KA, Pfeffer MA, Skene AM. Intensive versus moderate lipid lowering with statins after acute coronary syndromes. N Engl J Med. 2004;350(15): 1495–504.
12. LaRosa JC, Grundy SM, Waters DD, Shear C, Barter P, Fruchart JC, Gotto AM, Greten H, Kastelein JJ, Shepherd J, et al. Intensive lipid lowering with atorvastatin in patients with stable coronary disease. N Engl J Med. 2005; 352(14):1425–35.
13. Liu J, Sempos CT, Donahue RP, Dorn J, Trevisan M, Grundy SM. Non-high-density lipoprotein and very-low-density lipoprotein cholesterol and their risk predictive values in coronary heart disease. Am J Cardiol. 2006;98(10): 1363–8.
14. Iannaccone M, D'Ascenzo F, Templin C, Omede P, Montefusco A, Guagliumi G, Serruys PW, Di Mario C, Kochman J, Quadri G et al. Optical coherence tomography evaluation of intermediate-term healing of different stent types: systemic review and meta-analysis. Eur Heart J Cardiovasc Imaging. 2016;jew070. Epub ahead of print.
15. Diffenderfer MR, Schaefer EJ. The composition and metabolism of large and small LDL. Curr Opin Lipidol. 2014;25(3):221–6.

17

A new technique to salvage myocardium following the failure of thrombus aspiration in acute myocardial infarction

Daoyuan Si[†] [iD], Guohui Liu[†], Yaliang Tong, Cheng Zhang and Yuquan He[*]

Abstract

Background: The failure of aspiration thrombectomy may negatively impact outcomes in patients with acute myocardial infarction (AMI), but the available options are limited.

Case presentation: A 41-year-old man with chest pain for 2 h presented with ST-segment elevation myocardial infarction. Coronary angiography revealed a large filling defect extending from the distal left main (LM) coronary artery into the proximal left circumflex (LCX) coronary artery. The whole thrombus moved and occluded the proximal left anterior descending (LAD) artery, while the guidewire crossed the lesion. Dedicated manual aspiration thrombectomy (MAT) and balloon dilation failed to reduce thrombus burden. We considered thrombus extraction as impossible when it moved forward to occlude the middle LAD. To reduce infarct size, a new balloon-pushing technique was successfully performed to move the thrombus to the terminal LAD based on the actual condition of the LAD. The final angiogram demonstrated no stenosis in the LM artery and stent deployment was not performed. A 1-week follow-up coronary angiography revealed the complete resolution of thrombus and flow restoration in the left coronary artery. Intravascular ultrasound (IVUS) showed nonsignificant residual stenosis of the LM artery. No adverse events occurred during a 12-month follow-up period.

Conclusion: This case suggests that the new balloon-pushing technique is a useful remedy if repeated MAT fails during AMI.

Keywords: Acute myocardial infarction, Thromboembolism, Aspiration thrombectomy, Left main coronary artery

Background

Although thrombus aspiration in acute myocardial infarction (AMI) did not lead to clinical benefits according to two recent two large randomized clinical trials [1, 2], thrombus aspiration during the primary percutaneous coronary intervention (PCI) might decrease the risks of stent thrombosis and reinfarction [1, 3]. Thrombus aspiration remains in use in numerous patients with AMI because of its appealing effect regarding the reduc-tion of thrombus burden and no-reflow phenomena [4]. However, the available options are limited when manual aspiration thrombectomy (MAT) fails during primary PCI, especially among patients with thromboembolism. Here, we report a case of a successful myocardium salvage through a new balloon-pushing technique following the failure of repeated MAT in a patient receiving primary PCI.

Case presentation

A 41-year-old male heavy smoker with no specific medical history was admitted to our hospital with severe chest pain lasting 2 h. His blood pressure was 130/80 mmHg on admission, and he presented with no laterality in the upper extremities. Electrocardiography on arrival showed ST-segment elevation in leads II, III, and aVF.

* Correspondence: hyq2@sina.com
†Daoyuan Si and Guohui Liu contributed equally to this work.
Department of Cardiology, China-Japan Union Hospital of Jilin University, Jilin Provincial Engineering Laboratory for Endothelial Function and Genetic Diagnosis of Cardiovascular Disease, Jilin Provincial Cardiovascular Research Institute, Xiantai Street NO.126, Changchun, Jilin, China

The cardiac troponin I was 0.68 ng/ml. He was diagnosed with inferior ST-segment elevation myocardial infarction (STEMI) in Killip Class I and immediately brought to the cardiac catheterization laboratory. An emergency coronary angiography revealed a large filling defect extending from the distal LM artery into the proximal LCX artery (Fig. 1a and b). Otherwise, no significant lesions were found and thrombolysis in myocardial infarction (TIMI) III flows were observed in all coronary arteries. Therefore, PCI was performed using a 6Fr guiding catheter (EBU3.5, Medtronic). Unfortunately, while a 0.014-in. guidewire (Runthrough, Terumo) crossed the LM artery, the whole thrombus was extracted from the proximal LCX artery and pushed into the LAD artery. The proximal LAD artery was completely occluded by the thrombus (Fig. 1c). After crossing the lesion in the LAD artery with the guidewire (Runthrough, Terumo), thrombectomy was attempted several times using an aspiration catheter (Export, Medtronic), and the intracoronary administration of Glycoprotein IIbIIIa inhibitor was slowly infused. However, these treatments did not reduce the thrombus burden in the proximal LAD artery, and no visible thrombus was detected in the aspirate. Then, a 14-atm dilation of a semicompliant balloon (Ryujin 2.5 × 15 mm, Terumo) was performed in the lesion. However, the thrombus moved to the middle LAD artery with TIMI flow 0 (Fig. 1d). Following the failure of another attempt of aspiration using an Export catheter (Medtronic), thrombus

extraction from the LAD artery was considered as impossible. The initial angiogram showed no stenosis in the LAD artery, which had diameters above 2.5 mm and above 1.5 mm at the distal and terminal sites, respectively. To reduce the infarct size, we decided to try a new technique by pushing the thrombus to the terminal LAD artery. A dilated balloon with 6 atm (Ryujin 2.5 × 15 mm, Terumo) was used to push the thrombus carefully toward the distal LAD artery (Fig. 2a and b). Furthermore, the contracted balloon (Ryujin 2.5 × 15 mm, Terumo) successfully pushed the thrombus to the terminal LAD artery (Fig. 2c and d). The final angiogram demonstrated no other significant stenosis except the embolization in the terminal site of the LAD artery (Fig. 3a); thus, stent deployment was not performed.

The patient was transferred to the coronary intensive care unit in a hemodynamically stable condition, while his ST elevation subsided. He was started on low-molecular-weight heparin in addition to regular aspirin, ticagrelor and rosuvastatin. Glycoprotein IIbIIIa inhibitor administration was continued for 24 h. The immunological screen results were unremarkable. A follow-up coronary angiography was performed 1 week later, which revealed the restoration of TIMI 3 flow and the complete resolution of thrombus in the left coronary artery (Fig. 3b). Intravascular ultrasound (IVUS) showed nonsignificant residual stenosis of the LM artery (Fig. 3c). Echocardiography revealed the left ventricular ejection fraction (EF) was 61% with a slight apex hypokinesis,

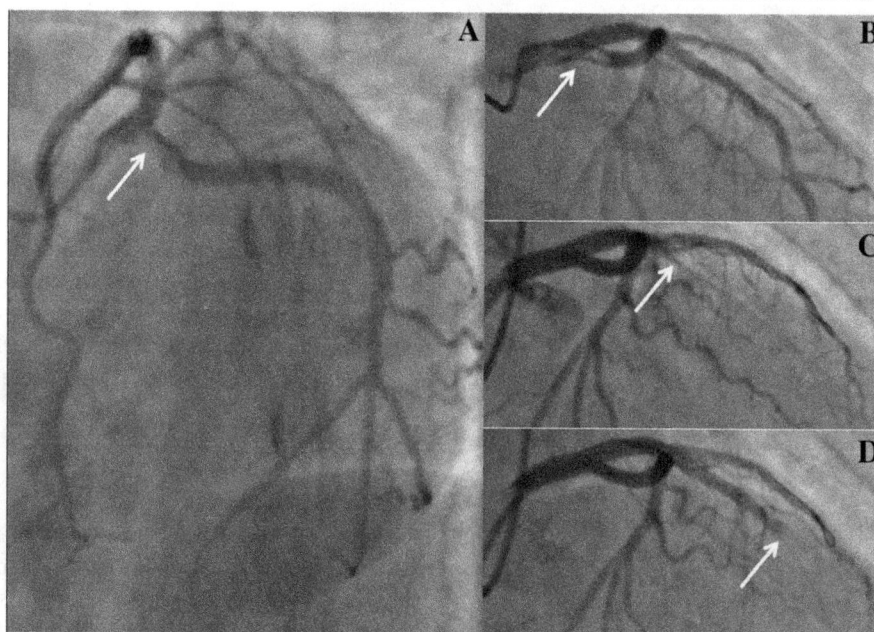

Fig. 1 Angiography and movement of thrombus. **a** and **b** Initial left coronary angiogram demonstrating a filling defect (white arrow) in the left main coronary artery extending into the left circumflex coronary artery. **c** The whole thrombus (white arrow) moved into the proximal left anterior descending artery while the guidewire crossed the lesion. **d** The thrombus (white arrow) moved toward the middle site

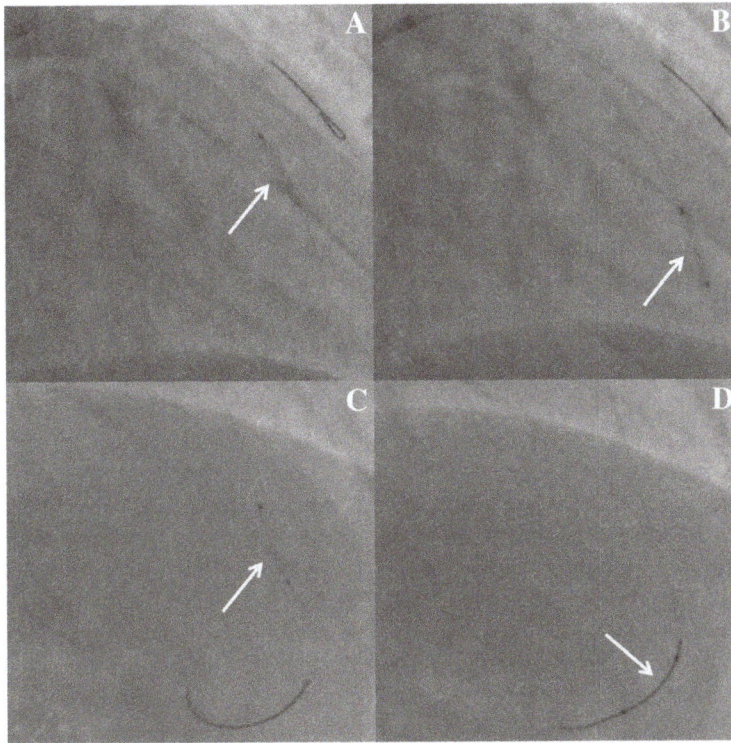

Fig. 2 Balloon pushing technique. **a** and **b** The dilated balloon (white arrow) pushing the thrombus toward the distal left anterior descending artery (LAD). **c** and **d** The undilated balloon (white arrow) pushing the thrombus to the terminal LAD

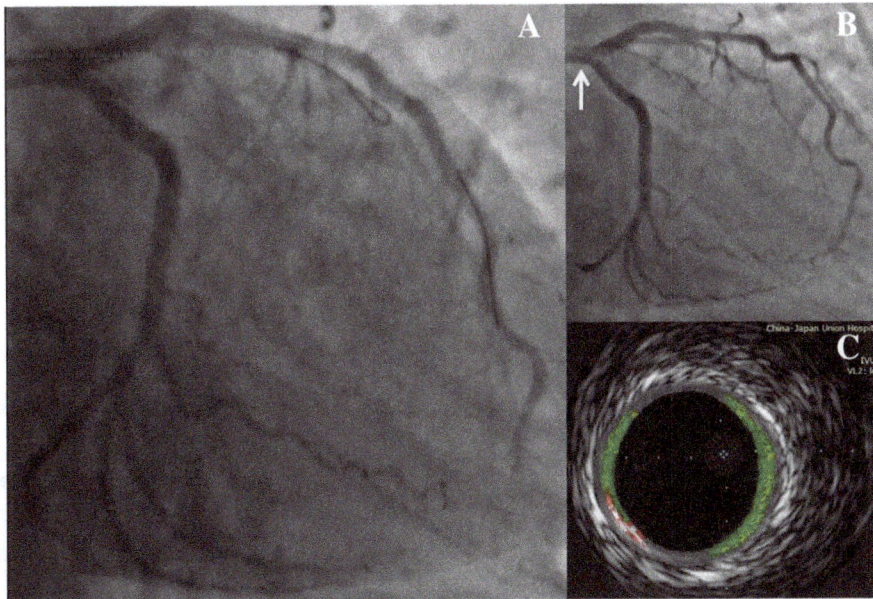

Fig. 3 Final result and follow-up. **a** The final angiogram showed that only the terminal left anterior descending artery (LAD) was occluded by the thrombus. **b**. No angiographic signs of the residual thrombus in LAD were revealed in follow-up angiography. **c** Intravascular ultrasound (IVUS) showed non-significant residual stenosis of the left main coronary artery

and the bubble study showed a negative result. The patient had an uncomplicated recovery and was discharged after 2 days. No adverse events occurred during a 12-month follow-up period.

Discussion and conclusions

LM artery thrombosis is rare and challenging in the context of AMI, with an estimated incidence of 0.8–1.7% [5]. The usual trigger is the fibrous cap rupture of an atherosclerotic plaque or plaque erosion without rupture. Other causes include coronary embolism, which has an incidence of 3% during AMI [6]. The pathophysiologic and anatomic substrates of coronary embolism are hypercoagulability, endothelial injury, blood stasis and anatomic predispositions such as patent foramen ovale and mitral stenosis [6]. However, no evidence of the above was found in the present case. Thus, the filling defect detected in the present case was estimated to be a thrombus formation, not an embolism; however, a 1-week follow-up IVUS did not reveal the absence of atherosclerotic plaque. Surface erosion might explain this finding because the angiogram demonstrated no residual stenosis in the LM artery, and the follow-up IVUS did not detect any sign of plaque rupture. As a consequence, additional balloon angioplasty or stent placement was not performed. Consistent with our case, several case series demonstrated that additional angioplasty and stenting might not be necessary if thrombectomy treatment results in the complete restoration of coronary flow without significant residual stenosis or signs of plaque disruption [7, 8]. A recent 1-year follow-up report within the EROSION study demonstrated that a majority (92.5%) of patients with acute coronary syndrome caused by plaque erosion managed with aspirin and ticagrelor without stenting remained free of major adverse cardiovascular events for ≤1 year [9]. Our case suggests that this concept is also appropriate for LM artery thrombosis. Following conservative enhanced antiplatelets treatment, repeat coronary angiography should be performed to check the thrombus resolution. Intravascular imageology might facilitate the evaluation of the residual plaque and the need for further intervention.

Several studies have not shown a substantial benefit regarding the routine use of MAT during primary PCI [1, 2, 10]. Of interest, aspiration thrombectomy was associated with a significant reduction in cardiovascular death in a subgroup of patients with large thrombus burden, suggesting that MAT is a valid option for certain patients [11]. MAT, which is also suggested by clinical guidelines, remains one of the most frequently used thrombectomy methods when intracoronary thrombi are encountered in the context of AMI. However, feasible alternative methods are limited when MAT failed during

AMI, despite improvements in the MAT technique [12]. In our case, the thrombus was pushed to occlude the proximal LAD artery accidentally. Several MAT attempts failed to reduce the thrombus burden, and the condition deteriorated when the thrombus moved to the middle LAD artery. Thus, we considered it as impossible to remove the thrombus quickly during this primary PCI. The primary goal of primary PCI is the reperfusion of the infarcted myocardium. Because rapid and complete reperfusion could not be achieved in this unexpected scenario, we tried a new technique to minimize the infarct size. According to the anatomic characteristic of the LAD artery, we successfully pushed the thrombus to the terminal LAD artery using a balloon. A 1-week follow-up coronary angiography revealed the restoration of TIMI 3 flow and the complete resolution of the thrombus in the LAD artery following conservative antiplatelets treatment. Echocardiography also showed slight apex hypokinesis with normal EF.

The technical characteristics of this method are described below. First, we must ensure the distal portion of the target artery is normal; otherwise, the pushing process will cause additional injury to the pre-existing lesions, such as dissection of the coronary artery. Second, the diameter of the balloon selected should be smaller than that of the distal artery. Third, if the angiography result is not satisfying after the thrombus has been pushed to the distal site via the dilated balloon, then a contracted balloon can be used to push the thrombus to the terminal site. The key point of this technique is switching the proximal thrombosis to the terminal thrombosis, minimizing the infarct size when it cannot be extracted. To the best of our knowledge, our report is the first to describe this alternative method of MAT in primary PCI.

This new balloon pushing technique proved to be effective and feasible in the current case. This procedure might represent a simple and viable remedy for patients with AMI unresponsive to conventional treatment. Although this technique is limited by its inherent characteristics, our experiences provided a practical alternative method for thrombus reduction in cases of primary PCI.

Abbreviations

AMI: Acute myocardial infarction; EF: Ejection fraction; IVUS: Intravascular ultrasound; LAD: Left anterior descending coronary artery; LCX: Left circumflex coronary artery; LM: Left main coronary artery; MAT: Manual aspiration thrombectomy; PCI: Percutaneous coronary intervention; STEMI: ST-elevation myocardial infarction; TIMI: Thrombolysis in myocardial infarction

Acknowledgments

Not applicable.

Funding

This work was supported by the grants from Excellent Youth Foundation of Science and Technology of Jilin Province (No.20180520054JH) and Project of Development and Reform Commission of Jilin Province (No. 2016C026).

Neither of these agencies was involved in collecting, analyzing, interpreting the data or writing the manuscript.

Authors' contributions

DS drafted the manuscript. YT contributed to data and images collection. DS, GL, DS and CZ performed the percutaneous coronary interventions. GL made critical revision of the manuscript. YH provided consultation, participated in the design and coordination of the manuscript. All authors read and approved the final manuscript.

Competing interests

The authors declare that they have no competing interests.

References

1. Jolly SS, Cairns JA, Yusuf S, Meeks B, Pogue J, Rokoss MJ, et al. Randomized trial of primary PCI with or without routine manual thrombectomy. N Engl J Med. 2015;372(15):1389–98.
2. Lagerqvist B, Frobert O, Olivecrona GK, Gudnason T, Maeng M, Alstrom P, et al. Outcomes 1 year after thrombus aspiration for myocardial infarction. N Engl J Med. 2014;371(12):1111–20.
3. Angeras O, Haraldsson I, Redfors B, Frobert O, Petursson P, Albertsson P, et al. Impact of Thrombus aspiration on mortality, stent thrombosis, and stroke in patients with ST-segment-elevation myocardial infarction: a report from the Swedish coronary angiography and angioplasty registry. J Am Heart Assoc. 2018;7(1).
4. Nishihira K, Shibata Y, Yamashita A, Kuriyama N, Asada Y. Relationship between thrombus age in aspirated coronary material and mid-term major adverse cardiac and cerebrovascular events in patients with acute myocardial infarction. Atherosclerosis. 2018;268:138–44.
5. Patel M, Bhangoo M, Prasad A. Successful percutaneous treatment of suspected embolic left main thrombosis in a patient with a mechanical aortic valve. J Invasive Cardiol. 2011;23(11):E263–6.
6. Raphael CE, Heit JA, Reeder GS, Bois MC, Maleszewski JJ, Tilbury RT, et al. Coronary embolus: an underappreciated cause of acute coronary syndromes. JACC Cardiovascular interventions. 2018;11(2):172–80.
7. Chong F, Cox N, Lim Y. Thrombus aspiration alone: a potential strategy in ST elevation myocardial infarction intervention. Heart Lung Circ. 2011;20(11):724–5.
8. Udayakumaran K, Subban V, Pakshirajan B, Lakshmanan A, Kalidoss L, Rajaram RS, et al. Primary percutaneous thrombus aspiration alone as definitive intervention for left main coronary artery occlusion presenting as acute anterior wall ST elevation myocardial infarction. Heart Lung Circ. 2014;23(2):166–70.
9. Xing L, Yamamoto E, Sugiyama T, Jia H, Ma L, Hu S, et al. EROSION study (effective anti-thrombotic therapy without stenting: intravascular optical coherence tomography-based Management in Plaque Erosion): a 1-year follow-up report. Circ Cardiovasc Interv. 2017;10(12).
10. Ge J, Schafer A, Ertl G, Nordbeck P. Thrombus aspiration for ST-segment-elevation myocardial infarction in modern era: still an issue of debate? Circ Cardiovasc Interv. 2017;10:10.
11. Mangiacapra F, Sticchi A, Barbato E. Thrombus aspiration in primary percutaneous coronary intervention: still a valid option with improved technique in selected patients! Cardiovasc Diagn Ther. 2017;7(Suppl 2):S110–S14.
12. Stiermaier T, de Waha S, Furnau G, Eitel I, Thiele H, Desch S. Thrombus aspiration in patients with acute myocardial infarction : scientific evidence and guideline recommendations. Herz. 2016;41(7):591–8.

18

Mortality and morbidity trends after the first year in survivors of acute myocardial infarction

Saga Johansson[1]*, Annika Rosengren[2,3], Kate Young[4] and Em Jennings[5]

Abstract

Background: Most studies of outcomes after myocardial infarction (MI) focus on the acute phase after the index event. We assessed mortality and morbidity trends after the first year in survivors of acute MI, by conducting a systematic literature review.

Methods: Literature searches were conducted in Embase, MEDLINE, and the Cochrane Database of Systematic Reviews to identify epidemiological studies of long-term (>10 years) mortality and morbidity trends in individuals who had experienced an acute MI more than 1 year previously.

Results: Thirteen articles met the inclusion criteria. Secular trends showed a consistent decrease in mortality and morbidity after acute MI from early to more recent study periods. The relative risk for all-cause death and cardiovascular outcomes (recurrent MI, cardiovascular death) was at least 30% higher than that in a general reference population at both 1–3 years and 3–5 years after MI. Risk factors leading to worse outcomes after MI included comorbid diabetes, hypertension and peripheral artery disease, older age, reduced renal function, and history of stroke.

Conclusions: There have been consistent improvements in secular trends for long-term survival and cardiovascular outcomes after MI. However, MI survivors remain at higher risk than the general population, particularly when additional risk factors such as diabetes, hypertension, or older age are present.

Keywords: Long-term, Morbidity, Mortality, Myocardial infarction, Risk factors

Background

The incidence of acute myocardial infarction (AMI) and case-fatality rates after AMI are declining in most countries, especially in those with high per capita incomes [1–3]. However, the aging world population, population growth, and the rising prevalence of long-term survivors of AMI mean that the burden of disease is generally increasing [1]. Secular trends in reduced morbidity and mortality in individuals with acute coronary syndromes, including AMI, are underpinned by advances in treatment and by the implementation of processes of care, such as networks for the treatment of ST-elevation MI (STEMI) [4, 5].

Survivors of AMI are at high risk of a recurrent myocardial infarction (MI), as well as other manifestations of cardiovascular (CV) disease such as stroke [6–8]. Most studies of post-MI outcomes focus on the acute phase after the index event, with few data available for follow-up beyond the first year. However, although the risk of CV events is highest in the first year post-index MI, it remains elevated in subsequent years [9, 10].

The objective of this systematic literature review was to assess whether morbidity and mortality in survivors of AMI after the first year mirror the general secular trend observed in survivors of MI, based on the results of epidemiological studies describing morbidity and mortality trends covering at least 10 years in long-term (>1 year) survivors of AMI.

* Correspondence: Saga.Johansson@astrazeneca.com
[1]AstraZeneca Gothenburg, Pepparedsleden 1, S-431 83 Mölndal, Sweden
Full list of author information is available at the end of the article

Methods

Systematic review

Literature searches were conducted in June 2015 in Embase, MEDLINE, and the Cochrane Database of Systematic Reviews to identify epidemiological studies of long-term (≥10-year) morbidity and mortality trends in individuals who had experienced an AMI more than 1 year previously. The following search string was used: ((acute coronary syndrome.mp.) OR ((myocardium OR myocardial) AND (ischemi* OR ischaemi*)).mp. OR (coronary heart disease.mp.) OR (coronary artery disease.mp.) OR (myocardial infarction.mp.) OR (unstable angina.mp.)) AND ((natural history.mp.) OR (longitudinal study.mp.) OR (survival.mp.) OR ((secular or time) adj1 trend*).mp. OR ((long term or long-term) adj1 prognosis).mp. OR (prognosis adj1 (following or after)).mp.) OR ((impact and (risk factor or model)).ab. OR (prognos* and model).ab. OR (attribut* risk.ab.)) NOT (clinical trial.mp.). Searches were limited to studies in adults that were published in the English language from 1 January 2010.

To be eligible for inclusion, studies needed to present 10-year data for trends analysis of mortality or other outcomes of atherosclerotic CV disease beyond the first year in survivors of AMI. A flow chart of the literature searches is depicted in Fig. 1.

Data collection

The following data were extracted: study characteristics (study region, data source, study years, study population, number of included individuals, mean age, proportion of men, and amount of follow-up time); and all-cause mortality and CV disease outcomes (incidence, risk analysis, and time trends).

Results

Study selection

The initial search identified 14,440 articles, of which 14,310 were excluded based on a review of the title and/or abstract and 130 underwent full-text review (Fig. 1). Following full-text review, a further 117 articles were excluded (Fig. 1 lists reasons for exclusion and the corresponding number of articles excluded). Thirteen articles fulfilled the inclusion criteria and did not meet the exclusion criteria [11–23].

Study characteristics

The characteristics of the included studies are summarized in Table 1. Four studies were conducted in Sweden [12, 13, 18, 21], one study (with several subgroups and follow-up times) was carried out in the Netherlands [11, 14–17, 22], and one study each took place in Denmark [19], Spain [23] and the United Kingdom [20]. National or regional registries were used as data sources in the four Swedish studies [12, 13, 18, 21], the Danish study

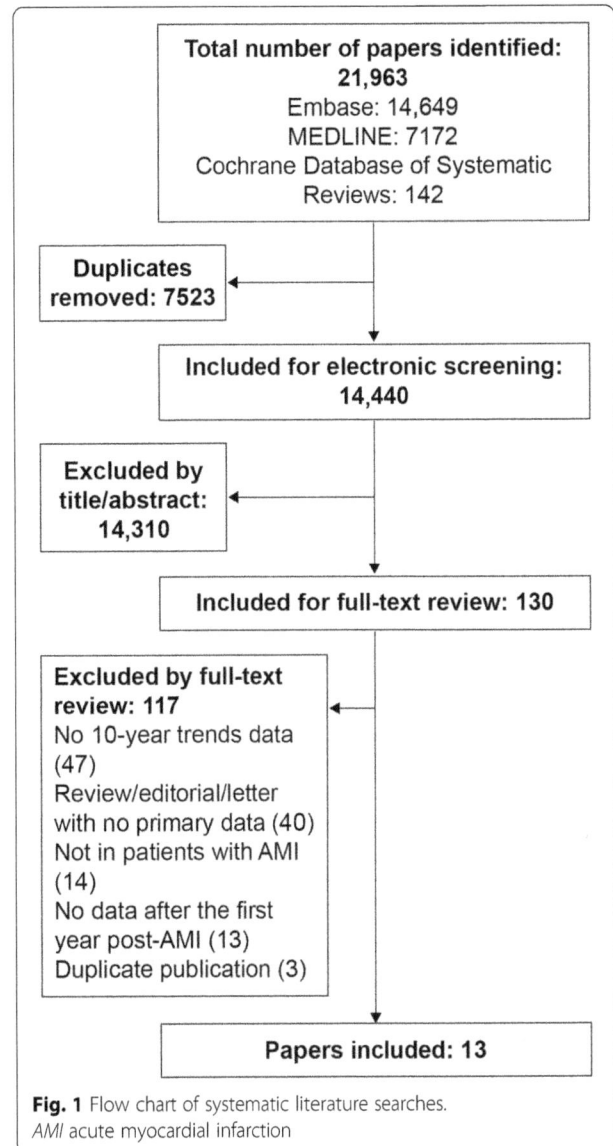

Fig. 1 Flow chart of systematic literature searches. *AMI* acute myocardial infarction

[19], and the study from the United Kingdom [20], whereas data from Spain [23] and the Netherlands [11, 14–17, 22] were from single-center studies. Study years covered ranged from 1985 to 2010. The number of included individuals in each study ranged from 1393 to 175,216, mean patient age ranged from 56 years to 81 years, and the proportion of men ranged from 49% to 81%.

All-cause mortality

Incidence

Data on all-cause mortality were provided for six study populations, described in 11 articles (Table 2) [11–18, 20, 22, 23]. Information on secular trends in all-cause mortality was provided for five study populations, all of which showed a consistent decrease when advancing

Table 1 Characteristics of included studies (eight study populations; 13 articles)

Study region	Data source(s)	Study years	Study population	Number	Mean age (years)	Men (%)	Follow-up (years)	Reference
Denmark	National Prescription Register, National Patient Register, Central Population Register	1997–2006	Individuals aged ≥30 years with first MI and without prior diabetes	77,147	70	61	Up to 5	Norgaard et al. 2010 [19]
Spain	Single center Coronary Care Unit Registry	1988–2008	Individuals aged ≥75 years with first STEMI	1393	81	49	1 and 5	Viana-Tejedor et al. 2015 [23]
Sweden	National Hospital Discharge Register, National Cause of Death Registry	1993–2004	Individuals admitted for first MI (no prior HF or CAD)	175,216	69	64	3	Shafazand et al. 2011 [21]
	RIKS-HIA	1996–2007	Individuals with first STEMI	61,238	70	65	Up to 15	Jernberg et al. 2011 [13]
	National Inpatient Register	1987–2006	Individuals with first MI aged 25–54 years	37,276	NR	81	4	Nielsen et al. 2014 [18]
	Northern Sweden MONICA MI Registry, Swedish National Cause of Death Registry	1985–2006	Individuals with first MI	8630	56	78	Median: 7.1	Isaksson et al. 2011 [12]
Netherlands	Thoraxcenter ICCU, Erasmus University Medical Center	1985–2008	Individuals hospitalized for MI					
			With NSTEMI[a]	7614	63	70	3	Nauta et al. 2011 [15]
			With STEMI[a]	6820	61	75	3	Nauta et al. 2011 [15]
							10	Snelder et al. 2013 [22]
			With renal impairment[b]	8632			Up to 20	Nauta et al. 2013 [17]
			With diabetes[a]	2015			Up to 20	Nauta et al. 2012 [14]
			With elevated blood glucose[c]	4671			Up to 20	Deckers et al. 2013 [11]
			Women[a]	4028			Up to 20	Nauta et al. 2012 [16]
United Kingdom	CALIBER (CPRD, MINAP, HES, and ONS)	2000–2010	Individuals with stable angina, other CHD, unstable angina, STEMI, NSTEMI, or unclassified MI	102,023 (STEMI: 4700; NSTEMI: 6818; unclassified MI: 9620)	STEMI: 66; NSTEMI: 72; unclassified MI: 69	STEMI: 72; NSTEMI: 63; unclassified MI: 65	Mean: 4.4[d]	Rapsomaniki et al. 2014 [20]

CAD coronary artery disease, *CALIBER* CArdiovascular disease research using LInked BEspoke studies and electronic health Records, *CHD* coronary heart disease, *CPRD* Clinical Practice Research Datalink, *HES* Hospital Episodes Statistics, *HF* heart failure, *ICCU* intensive coronary care unit, *MI* myocardial infarction, *MINAP* Myocardial Ischaemia National Audit Project registry, *MONICA* MONItoring trends and determinants in CArdiovascular disease, NR not reported, *NSTEMI* non-ST-elevation myocardial infarction, *ONS* Office for National Statistics, *RIKS-HIA* Register of Information and Knowledge about Swedish Heart Intensive care Admissions, *STEMI* ST-elevation myocardial infarction

[a]Of 14,434 individuals hospitalized for MI
[b]Of 12,087 individuals hospitalized for MI
[c]Of 11,324 individuals hospitalized for MI
[d]Follow-up started 6 months after the event

from early to more recent study periods (Table 2) [12–15, 18, 22, 23]. Data for time periods starting 1 year after the event were shown graphically and were not reported separately.

Relative risk

Relative risk analyses for all-cause death from 1 year after the AMI were reported in one study, conducted in Denmark (Table 3) [19]. The reference population

Table 2 All-cause mortality (six study populations; 11 articles)

Reference	Assessment	Mortality/survival
Viana-Tejedor et al. 2015 [23]	Mortality in years 1–5 in patients alive 1 year after MI[a]	• Mortality 1988–1993: 26.9% (42/156); 1994–1998: 32.5% (66/203); 1999–2003: 23.7% (57/241); 2004–2008: 15.4% (48/311) • 1-year and 5-year mortality decreased significantly over the 20-year period of study ($p < 0.001$)
Jernberg et al. 2011 [13]	Risk of death up to 12 years after event	• Time trends show risk of death 1996–1997 > 1998–1999 > 2000–2001 > 2002–2003 > 2004–2005 > 2006–2007[b]
Nielsen et al. 2014 [18]	Survival probability for 4 years after event	• For men, time trends show survival probability 1987–1991 < 1992–1996 < 1997–2001 < 2002–2006[b] • For women, time trends show survival probability 1987–1991 < 1992–1996 < 1997–2001, but levels for 2002–2006 were similar to those for 1997–2001[b]
Isaksson et al. 2011 [12]	Survival up to 24 years after event	• Time trends show survival 1985–1988 < 1989–1994 < 1995–2000 < 2001–2006[b] • Survival in women was generally higher than that for men before 2000, but similar for men and women after 2000
Nauta et al. 2011 [15]	Survival for 3 years after event in patients with NSTEMI	• Time trends show survival 1985–1990 < 1990–2000 < 2000–2008[b]
Snelder et al. 2013 [22]	Mortality for up to 10 years after event in patients with STEMI	• Time trends show mortality 1985–1990 > 1990–2000 > 2000–2008[b]
Nauta et al. 2013 [17]	Mortality for up to 20 years after event according to renal function	• Time trends for mortality stage 4–5 chronic kidney disease > stage 3 > stage 2 > normal kidney function[b]
Nauta et al. 2012 [14]	Mortality for up to 20 years after event according to diabetes status	• Mortality was higher in patients with diabetes than in those without • There was an increase in the risk of presenting with diabetes during the study period • Time trends show mortality 1985–1989 > 1990–1999 > 2000–2008 in patients with diabetes, and 1985–1989 ≈ 1990–1999 > 2000–2008 in patients without diabetes[b]
Deckers et al. 2013 [11]	Mortality for up to 20 years after event according to glucose levels	• Mortality was highest in patients with severe hyperglycemia, followed by those with mild hyperglycemia, and was lowest in those with normal glucose levels[b]
Nauta et al. 2012 [16]	Mortality for up to 20 years after event according to sex	• From 1985 to 2008, age at presentation increased and patients were more likely to have diabetes or anemia at presentation • Adjusted 20-year mortality was significantly lower in women than in men
Rapsomaniki et al. 2014 [20]	Cumulative all-cause mortality up to 5.5 years after event[c]	• Mortality in stable patients after NSTEMI > after STEMI[b]

MI myocardial infarction, *NSTEMI* non-ST-elevation myocardial infarction, *STEMI* ST-elevation myocardial infarction

[a]Calculated from data reported in the study
[b]All shown on curve; actual values not reported for time starting 1 year after the event
[c]Follow-up started 6 months after the event

Table 3 All-cause death: relative risk analysis (one study population; one article)

Reference	Assessment	Relative risk analysis
Norgaard et al. 2010 [19]	Relative risk (95% CI) versus reference population at 1–3 years and 3–5 years after MI during time periods 1997–2001 and 2001–2006	Men
		1997–2001: 1–3 years, 1.42 (1.36–1.49); 3–5 years, 1.38 (1.31–1.45)
		2001–2006: 1–3 years, 1.47 (1.39–1.55); 3–5 years, 1.46 (1.32–1.62)
		Women
		1997–2001: 1–3 years, 1.90 (1.81–2.00); 3–5 years, 1.84 (1.74–1.94)
		2001–2006: 1–3 years, 2.02 (1.91–2.15); 3–5 years, 1.80 (1.60–2.02)

CI confidence interval, *MI* myocardial infarction

comprised inhabitants of Denmark aged 30 years and above, with no prior prescriptions for glucose-lowering drugs and no history of MI [19]. The relative risk of all-cause death was increased at 1–3 years and 3–5 years after MI compared with the reference population, and was higher in women than in men (Table 3) [19]. Relative risk values for the time period January 1997–June 2001 were similar to those for the time period July 2001– December 2006 [19].

Another study compared estimated mortality in the study population (aged 25–54 years) in the 4 years after the index AMI with that expected in the general population, but data from 1 year after the event were not reported separately [18]. The excess in observed versus expected mortality decreased from early to more recent study periods in men, but less so in women [18].

Risk factors

Several risk factors were identified that led to worse outcomes, as follows. Mortality was higher in individuals with diabetes than in those without diabetes across study periods [14]. Mortality increased with increasing severity of hyperglycemia [11] and with decreasing renal function [17]. It was lower in women than in men [12, 16], but the rates became more similar between the sexes in more recent years [12, 18]. As expected, mortality increased with age [12]. Significant risk factors for all-cause death in patients who had experienced STEMI and non-ST-elevation myocardial infarction (NSTEMI) included increasing age, smoking, hypertension, diabetes, peripheral artery disease, history of stroke, chronic kidney disease, chronic obstructive pulmonary disease, chronic liver disease, and history of cancer [20]. Primary percutaneous coronary intervention was shown to lower all-cause mortality in patients with STEMI [23].

CV outcomes
Incidence

Incidence data for CV outcomes (heart failure [21], non-fatal MI/coronary death [20]) were provided in two studies (Table 4) [20, 21]. The incidence of heart failure at 1–3 years in patients surviving 1 year without heart failure decreased over time, ranging from 2.32% in the earliest study period (1993–1995) to 1.47% in the most recent study period (2002–2004) in the 35–64-year age group, and from 5.03% in the earliest to 4.28% in the most recent study period in the 65–84-year age group (p for trend <0.001 in both age groups) [21]. No data were provided that compared the incidence of CV outcomes or mortality with those in the general population.

Relative risk

Relative risk analyses for CV outcomes (recurrent MI, CV death) were reported in one study, conducted in Denmark (Table 5) [19]. The relative risks of recurrent MI and CV death increased at 1–3 years and 3–5 years after MI compared with the reference population, and were higher in women than in men (Table 5) [19]. Relative risks for the time period 1997–2001 were similar to those for 2001–2006 [19].

Risk factors

Several risk factors were identified that led to worse outcomes, as follows. The incidence of non-fatal MI/coronary death 1 year to 5.5 years after acute coronary syndromes in stable patients was highest after NSTEMI, followed by unspecified MI and then STEMI [20]. Identified significant risk factors for non-fatal MI/coronary death in patients with STEMI and NSTEMI included increasing age, smoking, hypertension, diabetes, peripheral artery disease, history of stroke, chronic kidney disease, and chronic obstructive pulmonary disease [20].

Table 4 Cardiovascular outcomes: incidence (two study populations; two articles)

Reference	Assessment	Incidence
Shafazand et al. 2011 [21]	HF at 1–3 years in patients surviving 1 year without HF	35–64-year age group 1993–1995: 2.32% 1996–1998: 1.82% 1999–2001: 1.79% 2002–2004: 1.47% $p < 0.001$ 65–84-year age group 1993–1995: 5.03% 1996–1998: 4.44% 1999–2001: 4.45% 2002–2004: 4.28% $p < 0.001$
Rapsomaniki et al. 2014 [20]	Cumulative non-fatal MI/coronary death risk up to 5.5 years after event[a]	Cumulative risk of non-fatal MI/coronary death was shown to increase further after 1 year for up to 5.5 years; cumulative risk of death in stable patients after NSTEMI > MI (type unspecified) > after STEMI[b]

HF heart failure, *MI* myocardial infarction, *NSTEMI* non-ST-elevation myocardial infarction, *STEMI* ST-elevation myocardial infarction
[a]Follow-up started 6 months after the event
[b]All shown on curve; actual values not reported for time starting 1 year after the event

Table 5 Cardiovascular outcomes: relative risk (one study population; one article)

Reference	Assessment	Risk analysis
Norgaard et al. 2010 [19]	Relative risk (95% CI) of recurrent MI versus reference population at 1–3 years and 3–5 years after MI during time periods 1997–2001 and 2001–2006	Men
		1997–2001: 1–3 years, 2.99 (2.80–3.18); 3–5 years, 2.67 (2.48–2.87)
		2001–2006: 1–3 years, 2.92 (2.69–3.17); 3–5 years, 2.70 (2.30–3.17)
		Women
		1997–2001: 1–3 years, 5.67 (5.25–6.11); 3–5 years, 4.33 (3.93–4.78)
		2001–2006: 1–3 years, 5.64 (5.13–6.21); 3–5 years, 5.15 (4.24–6.25)
	Relative risk (95% CI) of CV death versus reference population at 1–3 years and 3–5 years after MI during time periods 1997–2001 and 2001–2006	Men
		1997–2001: 1–3 years, 2.11 (2.00–2.23); 3–5 years, 1.99 (1.88–2.11)
		2001–2006: 1–3 years, 2.14 (2.00–2.28); 3–5 years, 2.10 (1.86–2.34)
		Women
		1997–2001: 1–3 years, 2.80 (2.64–2.97); 3–5 years, 2.63 (2.46–2.81)
		2001–2006: 1–3 years, 2.92 (2.72–3.13); 3–5 years, 2.77 (2.42–3.17)

CI confidence interval, *CV* cardiovascular, *MI* myocardial infarction

Discussion

This systematic literature review reveals consistent improvements from early to more recent periods in secular trends for long-term survival and CV outcomes after MI. However, compared with the general population, MI survivors remain at higher risk, particularly older individuals and patients with comorbid hypertension, diabetes, peripheral artery disease, or history of stroke. In the single study that compared survival after the first year with that of the general population, there was a lack of improvement between the time periods 1997–2001 and 2001–2006; most of the decrease in mortality would therefore seem to occur during the first year [19].

Secular trends data focusing on outcomes specifically in survivors of MI after 1 year are scarce, with only one study in this review reporting such information [19]. In that study, a general population of similar age was included as a reference, and the relative risk of all-cause death was shown to be increased at both 1–3 years and 3–5 years after MI compared with the reference population [19]. These data are supported by those of a recently published, large, four-country analysis, which showed an annual risk of death 1 year onwards after MI that was more than double that of a similar general population age group, with about half of deaths due to CV disease [10]. The four-country analysis used "big data" from hospital health records to assess long-term CV disease outcomes starting 1 year after the most recent discharge following AMI. It was conducted in the United States and three European countries, and included more than 100,000 survivors of MI aged 65 years and older.

Studies have shown the increased risk of CV events in individuals after MI to be higher in the first year following the index MI than in subsequent years [9, 10]. In a large Swedish registry study that formed part of the

four-country analysis which included 97,254 patients discharged after MI, the risk of non-fatal MI, non-fatal stroke, or CV death (primary composite end point) during the first year after the index MI was 18.3% [9]. Although the risk was lower in the subsequent 3 years than in the first year, it remained relatively high with about one in five patients without a combined end point during the first year having a non-fatal MI, non-fatal stroke, or CV death during the following 3 years [9]. Similarly, in the four-country analysis, death, stroke, or further MI after the first year following an MI occurred in about one-third of patients during the subsequent 3 years [10].

The high risk of vascular events after 1 year post-MI suggests that prolonged surveillance beyond 12 months is required in this patient group. Results from a recent clinical trial suggest that prolonged dual antiplatelet therapy (DAPT) beyond the first year after an AMI is beneficial in terms of preventing vascular events [24]. In the DAPT study in patients treated with a drug-eluting stent, of whom 31% presented with AMI, prolonged DAPT beyond 12 months significantly lowered the cumulative incidence of stent thrombosis and of major CV and cerebrovascular events during the subsequent 18 months compared with acetylsalicylic acid alone [25]. Current guidelines recommend DAPT for 12 months for secondary prevention [26–29], with European Society of Cardiology guidelines noting that the duration may be extended (up to 30 months) in selected patients, if required [27]. In patients stable 1 year after an AMI, validated prognostic models based on individual patient risk profiles can help to inform a decision of whether or not to prolong DAPT [30].

Studies in the current review show a particularly high risk of vascular events after MI in older individuals and in patients with hypertension, diabetes, peripheral artery disease, or history of stroke [14, 20]. Strong associations between the risk of subsequent MI, stroke, or death and the presence of diabetes, peripheral artery disease, and history of stroke were also revealed by the four-country analysis, which further identified comorbid heart failure, renal disease, and chronic obstructive pulmonary disease as risk factors [10]. These results indicate a particular need for better treatment options in these high-risk patient groups.

The current review highlights large information gaps for outcomes that occur 1 year or more after the index MI. Although most studies show time trends graphically, they do not report actual data values separately for the time period starting from 1 year post-MI. Thus, it is difficult to attribute differences and trends in longer-term survival to specific time periods after the index event. In addition, studies that report mortality and incidence data for the time period starting 1 year after the index event mostly present these as absolute values rather than values relative to a control population, making it difficult to assess to what extent the data from 1 year after the event differ from those in the general population.

Conclusions

In conclusion, there have been consistent improvements in secular trends for long-term survival and CV outcomes after MI. However, MI survivors remain at higher risk than the general population, particularly if there are additional risk factors such as older age, hypertension, or diabetes, all of which lead to worse outcomes.

Abbreviations

AHA: American Heart Association; AMI: Acute myocardial infarction; CAD: Coronary artery disease; CALIBER: CArdiovascular disease research using LInked BEspoke studies and electronic health Records; CHD: Coronary heart disease; CI: Confidence interval; CPRD: Clinical Practice Research Datalink; CV: Cardiovascular; DAPT: Dual antiplatelet therapy; ESC: European Society of Cardiology; HES: Hospital Episodes Statistics; HF: Heart failure; ICCU: Intensive coronary care unit; MI: Myocardial infarction; MINAP: Myocardial Ischaemia National Audit Project registry; MONICA: MONItoring trends and determinants in CArdiovascular disease; NR: Not responsive; NSTEMI: Non-ST-elevation myocardial infarction; ONS: Office for National Statistics; RIKS-HIA: Register of Information and Knowledge about Swedish Heart Intensive care Admissions; STEMI: ST-elevation myocardial infarction

Acknowledgements

Writing support was provided by Dr Anja Becher, from Oxford PharmaGenesis, Oxford, UK, and was funded by AstraZeneca Gothenburg, Mölndal, Sweden.

Funding

This analysis was funded by AstraZeneca Gothenburg, Mölndal, Sweden.

Authors' contributions

KY performed the systematic literature searches. SJ, AR, KY, and EJ analyzed the data and were major contributors in writing the manuscript. All authors read and approved the final manuscript.

Competing interests

Saga Johansson is an employee of AstraZeneca Gothenburg, Mölndal, Sweden. Annika Rosengren reports no disclosures. At the time the analysis was conducted, Kate Young was an employee of Oxford PharmaGenesis, Newtown, PA, USA, which has received funding from AstraZeneca. Em Jennings is an employee of AstraZeneca R&D, Cambridge, UK.

Author details

[1]AstraZeneca Gothenburg, Pepparedsleden 1, S-431 83 Mölndal, Sweden. [2]Department of Molecular and Clinical Medicine, Sahlgrenska Academy, University of Gothenburg, Gothenburg, Sweden. [3]Sahlgrenska University Hospital, Gothenburg, Sweden. [4]Research Evaluation Unit, Oxford PharmaGenesis, 503 Washington Ave, Newtown, PA 18940, USA. [5]AstraZeneca R&D, 132 Hills Rd, Cambridge CB2 1PG, UK.

References

1. Moran AE, Forouzanfar MH, Roth GA, Mensah GA, Ezzati M, Flaxman A, Murray CJ, Naghavi M. The global burden of ischemic heart disease in 1990 and 2010: the Global Burden of Disease 2010 study. Circulation. 2014;129(14):1493–501.
2. Mozaffarian D, Benjamin EJ, Go AS, Arnett DK, Blaha MJ, Cushman M, de Ferranti S, Despres JP, Fullerton HJ, Howard VJ, et al. Heart disease and stroke statistics – 2015 update: a report from the American Heart Association. Circulation. 2015;131(4):e29–322.
3. Nichols M, Townsend N, Scarborough P, Rayner M. Cardiovascular disease in Europe 2014: epidemiological update. Eur Heart J. 2014;35(42):2929.
4. Jokhadar M, Jacobsen SJ, Reeder GS, Weston SA, Roger VL. Sudden death and recurrent ischemic events after myocardial infarction in the community. Am J Epidemiol. 2004;159(11):1040–6.
5. Wallentin L, Kristensen SD, Anderson JL, Tubaro M, Sendon JL, Granger CB, Bode C, Huber K, Bates ER, Valgimigli M, et al. How can we optimize the processes of care for acute coronary syndromes to improve outcomes? Am Heart J. 2014;168(5):622–31.
6. Smolina K, Wright FL, Rayner M, Goldacre MJ. Long-term survival and recurrence after acute myocardial infarction in England, 2004 to 2010. Circ Cardiovasc Qual Outcomes. 2012;5(4):532–40.
7. Witt BJ, Brown Jr RD, Jacobsen SJ, Weston SA, Yawn BP, Roger VL. A community-based study of stroke incidence after myocardial infarction. Ann Intern Med. 2005;143(11):785–92.
8. Campo G, Saia F, Guastaroba P, Marchesini J, Varani E, Manari A, Ottani F, Tondi S, De Palma R, Marzocchi A. Prognostic impact of hospital readmissions after primary percutaneous coronary intervention. Arch Intern Med. 2011;171(21):1948–9.
9. Jernberg T, Hasvold P, Henriksson M, Hjelm H, Thuresson M, Janzon M. Cardiovascular risk in post-myocardial infarction patients: nationwide real world data demonstrate the importance of a long-term perspective. Eur Heart J. 2015;36(19):1163–70.
10. Rapsomaniki E, Thuresson M, Yang E, Blin P, Hunt P, Chung SC, Stogiannis D, Pujades-Rodriguez M, Timmis A, Denaxas SC, et al. Using big data from health records from four countries to evaluate chronic disease outcomes: a study in 114 364 survivors of myocardial infarction. Eur Heart J Qual Care Clin Outcomes. 2016;2(3):172–83.
11. Deckers JW, van Domburg RT, Akkerhuis M, Nauta ST. Relation of admission glucose levels, short- and long-term (20-year) mortality after acute myocardial infarction. Am J Cardiol. 2013;112(9):1306–10.
12. Isaksson RM, Jansson JH, Lundblad D, Naslund U, Zingmark K, Eliasson M. Better long-term survival in young and middle-aged women than in men after a first myocardial infarction between 1985 and 2006. An analysis of 8630 patients in the northern Sweden MONICA study. BMC Cardiovasc Disord. 2011;11:1.
13. Jernberg T, Johanson P, Held C, Svennblad B, Lindback J, Wallentin L. Association between adoption of evidence-based treatment and survival for patients with ST-elevation myocardial infarction. JAMA. 2011;305(16):1677–84.
14. Nauta ST, Deckers JW, Akkerhuis KM, van Domburg RT. Short- and long-term mortality after myocardial infarction in patients with and without diabetes: changes from 1985 to 2008. Diabetes Care. 2012;35(10):2043–7.
15. Nauta ST, Deckers JW, Akkerhuis M, Lenzen M, Simoons ML, van Domburg RT. Changes in clinical profile, treatment, and mortality in patients hospitalised for acute myocardial infarction between 1985 and 2008. PLoS One. 2011;6(11):e26917.

16. Nauta ST, Deckers JW, van Domburg RT, Akkerhuis KM. Sex-related trends in mortality in hospitalized men and women after myocardial infarction between 1985 and 2008: equal benefit for women and men. Circulation. 2012;126(18):2184–9.

17. Nauta ST, van Domburg RT, Nuis RJ, Akkerhuis M, Deckers JW. Decline in 20-year mortality after myocardial infarction in patients with chronic kidney disease: evolution from the prethrombolysis to the percutaneous coronary intervention era. Kidney Int. 2013;84(2):353–8.

18. Nielsen S, Bjorck L, Berg J, Giang KW, Zverkova Sandstrom T, Falk K, Maatta S, Rosengren A. Sex-specific trends in 4-year survival in 37 276 men and women with acute myocardial infarction before the age of 55 years in Sweden, 1987–2006: a register-based cohort study. BMJ Open. 2014;4(5):e004598.

19. Norgaard ML, Andersen SS, Schramm TK, Folke F, Jorgensen CH, Hansen ML, Andersson C, Bretler DM, Vaag A, Kober L, et al. Changes in short- and long-term cardiovascular risk of incident diabetes and incident myocardial infarction–a nationwide study. Diabetologia. 2010;53(8):1612–9.

20. Rapsomaniki E, Shah A, Perel P, Denaxas S, George J, Nicholas O, Udumyan R, Feder GS, Hingorani AD, Timmis A, et al. Prognostic models for stable coronary artery disease based on electronic health record cohort of 102 023 patients. Eur Heart J. 2014;35(13):844–52.

21. Shafazand M, Rosengren A, Lappas G, Swedberg K, Schaufelberger M. Decreasing trends in the incidence of heart failure after acute myocardial infarction from 1993–2004: a study of 175,216 patients with a first acute myocardial infarction in Sweden. Eur J Heart Fail. 2011;13(2):135–41.

22. Snelder SM, Nauta ST, Akkerhuis KM, Deckers JW, van Domburg RT. Weekend versus weekday mortality in ST-segment elevation acute myocardial infarction patients between 1985 and 2008. Int J Cardiol. 2013;168(2):1576–7.

23. Viana-Tejedor A, Loughlin G, Fernandez-Aviles F, Bueno H. Temporal trends in the use of reperfusion therapy and outcomes in elderly patients with first ST elevation myocardial infarction. Eur Heart J Acute Cardiovasc Care. 2015;4(5):461–7.

24. Bonaca MP, Bhatt DL, Cohen M, Steg PG, Storey RF, Jensen EC, Magnani G, Bansilal S, Fish MP, Im K, et al. Long-term use of ticagrelor in patients with prior myocardial infarction. N Engl J Med. 2015;372(19):1791–800.

25. Mauri L, Kereiakes DJ, Yeh RW, Driscoll-Shempp P, Cutlip DE, Steg PG, Normand SL, Braunwald E, Wiviott SD, Cohen DJ, et al. Twelve or 30 months of dual antiplatelet therapy after drug-eluting stents. N Engl J Med. 2014;371(23):2155–66.

26. Amsterdam EA, Wenger NK, Brindis RG, Casey Jr DE, Ganiats TG, Holmes Jr DR, Jaffe AS, Jneid H, Kelly RF, Kontos MC, et al. 2014 AHA/ACC guideline for the management of patients with non-ST-elevation acute coronary syndromes: a report of the American College of Cardiology/American Heart Association Task Force on Practice Guidelines. J Am Coll Cardiol. 2014;64(24):e139–228.

27. Roffi M, Patrono C, Collet JP, Mueller C, Valgimigli M, Andreotti F, Bax JJ, Borger MA, Brotons C, Chew DP, et al. 2015 ESC Guidelines for the management of acute coronary syndromes in patients presenting without persistent ST-segment elevation: Task Force for the management of acute coronary syndromes in patients presenting without persistent ST-segment elevation of the European Society of Cardiology (ESC). Eur Heart J. 2016;37:267–315.

28. Steg PG, James SK, Atar D, Badano LP, Blomstrom-Lundqvist C, Borger MA, Di Mario C, Dickstein K, Ducrocq G, Fernandez-Aviles F, et al. ESC Guidelines for the management of acute myocardial infarction in patients presenting with ST-segment elevation. Eur Heart J. 2012;33(20):2569–619.

29. Windecker S, Kolh P, Alfonso F, Collet JP, Cremer J, Falk V, Filippatos G, Hamm C, Head SJ, Juni P, et al. 2014 ESC/EACTS guidelines on myocardial revascularization: the Task Force on Myocardial Revascularization of the European Society of Cardiology (ESC) and the European Association for Cardio-Thoracic Surgery (EACTS) developed with the special contribution of the European Association of Percutaneous Cardiovascular Interventions (EAPCI). Eur Heart J. 2014;35(37):2541–619.

30. Pasea L, Chung SC, Pujades Rodriguez M, Jennings E, Emmas C, Westergaard M, Johansson S, Hemingway H. Development and validation of prognostic models for myocardial infarction, stroke and cardiovascular death and hospitalised bleeding in stable myocardial infarction survivors. J Am Coll Cardiol. 2015;65(10S):A1382.

19

Admission serum potassium concentration and long-term mortality in patients with acute myocardial infarction: results from the MONICA/KORA myocardial infarction registry

Miriam Giovanna Colombo[1,2]*, Inge Kirchberger[1,2], Ute Amann[1,2], Margit Heier[1,2], Christian Thilo[3], Bernhard Kuch[3,4], Annette Peters[2] and Christa Meisinger[1,2]

Abstract

Background: Conflicting with clinical practice guidelines, recent studies demonstrated that serum potassium concentrations (SPC) of ≥4.5 mEq/l were associated with increased mortality in patients with acute myocardial infarction (AMI). This study examined the association between SPC and long-term mortality following AMI in patients recruited from a population-based registry.

Methods: Included in the study were 3347 patients with AMI aged 28–74 years consecutively hospitalized between 1 January 2000 and 31 December 2008 and followed up until 31 December 2011. Patients were categorized into five SPC groups (<3.5, 3.5 to <4.0, 4.0 to <4.5, 4.5 to <5.0, and ≥5.0 mEq/l). The outcome of the study was all-cause mortality. Cox regression models adjusted for risk factors, co-morbidities and in-hospital treatment were constructed.

Results: In our study population, 249 patients (7.4%) had a low SPC (<3.5 mEq/l) and 134 (4.0%) patients had a high SPC (≥5.0 mEq/l). Patients with SPC of ≥5.0 mEq/l had the highest long-term mortality (29.9%) and in the adjusted model, their risk of dying was significantly increased (HR 1.46, 95% CI 1.03 to 2.07) compared to patients with SPC between 4.0 and <4.5 mEq/l. Analyses of increasing observation periods showed a trend towards a higher risk of dying in patients with SPC between 4.5 and <5.0 mEq/l.

Conclusion: An admission SPC of ≥5.0 mEq/l might be associated with an increased mortality risk in patients with AMI. Patients with an admission SPC between 4.5 and <5.0 mEq/l might have an increased mortality risk in the first few years following AMI.

Keywords: Myocardial Infarction, Potassium, Hypokalemia, Hyperkalemia, Mortality

Background

Hypo- and hyperkalemia have been shown to increase cardiovascular and total mortality in patients with acute myocardial infarction (AMI) [1–3]. Hypokalemia refers to a serum potassium concentration (SPC) of <3.5 mEq/l,

occurs frequently in hospitalized patients [1] and is associated with ventricular arrhythmias as well as an overall poor prognosis after cardiovascular events [2, 4]. Hyperkalemia is defined as a SPC of >5.0 mEq/l and can have a variety of adverse consequences, such as cardiac arrhythmias, in patients hospitalized after a cardiovascular event [3]. In patients with AMI recommended SPC are between 4.0 and 5.0 mEq/l [5, 6] or above 4.5 mEq/l [7].

In contrast to clinical practice guidelines [4–7], recent studies in patients with AMI concluded that a SPC of ≥4.5 mEq/l was associated with an increased in-hospital

* Correspondence: miriam.colombo@helmholtz-muenchen.de
[1]MONICA/KORA Myocardial Infarction Registry, Central Hospital of Augsburg, Augsburg, Germany
[2]Institute of Epidemiology II, Helmholtz Zentrum München, German Research Center for Environmental Health (GmbH), Neuherberg, Germany
Full list of author information is available at the end of the article

and 3-year mortality, respectively [8–10]. To examine whether these findings are valid for a longer observation period, we analyzed the association between SPC and long-term mortality in patients recruited from a population-based myocardial infarction registry.

Methods
Data source and study population
As part of the World Health Organization (WHO) project MONICA (Monitoring Trends and Determinants in Cardiovascular disease) the population-based Augsburg Myocardial Infarction Registry was established in 1984 [11]. MONICA was terminated in 1995 and the registry became part of the KORA (Cooperative Health Research in the Region of Augsburg) framework. Since the registry commenced, all cases of coronary death and non-fatal AMI of the 25- to 74-year old study population in the city of Augsburg and two adjacent counties (about 600,000 inhabitants) have been continuously registered. Patients admitted to one of the eight hospitals in the study area were included. Methods of case identification, diagnostic classification of events as well as data quality control have been described in detail elsewhere [11, 12]. Data collection and follow-up questionnaires have been approved by the ethics committee of the Bavarian Medical Association (Bayerische Landesärztekammer) and have been performed in accordance with the Declaration of Helsinki. All study participants gave written informed consent.

Included in our cohort study were all patients with a first ever AMI consecutively registered between 1 January 2000 and 31 December 2008, whose survival time exceeded 28 days after AMI. Patients were followed up until December 2011. From 4429 patients, we excluded those with missing SPC (n = 164) as well as those with incomplete data on any of the covariates included in our Cox regression models (n = 918). The final study population comprised 3347 male and female patients aged 28–74 years with a first ever AMI, who survived more than 28 days after the event.

Data collection
Interviews with study participants were conducted by trained study nurses during hospital stay using a standardized questionnaire [13, 14]. Patient demographics, risk factors and co-morbidities were covered during the interviews. Laboratory values, AMI characteristics, medical and drug treatment as well as in-hospital complications were obtained from the patients' medical record.

Patients' SPC was determined at hospital admission and expressed in mEq/l. Patients were divided into five groups according to their SPC: < 3.5, 3.5 to <4.0, 4.0 to <4.5, 4.5 to <5.0, ≥5.0 mEq/l.

Renal function was assessed by calculating the estimated glomerular filtration rate (eGFR) using the Modification of Diet in Renal Disease (MDRD) study equation (eGFR (ml/min/1.73 m^2) = 186.3 × (serum creatinine$^{-1.154}$) × (age$^{-0.203}$) × 0.742 (if female) × 1.212 (if black)) [15]. Since creatinine values were only available from 2005 onwards, missing values were incorporated in the analyses as part of a dummy-coded variable. An eGFR of <60 ml/min/1.73m^2 indicates renal impairment and is independently associated with increased all-cause as well as cardio-vascular mortality [16, 17]. Therefore, eGFR values were classified into three categories: <60, ≥60 ml/min/1.73m^2, and missing values.

Whether patients had been previously diagnosed with angina pectoris, hypertension, hyperlipidemia, diabetes and stroke (yes/no) as well as patients' smoking status (smoker/ex-smoker/never-smoker) was determined during the interviews and, with the exception of stroke and smoking status, confirmed by chart review. Hemoglobin and glucose concentration were measured at hospital admission. The highest value of creatine kinase-myocardial band (CK-MB) measured during hospital stay was included in our analyses to serve as a marker for the extent of myocardial injury [18]. Whether any in-hospital revascularization (coronary artery bypass surgery, percutaneous coronary intervention (PCI) or thrombolysis) was performed during hospital stay was included in the analysis as a single covariate (yes/no). Furthermore, treatment with the following medications at hospital discharge were documented (yes/no): antiplatelet agents, beta-blockers, angiotensin-converting enzyme inhibitors (ACEIs) or angiotensin-receptor blockers (ARBs), statins, diuretics, calcium channel blockers, nitrates, insulin and other antidiabetic agents. Administering four evidence-based medications (EBMs; antiplatelet agents, beta-blockers, ACEIs/ARBs, statins) after AMI is considered a standard of care since 2004 and was included as a covariate in our analyses (yes/no). A variable was created summarizing the occurrence of in-hospital complications, such as cardiac arrest, pulmonary edema, bradycardia, re-infarction, ventricular tachycardia, ventricular fibrillation or cardiogenic shock (yes/no). A reduced left ventricular ejection fraction (LVEF) was noted if echocardiography, ventriculography or radionuclide ventriculography revealed a LVEF of < 30% (yes/no).

The outcome of this study was all-cause mortality after more than 28 days following AMI. It was determined by monitoring the vital status of study participants through population registries in- and outside the study region until 31 December 2011.

Statistical analyses
Categorical variables were expressed as percentages, continuous variables as mean value with standard deviation (SD) and continuous variables that proved not to be normally distributed as median with interquartile

range (IQR). Potential covariates were cross-tabulated with the five SPC groups. Differences in frequencies were tested using Chi^2 or Kruskal-Wallis rank-sum test. To evaluate age differences among the SPC groups, a one-way ANOVA (analysis of variance) was performed. Kaplan-Meier plots were generated along with bivariate log-rank tests against survival to test for statistical significance.

To analyze the association between SPC and long-term mortality, Cox proportional hazards regression models were constructed. Patients with a SPC of 4.0 to <4.5 mEq/l served as reference group. An unadjusted model followed by a minimally adjusted model, additionally including the covariates sex and age, were calculated. A parsimonious model was created using backward elimination. Covariates that proved to be significantly associated with mortality in the univariate analysis were entered into the full model. Covariates were only included into the parsimonious model if they made a statistically significant contribution ($p < 0.05$) to the model. The final model was adjusted for prior angina pectoris, hypertension, hyperlipidemia, stroke, smoking status, peak CK-MB, any revascularization treatment and all four EBMs at discharge as well as the following discharge medications: diuretics, calcium channel blockers and insulin. The assumption of proportional hazards (parallel lines of log (–log(event)) versus log of event times) was tested graphically. Covariates violating the proportional hazards assumption were included as time-dependent covariates into the full model prior to backwards elimination. The covariates sex and age were forced to stay in the models. Multicollinearity among the independent variables was examined by assessing variance inflation factors (VIF) in the full model prior to backward selection [19].

Additionally, parsimonious models were calculated for observation periods of one, three, five and ten years in order to detect potential changes in HRs. A Cox regression model was calculated for patients excluded from the study due to missing data on covariates as a sensitivity analysis. To ensure comparability with the results of our study population, we adjusted this model for all covariates that were included in our main parsimonious model. Covariates providing information on stroke prior to AMI, smoking status and peak CK-MB were responsible for 95.3% ($n = 875$) of all missing values ($n = 918$) and, thus, could not be included in this model. Finally, since information on eGFR were only available from 2005 onwards, we calculated a separate Cox regression model using backward elimination and only including patients who were enrolled from 2005 onwards.

Statistical test results were considered significant if the p value was <0.05. All statistical analyses were performed using SAS software, version 9.2 (SAS Institute).

Results

The study sample comprised 3347 patients with a first ever AMI and a mean age of 59.9 years (SD 9.8). Male patients accounted for 75.6% ($n = 2531$) of the sample. The median follow-up time was 6.1 years (IQR 4.2).

Baseline characteristics

Baseline characteristics according to SPC are shown in Table 1. On average, patients with AMI had a SPC of 4.1 mEq/l (SD 0.5). The five SPC groups significantly differed from each other in terms of sex, history of diabetes and hypertension, smoking status, AMI type, laboratory values, medications received at hospital discharge (diuretics, insulin and other antidiabetic agents) and occurrence of any in-hospital complications (see Table 1).

Serum potassium concentration and long-term mortality

Long-term mortality in the whole study population was 14.3% ($n = 481$). The highest mortality of 29.9% ($n = 40$) was observed in patients with SPC of ≥5.0 mEq/l and the lowest (12.6%, $n = 134$) in patients with SPC of 3.5 to <4.0 mEq/l. Kaplan-Meyer survival curves along with the corresponding log-rank test demonstrated statistically significant differences in survival between the five serum potassium groups (see Fig. 1).

Results of the Cox regression analyses are shown in Table 2. In the unadjusted model, patients with SPC of ≥5.0 mEq/l had a significantly increased mortality risk compared to the reference group (unadjusted HR 2.49, 95% CI 1.77–3.50). Adjusting for sex and age resulted in a slight decrease of the HRs. Further adjusting for hypertension, hyperlipidemia, stroke, smoking status, peak CK-MB, any in-hospital revascularization, all four EBMs at discharge as well as diuretics, calcium channel blockers and insulin treatment at discharge, patients with SPC of ≥5.0 mEq/l still were at an increased risk of dying (adjusted HR 1.46, 95% CI 1.03 to 2.07). Patients with SPC of 3.5 to <4.5 mEq/l and <3.5 mEq/l showed the lowest long-term mortality risk compared to the reference group. However, these results did not prove to be statistically significant.

In the analysis of patients who were enrolled from 2005 onwards, those with a SPC of 4.5 - <5.0 mEq/l and those with a SPC ≥5.0 mEq/l did not have significantly increased HRs. Additionally, patients with a SPC of 3.5 - <4.0 mEq/l had a significantly decreased mortality risk compared to the reference group (data not shown). Except for the hypertension and angina pectoris, the same covariates remained in the model as in the parsimonious model shown in Table 2.

1-, 3-, 5- and 10-year mortality risks

Table 3 shows the results of the parsimonious regression models calculated for different observation periods as well as the corresponding mortality for each SPC group.

Table 1 Baseline characteristics of patients with acute myocardial infarction by admission serum potassium concentration (n = 3347)

	Admission SPC, mEq/l					p Value
	<3.5 (n = 249)	3.5 - <4.0 (n = 1060)	4.0 - <4.5 (n = 1406)	4.5 - <5.0 (n = 498)	≥5.0 (n = 134)	
Sociodemographic characteristics						
Female, n (%)	99 (39.8)	276 (26.0)	306 (21.8)	103 (20.7)	32 (23.9)	<0.0001
Age (years), mean ± SD	60.1 ± 9.6	59.9 ± 9.9	59.6 ± 9.7	60.4 ± 9.8	61.1 ± 9.1	0.3156
Risk factors and co-morbidities, n (%)						
Angina pectoris	31 (12.5)	135 (12.7)	196 (13.9)	72 (14.5)	23 (17.2)	0.5858
Hypertension	199 (79.9)	813 (76.7)	1033 (73.5)	383 (76.9)	111 (82.8)	0.0278
Hyperlipidemia	173 (69.5)	737 (69.5)	998 (71.0)	336 (67.5)	99 (73.9)	0.5139
Stroke	12 (4.8)	56 (5.3)	77 (5.5)	29 (5.8)	14 (10.5)	0.1640
Diabetes mellitus[a]	59 (23.8)	273 (25.8)	376 (26.7)	172 (34.5)	58 (43.3)	<0.0001
Smoking status						
Current smoker	83 (33.3)	404 (38.1)	552 (39.3)	203 (40.8)	52 (38.8)	0.0140
Ex-smoker	71 (28.5)	318 (30.0)	423 (30.1)	156 (31.3)	55 (41.0)	
Never-smoker	95 (38.2)	338 (31.9)	431 (30.7)	139 (27.9)	55 (20.2)	
Clinical characteristics, n (%)						
AMI type[b]						
STEMI	125 (50.4)	489 (46.5)	555 (39.8)	187 (28.3)	47 (35.3)	0.0007
NSTEMI	114 (46.0)	516 (49.1)	768 (55.1)	267 (54.7)	79 (59.4)	
Bundle branch block	9 (3.6)	46 (4.4)	70 (5.0)	34 (7.0)	7 (5.3)	
LVEF <30%[c]	16 (9.5)	84 (10.9)	104 (10.5)	49 (13.7)	13 (14.6)	0.3453
Laboratory values, median (IQR)						
Admission creatinine (mg/dl)[d]	0.96 (0.8–1.2)	0.97 (0.8–1.1)	0.97 (0.8–1.1)	1.01 (0.8–1.2)	1.14 (1.0–1.5)	<0.0001
Admission hemoglobin (g/l)[d]	141 (131–151)	145 (136–155)	146 (137–156)	145 (135–154)	145 (129–158)	0.0079
Admission troponin-I (ng/ml)[e]	0.32 (0.1–2.7)	0.41 (0.1–3.2)	0.66 (0.1–3.8)	0.73 (0.2–5.9)	1.21 (0.2–4.9)	<0.0001
Peak CK-MB (U/l)	51 (15–122)	48 (18–119)	41 (16–105)	38 (15–99)	41 (15–84)	0.0462
Admission glucose (mg/dl)	143 (119–168)	130 (112–162)	126 (108–161)	131 (112–179)	152 (121–224)	<0.0001
eGFR (ml/min/1.73m²)[d]	76.2 (61.2–96.8)	78.9 (66.2–94.0)	80.4 (67.3–95.1)	77.3 (61.1–91.7)	65.8 (47.2–80.3)	<0.0001
eGFR <60 (ml/min/1.73m²), n (%)[d]	29 (23.6)	69 (14.2)	96 (15.3)	56 (23.5)	24 (40.0)	<0.0001
In-hospital treatment, n (%)						
Coronary angiography	237 (95.2)	1002 (94.5)	1331 (94.7)	458 (92.0)	120 (89.6)	0.0306
PCI[f]	170 (68.3)	757 (71.4)	970 (69.0)	339 (68.1)	84 (62.7)	0.2392
CABG	37 (14.9)	153 (14.4)	247 (17.6)	87 (17.5)	22 (16.4)	0.2638
Thrombolysis[g]	38 (18.9)	137 (18.0)	130 (14.0)	46 (13.7)	8 (9.2)	0.0338
Any revascularization treatment	212 (85.1)	934 (88.1)	1225 (87.1)	427 (85.7)	108 (80.6)	0.1199
Medication at hospital discharge						
Antiplatelet agents	236 (94.8)	1028 (97.0)	1357 (96.5)	484 (97.2)	128 (95.5)	0.4053
Beta-blockers	236 (94.8)	1023 (96.5)	1350 (96.0)	474 (95.2)	124 (92.5)	0.1863
ACEIs/ARBs	217 (87.2)	883 (83.3)	1151 (81.9)	425 (85.3)	108 (80.6)	0.1436
Statins	219 (88.0)	949 (89.5)	1263 (89.8)	443 (89.0)	115 (85.8)	0.6086
All four EBMs	176 (70.7)	763 (72.0)	1004 (71.4)	364 (73.1)	85 (63.4)	0.2770
Diuretics	147 (59.0)	533 (50.3)	643 (45.7)	247 (49.6)	86 (64.2)	<0.0001
Calcium channel blockers	41 (16.5)	120 (11.3)	174 (12.4)	51 (10.2)	22 (16.4)	0.0598
Nitrates	3 (1.2)	38 (3.6)	61 (4.3)	22 (4.4)	8 (6.0)	0.1066

Table 1 Baseline characteristics of patients with acute myocardial infarction by admission serum potassium concentration ($n = 3347$)
(Continued)

Insulin	19 (7.6)	66 (6.2)	128 (9.1)	56 (11.2)	27 (20.2)	<0.0001
Other antidiabetic agents	11 (4.4)	103 (9.7)	149 (10.6)	84 (16.9)	23 (17.2)	<0.0001
Any In-hospital complications[h, i], n (%)	53 (21.5)	162 (15.4)	201 (14.4)	89 (17.9)	24 (18.3)	0.0340

SPC, Serum potassium concentration; SD, Standard deviation; AMI, Acute myocardial infarction; STEMI, ST-elevation myocardial infarction; NSTEMI, non-ST-elevation myocardial infarction; LVEF,
Left-ventricular ejection fraction; IQR, Interquartile range, CK-MB, Creatine kinase-myocardial band; eGFR, Estimated glomerular filtration rate; PCI, Percutaneous coronary intervention; CABG, Coronary artery bypass graft; ACEIs, Angiotensin-converting enzyme inhibitors; ARBs, Angiotensin-receptor blockers; EBMs, Evidence-based medications (antiplatelet agents, beta-blockers, ACEIs/ARBs, statins)
[a] $n = 3346$
[b] $n = 3313$
[c] $n = 2382$
[d] $n = 1534$
[e] $n = 2503$
[f] $n = 3346$
[g] $n = 2317$
[h] Including cardiac arrest, pulmonary edema, bradycardia, re-infarction, ventricular tachycardia, ventricular fibrillation and cardiogenic shock occurring during hospital stay
[i] $n = 3317$

The highest mortality was found in patients with a SPC of ≥5.0 mEq/l across all observation periods, whereas the lowest mortality was mainly found in patients with a SPC between 3.5 and <4.0 mEq/l. After a one-year observation period, the mortality risk of patients with a SPC between 4.5 and <5.0 mEq/l was increased by 96% (adjusted HR 1.96, 95% CI 1.10 to 3.48). Although the results for three- and five-year observation periods did not meet statistical significance, a trend towards an increased mortality risk in patients with SPC between 4.5 and <5.0 mEq/l could be identified (Table 3). After a ten-year observation period, only the HRs of patients with a SPC of ≥5.0 mEq/l were significantly increased.

Mortality in patients excluded from the study
In patients excluded from the study due to partly missing data on relevant covariates, an increased long-term mortality risk was found in patients with SPC between 4.5 and <5.0 mEq/l (adjusted HR 1.43, 95% CI 1.00 to 2.04) and ≥5.0 mEq/l (adjusted HR 2.40, 95% CI 1.55 to 3.67) compared to the reference group (see Table 4).

Discussion
In the present study, we analyzed the association between admission SPC and long-term all-cause mortality in patients with AMI. Mortality risks were significantly increased in the highest SPC group (≥5.0 mEq/l).

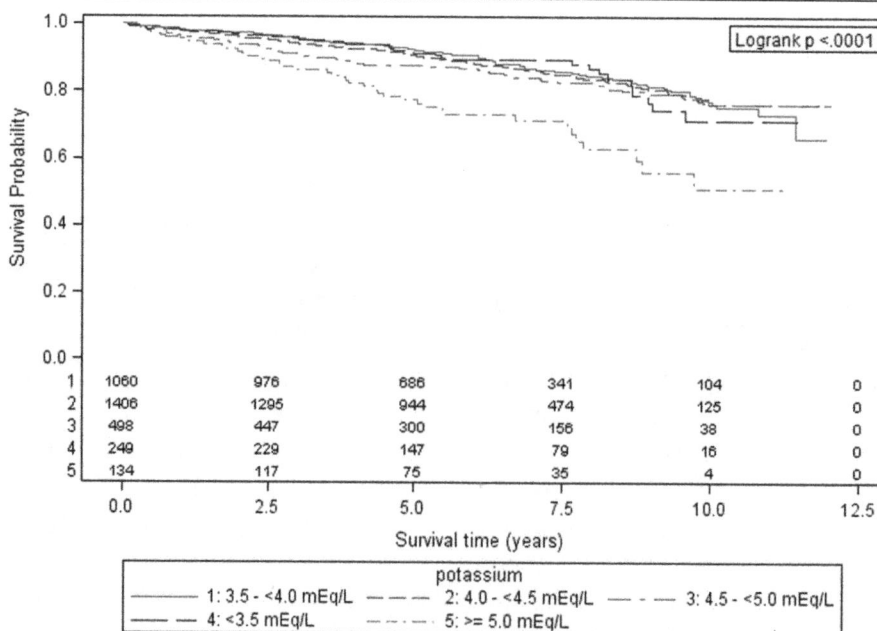

Fig. 1 Kaplan-Meier curves of 12-year survival for the five admission serum potassium concentration groups

Table 2 Cox regression models for long-term mortality following acute myocardial infarction by admission serum potassium concentration (n = 3347)

Admission SPC, mEq/l	Unadjusted Model		Minimal Model[a]		Parsimonious Model[b]	
	HR (95% CI)	p Value	HR (95% CI)	p Value	HR (95% CI)	p Value
<3.5	0.98 (0.67–1.42)	0.9125	0.97 (0.68–1.44)	0.9420	0.92 (0.63–1.34)	0.6686
3.5 - <4.0	0.93 (0.74–1.15)	0.4871	0.88 (0.71–1.10)	0.2593	0.87 (0.70–1.09)	0.2297
4.0 - <4.5	1 (Ref.)		1 (Ref.)		1 (Ref.)	
4.5 - <5.0	1.18 (0.91–1.53)	0.2176	1.15 (0.88–1.49)	0.3038	1.08 (0.83–1.41)	0.5582
≥5.0	2.49 (1.77–3.50)	<0.0001	2.31 (1.64–3.25)	<0.0001	1.46 (1.03–2.07)	0.0360

SPC, Serum potassium concentration; HR, Hazard Ratio; CI, Confidence Interval
[a]Adjusted for sex and age
[b]Adjusted for sex, age, angina pectoris, hypertension, hyperlipidemia, stroke, smoking status, peak creatine kinase - mycoardial band (CK-MB), any revascularization treatment (coronary artery bypass surgery, percutaneous coronary intervention (PCI) or thrombolysis), all four evidence-based medications (EBMs) at discharge (antiplatelet agents, beta-blockers, ACEIs/ARBs (Angiotensin-converting enzyme inhibitors/Angiotensin receptor blockers), statins, diuretics at discharge, calcium channel blockers at discharge, insulin at discharge

Table 3 Adjusted Cox regression models for observation periods of one, three, five and ten years (n = 3347)

	Admission SPC, mEq/l	Parsimonious model[a]	
		HR (95% CI)	p Value
1-year observation period (>28 days to one year)	< 3.5	1.04 (0.43–2.55)	0.9269
	3.5 - <4-0	0.92 (0.51–1.67)	0.7924
	4.0 - <4.5	1 (Ref.)	
	4.5 - <5.0	1.96 (1.10–3.48)	0.0230
	≥5.0	1.22 (0.49–3.04)	0.6638
3-year observation period (>28 days to 3 years)	<3.5	0.60 (0.31–1.16)	0.1268
	3.5 - <4-0	0.72 (0.50–1.04)	0.0780
	4.0 - <4.5	1 (Ref.)	
	4.5 - <5.0	1.39 (0.96–2.00)	0.0799
	≥5.0	1.29 (0.75–2.21)	0.3560
5-year observation period (>28 days to 5 years)	<3.5	0.79 (0.49–1.29)	0.3423
	3.5 - <4-0	0.78 (0.58–1.04)	0.0901
	4.0 - <4.5	1 (Ref.)	
	4.5 - <5.0	1.32 (0.97–1.80)	0.0811
	≥5.0	1.40 (0.91–2.14)	0.1232
10-year observation period (>28 days to 10 years)	<3.5	0.92 (0.63–1.34)	0.6527
	3.5 - <4-0	0.85 (0.68–1.06)	0.1463
	4.0 - <4.5	1 (Ref.)	
	4.5 - <5.0	1.08 (0.83–1.41)	0.5650
	≥5.0	1.44 (1.02–2.05)	0.0218

SPC, Serum potassium concentration; HR, Hazard ratio; CI, Confidence interval
[a]Adjusted for sex, age, angina pectoris, hypertension, hyperlipidemia, stroke, smoking status, peak creatine kinase -myocardial band (CK-MB), any revascularization treatment (coronary artery bypass surgery, percutaneous coronary intervention (PCI) or thrombolysis), all four medications at discharge (antiplatelet agents, beta-blockers, ACEIs/ARBs (Angiotensin-converting enzyme inhibitors/Angiotensin receptor blockers), statins, diuretics at discharge, calcium channel blockers at discharge, insulin at discharge

Analyses covering different observation periods showed a trend towards increased mortality risks in patients with SPC between 4.5 and <5.0 mEq/l as well as a significant association between a SPC of ≥5.0 mEq/l and increased mortality after a ten-year observation period.

In contrast to recent observational studies [8–10], our results for the total observation period do not suggest changing current clinical practice guidelines regarding desirable SPC in patients with AMI. A significantly increased long-term mortality risk was found only in patients with SPC of ≥5.0 mEq/l. However, our findings for shorter observation periods are partly comparable to the ones reported in recent studies. A study in 38,689 patients with AMI recruited from the Cerner Health Facts database and a Korean study in 1924 patients with AMI reported U-shaped associations between mean SPC and in-hospital and three-year mortality and found significantly increased risks in both patients with mean SPC of <3.5 mEq/l and ≥4.5 mEq/l [8, 9]. In addition to mean SPC, Goyal et al. analyzed the association between SPC

Table 4 Adjusted Cox regression model for patients excluded from the study due to missing covariates (n = 875)

Admission SPC, mEq/l	Parsimonious Model [a,b]	
	HR (95% CI)	p Value
<3.5	1.37 (0.80–2.33)	0.2481
3.5 - <4-0	1.03 (0.73–1.44)	0.8840
4.0 - <4.5	1 (Ref.)	
4.5 - <5.0	1.43 (1.00–2.04)	0.0486
≥5.0	2.40 (1.55–3.67)	<0.0001

SPC, Serum potassium concentration; HR, Hazard ratio; CI, Confidence interval
[a]Adjusted for age, sex, angina pectoris, hypertension, hyperlipidemia, any revascularization therapy (coronary artery bypass surgery, percutaneous coronary intervention (PCI) or thrombolysis), all four evidence-based medications (EBMs) at discharge (antiplatelet agents, beta-blockers, ACEIs/ARBs (Angiotensin-converting enzyme inhibitors/Angiotensin receptor blockers), statins, diuretics at discharge, calcium channel blockers at discharge, insulin at discharge
[b] Not adjusted for stroke, smoking status and peak creatine kinase - myocardial band (CK-MB)

measured at hospital admission and in-hospital mortality [8]. The HRs were attenuated yet still significantly increased in patients with SPC ≥4.5 mEq/l. In line with those findings, patients with SPC between 4.5 and <5.0 mEq/l had an increased mortality risk in our study population after a one-year observation period. A similar trend, yet not statistically significant, was found for three- and five-year observation periods. Our analysis of patients excluded from the study also suggests that an increased risk of dying might already be present in patients with SPC between 4.5 and <5.0 mEq/l. In patients with AMI, SPC between 4.5 and <5.0 mEq/l might therefore negatively affect survival during the first few years following the event, whereas in the long run, SPC of ≥5.0 mEq/l might be more harmful. A similar trend was demonstrated in another study in AMI patients [10]. In this study, the odds ratios of patients with SPC between 4.5 and ≤5.0 mEq/l were significantly increased after one and five years of follow-up. However, the OR deviated only marginally from the reference group after a ten-year follow-up [10].

Studies conducted in prior years examined in-hospital outcomes associated with SPC, but had low statistical power to detect higher mortality risks due to small study populations. These studies concluded that patients with AMI and hypokalemia had an increased risk for cardiac arrhythmias [20, 21] and a higher in-hospital mortality [22]. One study found no significant difference in in-hospital mortality in patients with AMI and hypo- or normokalemia [23]. Comparability with these studies is limited not only because they focused on in-hospital outcomes, but also due to methodological differences and the fact that AMI treatment has changed substantially both in terms of revascularization and drug treatment.

In contrast to earlier studies [7–9, 22, 24], we did not detect increased mortality risks in patients with low SPC. These results might be explained by an improved treatment of patients with AMI counteracting hypokalemia. Apart from beneficial effects on survival, medications routinely administered after AMI, such as beta-blockers, prevent hypokalemia [8, 23]. Furthermore, hypokalemia affects morbidity and mortality in patients with an established cardiovascular event [7, 22, 25, 26]. Especially patients with AMI had an increased risk for ventricular arrhythmias even if their SPC was only mildly decreased [1, 3, 7]. Additionally, changes in SPC subsequent to hospital admission occur frequently. A recent study in patients with heart failure concluded that the SPC measured within 48 h after hospital admission is often abnormal and increases during hospitalization [27]. SPC in our study was only measured at hospital admission and we did not know if and how hypo-or hyperkalemia were treated during hospital stay. Improved medical treatment of AMI and of hypokalemia in AMI patients might have positively influenced long-term survival in our study population with low SPC at hospital admission.

Potassium homeostasis primarily depends on a normal renal function [7] and both hypo- and hyperkalemia can occur due to impaired renal excretion [1, 2]. According to a large-scale study in 118,753 patients with AMI, renal impairment is an important long-term predictor of mortality [28]. Furthermore, hyperkalemia has been demonstrated to be one of the largest risk factors for all-cause mortality in patients with an established cardiovascular disease and impaired renal function [29]. In our study population, patients with high SPC had a lower eGFR than the reference group, indicating renal impairment. However, the corresponding covariate did not make it into the final parsimonious model. Nevertheless, we cannot rule out the possibility of bias since the admission creatinine level, and consequently the eGFR, was only available from 2005 onwards in our data set. In the analysis including only patients enrolled from 2005 onwards, we did not find significantly increased mortality risks in those with a SPC of 4.5- <5.0 mEq/l and ≥5.0 mEq/l, respectively.

In the present study we focused on long-term mortality and, therefore, patients who died within 28 days after AMI were excluded. The excluded patients had a SPC of 4.4 mEq/l (SD 0.8), while the actual study population had a mean SPC of 4.1 mEq/l (SD 0.5) (data not shown). Patients who died within 28 days were more likely to have extreme SPC (<3.5 mEq/l and ≥5.0 mEq/l), they were overall sicker and older than the included patients (data not shown). Therefore, including them into the analysis would have further increased the mortality risk estimates for patients with high SPC.

This study is characterized by several strengths. To our knowledge this is the first longitudinal study with an observation period of more than three years. Data were collected in the framework of a population-based registry with consecutive enrollment. Important covariates such as in-hospital treatment and complications, medication received at hospital discharge as well as risk factors and co-morbidities were included.

The following limitations should be considered. We did not have the possibility to distinguish between potassium-sparing versus non-potassium-sparing diuretics. In addition, our results do not apply to patients with AMI who are older than 74 years. Data on ethnicity was not collected in the framework of the registry and, therefore, the results might not be generalizable to all ethnic groups. Patients with AMI were enrolled between 2000 and 2008 for this study and treatment strategies most likely improved during this time span both for hypo- or hyperkalemia after AMI as well as AMI itself.

Data on the treatment of AMI was included in the analysis; however, data on the treatment of abnormal SPC was not collected in the framework of the registry. Finally, due to the observational design of our study we might not have considered all relevant confounders and we cannot exclude the possibility of reverse causation.

Conclusion

Based on our analysis, an admission SPC of ≥5.0 mEq/l might be associated with an increased mortality risk in patients with AMI. Furthermore, our results indicate that also patients with admission SPC between 4.5 and <5.0 mEq/l may experience a higher mortality risk in the first few years following AMI. Due to the limited data on renal function in our study, further long-term studies are needed to provide evidence on the relevance of admission SPC in patients with AMI.

Abbreviations

ACEI: Angiotensin-converting enzyme inhibitor; AMI: Acute myocardial infarction; ANOVA: Analysis of variance; ARB: Angiotensin-receptor blockers; CK-MB: Creatine kinase-myocardial band; EBM: Evidence-based medication; eGFR: Estimated glomerular filtration rate; HR: Hazard ratio; IQR: Interquartile range; KORA: Cooperative Health Research in the Region of Augsburg; LVEF: Left ventricular ejection fraction; MDRD: Modification of Diet in Renal Disease; MI: Myocardial infarction; MONICA: Monitoring Trends and Determinants in Cardiovascular disease; PCI: Percutaneous coronary intervention; SD: Standard deviation; SPC: Serum potassium concentration; VIF: Variance inflation factor; WHO: World Health Organization

Acknowledgments

We thank all members of the Helmholtz Zentrum München, Institute of Epidemiology II and the field staff in Augsburg who were involved in the planning and conduct of the study. We wish to thank the local health departments, the office-based physicians and the clinicians of the hospitals within the study area for their support. Finally, we express our appreciation to all study participants.

Funding

The KORA research platform and the MONICA Augsburg studies were initiated and financed by the Helmholtz Zentrum München, German Research Center for Environmental Health, which is funded by the German Federal Ministry of Education, Science, Research and Technology and by the State of Bavaria. Since the year 2000, the collection of MI data has been co-financed by the German Federal Ministry of Health to provide population-based MI morbidity data for the official German Health Report (see www.gbe-bund.de). Steering partners of the MONICA/KORA Infarction Registry, Augsburg, include the KORA research platform, Helmholtz Zentrum München and the Department of Internal Medicine I, Cardiology, Central Hospital of Augsburg.

Authors' contributions

MGC, IK and CM conceived the study. MGC performed the statistical analyses and drafted the manuscript. CM, MH, BK, CT and AP contributed to the interpretation of data. CM, MH, BK and CT contributed to data acquisition. IK, UA, MH, CT, BK, AP and CM read, critically revised and approved the final manuscript.

Competing interests

The authors declare that they have no competing interests.

Author details

[1]MONICA/KORA Myocardial Infarction Registry, Central Hospital of Augsburg, Augsburg, Germany. [2]Institute of Epidemiology II, Helmholtz Zentrum München, German Research Center for Environmental Health (GmbH), Neuherberg, Germany. [3]Department of Internal Medicine I – Cardiology, Central Hospital of Augsburg, Augsburg, Germany. [4]Department of Internal Medicine/Cardiology, Hospital of Nördlingen, Nördlingen, Germany.

References

1. Schaefer TJ, Wolford RW. Disorders of potassium. Emerg Med Clin North Am. 2005;23(3):723–47. viii-ix
2. Clausen T. Hormonal and pharmacological modification of plasma potassium homeostasis. Fundam Clin Pharmacol. 2010;24(5):595–605.
3. Alfonzo AV, Isles C, Geddes C, Deighan C. Potassium disorders–clinical spectrum and emergency management. Resuscitation. 2006;70(1):10–25.
4. Cohn JN, Kowey PR, Whelton PK, Prisant LM. New guidelines for potassium replacement in clinical practice: a contemporary review by the National Council on potassium in clinical practice. Arch Intern Med. 2000;160(16):2429–36.
5. Zipes DP, Camm AJ, Borggrefe M, Buxton AE, Chaitman B, Fromer M, Gregoratos G, Klein G, Moss AJ, Myerburg RJ et al. ACC/AHA/ESC 2006 guidelines for management of patients with ventricular arrhythmias and the prevention of sudden cardiac death: a report of the American College of Cardiology/American Heart Association Task Force and the European Society of Cardiology Committee for Practice Guidelines (Writing Committee to Develop guidelines for management of patients with ventricular arrhythmias and the prevention of sudden cardiac death) developed in collaboration with the European Heart Rhythm Association and the Heart Rhythm Society. Europace. 2006;8(9):746–837.
6. Antman EM, Anbe DT, Armstrong PW, Bates ER, Green LA, Hand M, Hochman JS, Krumholz HM, Kushner FG, Lamas GA, et al. ACC/AHA guidelines for the management of patients with ST-elevation myocardial infarction–executive summary. A report of the American College of Cardiology/American Heart Association task force on practice guidelines (writing committee to revise the 1999 guidelines for the management of patients with acute myocardial infarction). J Am Coll Cardiol. 2004;44(3):671–719.
7. Macdonald JE, Struthers AD. What is the optimal serum potassium level in cardiovascular patients? J Am Coll Cardiol. 2004;43(2):155–61.
8. Goyal A, Spertus JA, Gosch K, Venkitachalam L, Jones PG, Van den Berghe G, Kosiborod M. Serum potassium levels and mortality in acute myocardial infarction. JAMA. 2012;307(2):157–64.
9. Choi JS, Kim YA, Kim HY, Oak CY, Kang YU, Kim CS, Bae EH, Ma SK, Ahn YK, Jeong MH, et al. Relation of serum potassium level to long-term outcomes in patients with acute myocardial infarction. Am J Cardiol. 2014;113(8):1285–90.
10. Shiyovich A, Gilutz H, Plakht Y. Serum potassium levels and long-term post-discharge mortality in acute myocardial infarction. Int J Cardiol. 2014;172(2):e368–70.
11. Meisinger C, Hormann A, Heier M, Kuch B, Lowel H. Admission blood glucose and adverse outcomes in non-diabetic patients with myocardial infarction in the reperfusion era. Int J Cardiol. 2006;113(2):229–35.
12. Kuch B, Heier M, von Scheidt W, Kling B, Hoermann A, Meisinger C. 20-year trends in clinical characteristics, therapy and short-term prognosis in acute myocardial infarction according to presenting electrocardiogram: the MONICA/KORA AMI registry (1985-2004). J Intern Med. 2008;264(3):254–264.
13. Kirchberger I, Heier M, Goluke H, Kuch B, von Scheidt W, Peters A, Meisinger C. Mismatch of presenting symptoms at first and recurrent acute myocardial infarction. From the MONICA/KORA myocardial infarction registry. Eur J Prev Cardiol. 2016;23(4):377–84.
14. Lowel H, Meisinger C, Heier M, Hormann A. The population-based acute myocardial infarction (AMI) registry of the MONICA/KORA study region of Augsburg. Gesundheitswesen. 2005;67(Suppl 1):S31–7.
15. Levey AS, Bosch JP, Lewis JB, Greene T, Rogers N, Roth D. A more accurate method to estimate glomerular filtration rate from serum creatinine: a new prediction equation. Modification of diet in renal disease study group. Ann Intern Med. 1999;130(6):461–70.
16. Chronic Kidney Disease Prognosis Consortium, Matsushita K, Van Der Velde M, Astor BC, Woodward M, Levey AS, De Jong PE, Coresh J, Gansevoort RT. Association of estimated glomerular filtration rate and albuminuria with all-cause and cardiovascular mortality in general population cohorts: a collaborative meta-analysis. Lancet. 2010;375(9731):2073–81.

17. Bae EH, Lim SY, Cho KH, Choi JS, Kim CS, Park JW, Ma SK, Jeong MH, Kim SW. GFR and cardiovascular outcomes after acute myocardial infarction: results from the Korea acute myocardial infarction registry. Am J Kidney Dis. 2012;59(6):795–802.

18. Chin CT, Wang TY, Li S, Wiviott SD, DeLemos JA, Kontos MC, Peterson ED, Roe MT. comparison of the prognostic value of peak creatine kinase-MB and troponin levels among patients with acute myocardial infarction: a report from the acute coronary treatment and intervention outcomes network registry-get with the guidelines. Clin Cardiol 2012;35(7):424–429.

19. Allison P. When can you safely ignore multicollinearity? 2012. http://statisticalhorizons.com/multicollinearity. Accessed 5 Jun 2016.

20. Friedensohn A, Faibel HE, Bairey O, Goldbourt U, Schlesinger Z. Malignant arrhythmias in relation to values of serum potassium in patients with acute myocardial infarction. Int J Cardiol. 1991;32(3):331–8.

21. Nordrehaug JE, Johannessen KA, von der Lippe G. Serum potassium concentration as a risk factor of ventricular arrhythmias early in acute myocardial infarction. Circulation. 1985;71(4):645–9.

22. Dyckner T. Relation of cardiovascular disease to potassium and magnesium deficiencies. Am J Cardiol. 1990;65(23):44K–6K.

23. Madias JE, Shah B, Chintalapally G, Chalavarya G, Madias NE. Admission serum potassium in patients with acute myocardial infarction: its correlates and value as a determinant of in-hospital outcome. Chest. 2000;118(4):904–13.

24. Krijthe BP, Heeringa J, Kors JA, Hofman A, Franco OH, Witteman JC, Stricker BH. Serum potassium levels and the risk of atrial fibrillation: the Rotterdam study. Int J Cardiol. 2013;168(6):5411–5.

25. Hulting J. In-hospital ventricular fibrillation and its relation to serum potassium. Acta Med Scand Suppl. 1981;647:109–16.

26. Pourmoghaddas A, Shemirani H, Garakyaraghi M. Association of serum potassium level with ventricular tachycardia after acute myocardial infarction. ARYA Atheroscler. 2012;8(2):79–81.

27. Khan SS, Campia U, Chioncel O, Zannad F, Rossignol P, Maggioni AP, Swedberg K, Konstam MA, Senni M, Nodari S, et al. Changes in serum potassium levels during hospitalization in patients with worsening heart failure and reduced ejection fraction (from the EVEREST trial). Am J Cardiol. 2015;115(6):790–6.

28. Smith GL, Masoudi FA, Shlipak MG, Krumholz HM, Parikh CR. Renal impairment predicts long-term mortality risk after acute myocardial infarction. J Am Soc Nephrol. 2008;19(1):141–50.

29. Jain N, Kotla S, Little BB, Weideman RA, Brilakis ES, Reilly RF, Banerjee S. Predictors of hyperkalemia and death in patients with cardiac and renal disease. Am J Cardiol. 2012;109(10):1510–3.

Association of sleep problems with neuroendocrine hormones and coagulation factors in patients with acute myocardial infarction

Roland von Känel[1]*[iD], Mary Princip[1], Jean-Paul Schmid[2], Jürgen Barth[3], Hansjörg Znoj[4], Ulrich Schnyder[5] and Rebecca E. Meister-Langraf[6]

Abstract

Background: Obstructive sleep apnea (OSA) and insomnia are frequent sleep problems that are associated with poor prognosis in patients with coronary heart disease. The mechanisms linking poor sleep with an increased cardiovascular risk are incompletely understood. We examined whether a high risk of OSA as well as insomnia symptoms are associated with neuroendocrine hormones and coagulation factors in patients admitted with acute myocardial infarction.

Methods: We assessed 190 patients (mean age 60 years, 83% men) in terms of OSA risk (STOP screening tool for the assessment of high vs. low OSA risk) and severity of insomnia symptoms (Jenkins Sleep Scale for the assessment of subjective sleep difficulties) within 48 h of an acute coronary intervention. Circulating concentrations of epinephrine, norepinephrine, cortisol, fibrinogen, D-dimer, and von Willebrand factor were measured the next morning. The association of OSA risk and insomnia symptoms with neuroendocrine hormones and coagulation factors was computed using multivariate models adjusting for demographic factors, health behaviors, somatic and psychiatric comorbidities, cardiac disease-related variables, and OSA risk in the model for insomnia symptoms, respectively, for insomnia symptoms in the model for OSA risk.

Results: High OSA risk was identified in 41% of patients and clinically relevant insomnia symptoms were reported by 27% of patients. Compared to those with low OSA risk, patients with high OSA risk had lower levels of epinephrine ($p = 0.015$), norepinephrine ($p = 0.049$) and cortisol ($p = 0.001$). More severe insomnia symptoms were associated with higher levels of fibrinogen ($p = 0.037$), driven by difficulties initiating sleep, and with lower levels of norepinephrine ($p = 0.024$), driven by difficulties maintaining sleep.

Conclusions: In patients with acute myocardial infarction, sleep problems are associated with neuroendocrine hormones and coagulation activity. The pattern of these relationships is not uniform for patients with a high risk of OSA and those with insomnia symptoms, and whether they contribute to adverse cardiovascular outcomes needs to be established.

Keywords: Acute coronary syndrome, Biomarker , Blood coagulation , HPA axis, Insomnia, Sleep apnea, Sympathetic nervous system

* Correspondence: roland.vonkaenel@usz.ch
[1]Department of Consultation-Liaison Psychiatry and Psychosomatic Medicine, University Hospital Zurich, Culmannstrasse 8, CH-8091 Zurich, Switzerland
Full list of author information is available at the end of the article

Background

Obstructive sleep apnea (OSA) is a common sleep-related breathing disorder that is caused by repeated upper airway obstruction during sleep and characterized through symptoms of snoring, breathing cessations while sleeping, and daytime sleepiness and fatigue [1]. Insomnia disorders are characterized by subjective sleep initiating and maintaining problems in spite of adequate circumstances to sleep and daytime impairment, whereas insomnia symptoms alone do not merit a formal diagnosis of insomnia [2].

Obstructive sleep apnea and insomnia symptoms, including difficulty initiating sleep, difficulty maintaining sleep and non-restorative sleep, have been associated with an increased risk of incident coronary heart disease (CHD) events, independently of a range of other risk factors [3–7]. Sleep problems may also be associated with poor prognosis of CHD. In two meta-analyses, CHD patients with OSA had an almost two-fold higher risk of poor cardiovascular prognosis, including recurrent CHD events and stroke, than CHD patients without OSA [8, 9]. In terms of insomnia symptoms in patients with acute myocardial infarction (MI), not feeling well-rested was predictive of case fatality in the 4 weeks post-MI in men and of 10-year risk of new CVD events in women [10]. In women, assessed 3–6 months after acute coronary syndrome (ACS), a sleep quality index, defined by insomnia symptoms was a predictor of recurrent CHD events at 5-year follow-up, after controlling for CVD risk factors and depressive symptoms [11]. In men who had undergone percutaneous coronary angioplasty, a state of vital exhaustion, characterized by subjective sleep disturbances, including troubles falling asleep, waking up repeatedly during the night, and not feeling well rested, along with profound feelings of fatigue, was predictive of new CHD events after a follow-up of 1.5 years [12].

Different biological mechanisms, initiated by intermittent hypoxia, are thought to underpin the association of OSA with an increased risk of incident CHD, including sympathetic hyperactivity, systemic inflammation, oxidative stress, vascular endothelial dysfunction, and hypercoagulability [13, 14]. Likewise, sympathetic hyperactivity and systemic inflammation, but also elevated cortisol (COR) levels have been proposed to be biological mechanisms potentially linking insomnia with incident CVD [15]. Although these mechanisms might also link poor sleep with recurrent atherothrombotic events in patents with established CHD, this has not systematically been explored. In the present study, we focused on circulating neuroendocrine and coagulation markers in patients with sleep problems admitted with acute MI, as sleep studies in individuals without CVD suggest a role of neuroendocrine changes and coagulation activation in incident atherothrombotic events. For instance, in middle-aged and elderly subjects, objective sleep problems, including greater apnea-hypopnea index and oxygen desaturation, indicating OSA, as well as poor subjective sleep quality, were associated with increased plasma levels of fibrinogen, D-dimer, and von Willebrand factor (VWF) [16–20]. In patients with ACS, these prothrombotic markers were of prognostic value for major cardiovascular events and all-cause mortality [21–24].

In OSA, hyperactivity of the sympathetic nervous system (SNS) is evidenced by increased norepinephrine (NEPI) turnover [25], whereas findings on hypothalamic-pituitary adrenal (HPA) axis function, including COR levels, are contradictory [26]. In insomnia, HPA axis dysregulation is evidenced by high COR levels in the evening, affecting sleep architecture [27], and low morning COR levels, which relate to poor sleep quality, nightly awakenings and unrefreshing sleep [28]. The metabolic consequences of neuroendocrine dysregulation include hypertension, dyslipidemia, obesity, diabetes and a prothrombotic state, which are associated with the progression of atherothrombotic disease [29]. Secretion of epinephrine (EPI), NEPI, and COR has effects on coagulation, including increases in fibrinogen, D-dimer and VWF levels [30, 31], and neuroendocrine dysregulation might partially account for a link between sleep problems and coagulation activity [17].

Insomnia and OSA are often found together in the same patient, with up to 50% of OSA patients having insomnia symptoms; a similar prevalence of at least mild OSA is found in patients with insomnia [32]. However, in meta-analyses of prospective studies incident and recurrent CVD risk were not adjusted for the other sleep disorder nor were joint effects investigated [3–9]. As yet, except for hypertension [33], there is little evidence that OSA and insomnia together are associated with a greater risk of CVD or frequency of CVD risk factors than OSA alone [34]. However, such studies are still few in number and, to our knowledge, researchers did not investigate neuroendocrine and coagulation activity.

In this study we aimed to examine the association of a high risk of OSA and insomnia symptoms, independently of each other, with neuroendocrine hormones and coagulation factors in patients with acute MI. We specifically hypothesized that more sleep problems would be associated with higher levels of fibrinogen, D-dimer and VWF. We specified no a priori hypothesis regarding the direction of an association of sleep problems with EPI, NEPI and COR levels; this is because findings vary across studies, depending upon circadian factors, natural vs. experimental designs, confounding variables, and measures of sleep quantity and quality [26, 35, 36]. We predicted the hypothesized relationships to be independent of demographics, comorbidity, health behaviors, and cardiac-related variables. In complementary analyses we examined whether neuroendocrine hormones may account for the relation between sleep problems and coagulation factors, and whether there were joint effects of OSA risk and insomnia symptoms for neuroendocrine and coagulation outcomes.

Methods
Study participants and design
Rationale of the parent study
Data for this ancillary sleep study were collected from patients who participated in the Myocardial Infarction-Stress Prevention Intervention (MI-SPRINT) randomized controlled trial [37]. The primary aim of the parent study was to test whether a psychological first aid approach (i.e., one single 45-min session of psychological counseling at hospital referral) may prevent the incidence of ACS-induced posttraumatic stress at 3-month follow-up [37]. About 12% of ACS patients develop clinically significant levels of posttraumatic stress which is a predictor of poor cardiac prognosis [38]. Disrupted sleep could be one mechanism to explain this link [39]. The overarching hypothesis was that patients undergoing trauma-focused counseling would show better mental and physical health, including sleep, at follow-up than patients undergoing general stress counseling [37]. The intervention was not considered for the present study, as it showed no significant association with sleep, neuroendocrine and coagulation outcomes at hospital admission.

Patient recruitment
In brief, for MI-SPRINT, we recruited 190 patients with verified acute ST-elevation MI (STEMI) or non-STEMI and referred for acute coronary care intervention to the Bern University Hospital ("Inselspital") between January 2013 and September 2015. The diagnostic criteria and therapy for acute STEMI and non-STEMI followed the European Society of Cardiology guidelines on myocardial revascularization, including indications for primary percutaneous coronary intervention in non-STEMI, antithrombotic treatments, and treatments to establish stable hemodynamic conditions [40, 41]. Inclusion criteria were 18 years or older, stable hemodynamic conditions, and a high level of acute distress during MI defined by scores of at least 5 for chest pain plus at least 5 for fear of dying and/or helplessness on numeric rating scales from 0 to 10 [37]. Exclusion criteria were emergency coronary artery bypass grafting, comorbid diseases likely to cause death within 1 year, cognitive impairment, severe clinical depression, suicidal ideations in the prior 2 weeks, inadequate knowledge of German, or participation in another trial. The study protocol was approved by the ethics committee of the State of Bern (KEK-Nr. 170/12). All patients were informed and gave signed consent.

Data collection
Within 48 h after having reached stable hemodynamic conditions, all included patients underwent a structured clinical interview on the coronary care unit on which occasion a medical history, sleep-related data and information on health behaviors were collected. To limit patient burden in this acute clinical setting, we decided to assess sleep problems with just two short screening tools, one to rate OSA risk, and one to rate the severity of sleep difficulties in terms of insomnia symptoms (see below). Cardiac-related variables were additionally abstracted from hospital charts. Fasting venous blood samples were collected for the measurement of neuroendocrine hormones and coagulation factors the next morning at 6 am. For logistical reasons and reasons of patient care, blood was collected non-fasting in 12 cases and not at 6 am in 46 cases. Specific collection times were between 1 am and 5 am ($n = 14$), at 6 am ($n = 144$), between 7 am and 8 am ($n = 13$), between 9 am and 1 pm ($n = 10$), and between 2 pm and 6 pm ($n = 9$). Collection time (all p-values > 0.64) and fasting state (all p-values > 0.05) were not significantly associated with circulating levels of any neuroendocrine hormone or coagulation factor.

Measures
Sleep problems
To rate the risk of OSA, we applied a slightly modified version of the STOP questionnaire that is a tool to screen patients for OSA, asking for snoring (S); tiredness (T), observed (O) breathing cessations during sleep; and high blood pressure (P) [42]. The STOP questionnaire has been validated in patients with CHD [43] and in German [44]. The STOP questionnaire is particularly sensitive to identify patients with more severe forms of OSA [45], including in CHD patients [43]. Specific questions in our study (slight modifications from the original tool) asked about a history of snoring (irrespective of its loudness); history of breathing cessations while sleeping (although not necessarily observed); being often fatigued after sleep or while awake (sparing sleepiness); and history of hypertension (sparing treatment). Patients answering "yes" to at least two of these four questions were classified with a "high OSA risk", and all others with a "low OSA risk" [42]. To verify the accuracy of the STOP screening tool to a certain extent, we also inquired about a positive history of sleep apnea, predicting that patients who confirmed would largely fall into the group with a high OSA risk. We also asked patients whether they lived with someone to account for the fact that household members often notice and communicate signs of sleep-disordered

breathing. Patients identified with a high OSA risk were not treated for a presumed sleep disorder during their acute hospitalization.

Sleep difficulties in terms of insomnia symptoms in the previous 4 weeks were inquired with the 4-item Jenkins Sleep Scale with questions about difficulties initiating sleep, frequent awakenings during the night, difficulties maintaining sleep, and non-restorative sleep (i.e., feeling tired and worn out in the morning after a usual night's sleep) [46]. Response alternatives (scores) are: not at all (0), 1–3 days (1), 4–7 days (2), 8–14 days (3), 15–21 days (4), and 22–31 days (5), yielding an average total score of all sleep difficulties between 0 and 5. Lower scores are indicative of better sleep quality. For illustrative purposes, patients were categorized in those with poor (sore > 2) vs. good (score ≤ 2) sleep. Cronbach's alpha was 0.70 in the present study, suggesting acceptable internal consistency of the scale.

Neuroendocrine hormones

Serum COR (nmol/L) was determined with an electro-chemiluminescence immunoassay on a Cobas analyzer (Roche Diagnostics, Switzerland) at the Institute of Clinical Chemistry, Inselspital, Bern University Hospital, Switzerland. EPI and NEPI concentrations were quantified in EDTA plasma by high-pressure liquid chromatography using electrochemical detection [47] at the Laboratory for Stress Monitoring, Göttingen, Germany (inter–/intra-assay coefficients of variation < 10%; limit of detection 10 pg/mL). Undetectable EPI levels ($n = 16$) were assigned half the limit of detection (5 pg/mL).

Coagulation factors

Following a strict in-house protocol to ensure adequate preanalytical conditions, all coagulation factors were determined in citrate plasma at the haemostasis laboratory, Inselspital, Bern University Hospital, Switzerland. Fibrinogen measurements (g/L) were performed according to the Clauss method (Dade® Thrombin, Dade Behring, Liederbach, Germany). Plasma D-dimer levels (ng/mL) were determined with a quantitative sandwich enzyme immunoassay (VIDAS-D-Dimer, bioMérieux, Geneva, Switzerland), and from June 2015 on, with a particle-based immunoturbidimetric assay (Innovance® D-Dimer; Siemens AG, Munich, Germany). A highly significant correlation (Passing Bablock regression analysis: $r = 0.952$) between D-dimer values assessed with these two methods has previously been demonstrated, suggesting that their analytical performance is equally good [48]. Von Willebrand factor antigen concentration (IU/dL) was determined with vWF Ag® Kit (Siemens AG, Munich, Germany), an immunoturbidimetric method using polystyrene-based antibodies against VWF.

Covariates

In order to avoid overfitting of multivariate models, we included a selection of 16 potentially relevant predictors that might be confounders of the relationship between sleep problems and neuroendocrine measures and coagulation factors. We selected these covariates a priori based on the literature and on theoretical assumptions.

Demographic factors

Age and gender were abstracted from hospital charts. Socioeconomic status was based on the highest education level (high: high school graduation/matura, university graduation, including applied sciences; medium: apprenticeship or vocational school; low: lower than apprenticeship or vocational school) [49].

Comorbidities

We calculated the Charlson comorbidity index that provides an estimate of future mortality across several diseases [50]. Information on high cholesterol, hypertension, diabetes either with or without end organ damage, and lifetime depression was obtained through history taking.

Health behaviors

Patients disclosed their weight and height for the calculation of the body mass index. Smoking status was assessed in terms of current, former and never smokers, and physical activity ("that makes you sweat") in terms of the average frequency per week. Regarding alcohol consumption, we categorized patients into abstainers, moderate drinkers, and heavy drinkers (> 21 drinks/week for men, > 14 drinks/week for women).

Cardiac-related variables

These included the type of MI (STEMI/non-STEMI), previous MI (yes/no), and the number of coronary arteries with stenosis ≥50%. As an objective marker of MI severity, we calculated the Global Registry of Acute Coronary Events (GRACE) risk score from eight variables obtained at hospital admission: age, heart rate, systolic blood pressure, creatinine, Killip class, cardiac arrest, ST-segment deviation, and elevated cardiac enzymes [51]. The GRACE score is a robust predictor of the cumulative risk of death or death and recurrent MI from admission to 6 months after discharge [51].

Acute distress

The intensity of perceived distress during MI was assessed with three numeric rating scales (scores 0–10) for "pain intensity (during MI)", "fear of dying (until admission to the coronary care unit)" and "making sorrows and feeling helpless (when being told about having MI)" [37]. These measures were previously shown to predict CVD-related hospital readmissions in ACS patients after a 3-year follow-up [52]. The added sum score of the three numeric rating scales was divided by three to yield a severity index of acute distress.

Data analysis
Data were analyzed using SPSS 23.0 for Windows (SPSS Inc., Chicago, IL) with level of significance at $p < 0.05$. For technical and logistic reasons (e.g., early discharge of patients), EPI and NEPI were missing in 45 patients, COR in 16 patients, fibrinogen in 14 patients, and D-dimer and VWF in 15 patients each. Due to lacking information, the GRACE risk score could not be computed for 18 patients. Seven or less values were missing for all other measures. We replaced all missing values with the expectation maximization algorithm to make use of all the available information from the total sample of 190 study participants. Supporting the adequacy of this approach, the strength and significance of the associations between OSA risk and COR ($r = -0.16$, $p = 0.043$; $n = 170$) and between sleep difficulties and both fibrinogen ($r = 0.16$, $p = 0.032$; $n = 172$) and NEPI ($r = -0.18$, $p = 0.036$; $n = 141$) in the patients with complete data for these measures were similar to those shown in the result section for the whole sample. Values of neuroendocrine hormones and coagulation factors were log-transformed before analysis.

Pearson correlation analysis was used to estimate the univariate relationship between two variables. Multivariate regression analysis was employed to identify whether OSA risk (categorical variable: high vs. low) and sleep difficulties (continuously scaled variable) were independently associated with neuroendocrine hormones and coagulation factors, after controlling for demographics, comorbidity, health behaviors, and cardiac-related variables, all entered in one block. If the total sleep difficultly scale showed a significant association, we computed post hoc analyses on each individual item. Finally, to test for a possible joint effect of OSA risk and sleep difficulties on outcomes, we additionally entered the interaction between the STOP score and the sleep difficulties score total into the regression equation. We allowed a maximum of 19 independent predicting variables to protect against model overfitting. Cook's distance and variance inflation factor, respectively, were used to verify the absence of influential outliers in the set of predictor variables and critical multicollinearity between two predictor variables, respectively.

We did not adjust p-values for multiple comparisons because of the pre-established primary hypothesis of a significant association of sleep problems with neuroendocrine and coagulation measures, and because of the risk of deeming truly important differences non-significant in a still

nascent field of research [53]. However, partial correlation coefficients (r_p) from the regression output were used to interpret effect sizes as small (0.1), medium (0.3), or large (0.5), irrespective of p-values [54].

Results
Patient characteristics
Table 1 shows the characteristics of the 190 patients, all of Caucasian ethnicity. The majority of participants were well-educated men with a first-time STEMI and living together with someone. The Charlson index indicated low comorbidity; nevertheless, a history of hypertension and high cholesterol were reported by every other patient, and a history of depression by almost 30%. According to the GRACE score, the median (inter-quartile range) risk of 6-month death was 5% (3–9). Regarding health behaviors, patients were on average overweight, and a substantial portion were current smokers and physically inactive. Defining the group of poor sleepers, a total of 52 (27.4%) patients reported sleep difficulties on more than 7 days in the previous 4 weeks. A total of 77 (40.5%) patients could be identified with a high OSA risk; 15 (78.9%) of the 19 patients with a history of sleep apnea were in this group. Living with someone was not associated with OSA risk ($p = 0.98$), so it was not used as a covariate. The type of drugs delivered at admission and glucocorticoid use did not significantly differ between patients with high versus low OSA risk (all p-values > 0.06).

Unadjusted associations among sleep, neuroendocrine and coagulation measures
There were several significant bivariate relationships between sleep problems, neuroendocrine and coagulation measures. High OSA risk was associated with more sleep difficulties ($r = 0.20$, $p = 0.006$), with frequent nighttime awakenings ($r = 0.30$, $p < 0.001$) and nonrestorative sleep ($r = 0.19$, $p = 0.011$) driving this relationship. High OSA risk was also associated with lower COR levels ($r = -0.17$, $p = 0.022$), and more sleep difficulties were associated with higher fibrinogen levels ($r = 0.14$, $p = 0.048$), with difficulties initiating sleep driving this relationship ($r = 0.22$, $p = 0.003$).

Further expected direct associations were seen among all stress hormones (EPI and NEPI: $r = 0.51$; EPI and COR: $r = 0.30$; NEPI and COR: 0.29; p-values < 0.001) and among all coagulation factors (fibrinogen and D-dimer: $r = 0.35$; fibrinogen and VWF; $r = 0.38$; D-dimer and VWF: r = 0.38; p-values < 0.001). Direct associations also emerged for NEPI with D-dimer ($r = 0.17$, $p = 0.020$) and VWF ($r = 0.16$, $p = 0.033$) levels, and between COR and fibrinogen levels ($r = 0.21$, $p = 0.004$).

Table 1 Demographic and clinical characteristics of the 190 study participants

Age, yrs., M (SD)	59.9 (11.2)
Sex (men), n (%)	157 (82.6)
Education level	
High, n (%)	36 (18.9)
Medium, n (%)	136 (71.6)
Low, n (%)	18 (9.5)
Living with someone, n (%)	138 (72.6)
Charlson comorbidity index, M (SD)	1.80 (1.20)
Positive history of hypertension, n (%)	98 (51.6)
Positive history of high cholesterol, n (%)	86 (45.3)
Positive history of depression, n (%)	54 (28.4)
Body mass index, kg/m^2, M (SD)	27.7 (4.6)
Smoking status	
Current smoker, n (%)	83 (43.7)
Former smoker, n (%)	50 (26.3)
Never smoker, n (%)	57 (30.0)
Alcohol consumption (drinks per week)	
Abstainers, n (%)	33 (17.4)
Moderate drinkers, n (%)	147 (77.4)
Heavy drinkers, n (%)	10 (5.3)
Physical activity (number of times per week)	
3–7, n (%)	49 (25.8)
1–2, n (%)	52 (27.4)
< 1, n (%)	89 (46.8)
Previous myocardial infarction, n (%)	20 (10.5)
Previous percutaneous coronary intervention	27 (14.2)
Previous coronary artery bypass surgery	5 (2.6)
Type of confirmed acute infarction	
ST-elevation myocardial infarction, n (%)	136 (71.6)
Non-ST-elevation myocardial infarction, n (%)	54 (28.4)
Major coronary arteries with stenosis ≥50% (number), M (SD)	1.93 (0.86)
Left ventricular ejection fraction (angiography), %, M (SD)	47. 6 (11.8)
Vasopressant drugs at admission	
Epinephrine, n (%)	9 (4.7)
Norepinephrine, n (%)	6 (3.2)
Dobutamine, n (%)	8 (4.2)
Dopamine, n (%)	1 (0.5)
Antithrombotic therapy at admission	
Aspirin, n (%)	190 (100)
Clopidogrel, n (%)	57 (30.0)
Prasugrel, n (%)	99 (52.1)
Ticagrelor, n (%)	80 (42.1)
Fondaparinux, n (%)	154 (81.1)

Table 1 Demographic and clinical characteristics of the 190 study participants (Continued)

Unfractioned heparin, n (%)	145 (76.3)
Low molecular weight heparin, n (%)	13 (6.8)
Bivalirudin, n (%)	2 (1.1)
Abciximab, n (%)	46 (24.2)
Thrombolysis, n (%)	2 (1.1)
Beta-blocker therapy at admission, n (%)	173 (91.1)
Regular use of glucocorticoids, n (%)	13 (6.8)
Global Registry of Acute Coronary Events risk score, M (SD)	107 (27)
Acute distress during myocardial infarction, M (SD)	6.23 (1.40)
Sleep difficulties total, M (SD)	1.53 (1.29)
Difficulties initiating sleep, M (SD)	1.24 (1.62)
Nighttime awakenings, M (SD)	2.53 (2.10)
Difficulties maintaining sleep, M (SD)	1.17 (1.68)
Nonrestorative sleep, M (SD)	1.17 (1.67)
High risk of obstructive sleep apnea, n (%)	77 (40.5)

Independent associations of sleep measures with neuroendocrine hormones

Table 2 shows the fully adjusted multivariate model for the levels of neuroendocrine hormones. Compared to patients with low OSA risk, those with high OSA risk had significantly lower levels for all three hormones. Figure 1 shows absolute values of these group differences. More sleep difficulties (continuously scaled) were also significantly associated with lower NEPI levels (absolute values illustrated in Fig. 2 for poor vs. good sleepers). The relationship between sleep difficulties and NEPI was driven by difficulties initiating ($r_p = -0.15$, $p = 0.049$) and maintaining ($r_p = -0.20$, $p = 0.008$) sleep. Moreover, there was no significant interaction between OSA risk and sleep difficulties for stress hormones (p-values > 0.36).

Independent associations of sleep measures with coagulation factors

Table 3 shows the fully adjusted multivariate model for the three coagulation factors. More sleep difficulties were associated with greater fibrinogen levels (absolute values illustrated in Fig. 2 for poor vs. good sleepers), with difficulties initiating sleep driving this relationship ($r_p = 0.25$, $p = 0.001$). Risk of OSA was not significantly associated with any coagulation factor. Likewise, there was no significant interaction between OSA risk and sleep difficulties for coagulation factors (p-values > 0.35).

Role of stress hormones in the relation between sleep and coagulation factors

The positive association of sleep difficulties with fibrinogen levels was virtually unchanged when EPI ($r_p = 0.16$,

Table 2 Multivariate relations between sleep problems and neuroendocrine measures

Entered variables	Epinephrine		Norepinephrine		Cortisol	
	Partial corr.	P	Partial corr.	P	Partial corr.	P
Age	−0.183	0.016	0.050	0.516	−0.087	0.254
Male sex	−0.079	0.302	0.080	0.295	−0.031	0.690
Education	−0.092	0.230	−0.003	0.970	−0.051	0.504
Charlson index	−0.240	0.001	−0.126	0.098	−0.111	0.147
Hypertension history	0.159	0.037	0.088	0.247	0.139	0.068
High cholesterol history	0.130	0.089	−0.070	0.357	− 0.002	0.978
Depression history	0.070	0.360	0.054	0.479	0.007	0.928
Body mass index	−0.053	0.489	0.178	0.019	0.101	0.187
Smoking	−0.047	0.541	−0.021	0.786	0.030	0.693
Alcohol consumption	0.026	0.731	−0.126	0.098	0.025	0.747
Physical activity	−0.149	0.051	−0.031	0.688	0.043	0.572
Previous MI	0.140	0.067	0.001	0.994	0.074	0.333
ST-elevation MI	0.150	0.049	0.172	0.024	0.081	0.289
Stenotic coronary arteries	0.074	0.334	0.116	0.130	0.232	0.002
GRACE risk score	0.234	0.002	0.131	0.085	0.157	0.039
Acute distress	0.210	0.006	0.170	0.025	0.029	0.706
Sleep difficulties	−0.054	0.482	−0.172	0.024	0.094	0.217
High risk of OSA	−0.185	0.015	−0.150	0.049	−0.251	0.001
Model statistic	$R^2 = 0.295$ $F_{18,171} = 3.97$ $P < 0.001$		$R^2 = 0.212$ $F_{18,171} = 2.55$ $P = 0.001$		$R^2 = 0.174$ $F_{18,171} = 2.00$ $P = 0.012$	

Linear regression model with all variables entered in one block. Significant correlation coefficients (Partial corr.) and P-values are given in bold
GRACE Global Registry of Acute Cardiac Events, MI myocardial infarction, OSA obstructive sleep apnea

$p = 0.043$), NEPI ($r_p = 0.16$, $p = 0.031$) and COR ($r_p = 0.15$, $p = 0.055$) were separately added to the model in Table 3. Neuroendocrine hormones were not significantly predictive of fibrinogen (p-values > 0.06), D-dimer (p-values > 0.07) and VWF (p-values > 0.37) levels, independently of all other covariates. Also, OSA risk (p-values > 0.27) and sleep difficulties (p-values > 0.11) showed no significant interaction with neuroendocrine hormones for any coagulation factor.

Discussion

In patients admitted with acute MI, we found a high risk of OSA to be associated with decreased levels of EPI, NEPI, and COR, compared to when OSA risk was low, independent of covariates. Sleep difficulties in terms of insomnia symptoms were also independently associated with low NEPI levels, although not with EPI and COR levels. Less evidence was found for an independent relationship between sleep problems and coagulation factors. Whereas insomnia symptoms were associated with higher levels of fibrinogen, although not with D-dimer and VWF, OSA risk did not show a significant association with any coagulation factor. The size of these associations was similar to that observed for several

covariates with neuroendocrine and coagulation outcomes, including the prognostic GRACE score, implying not only statistical, but also clinical significance with small-to-moderate effects of sleep problems.

In our sample, 40.5% of patients had a high OSA risk, a prevalence similar to previous studies showing that close to a half of patients with ACS have moderate or severe OSA (apnea-hypopnea index ≥15) [55]. Also comparable to a previous study showing that 37.3% of hospitalized patients with ACS have clinically relevant insomnia symptoms [56], 27.4% of our patients were poor sleepers. In agreement with previous studies on CVD outcomes [34], we did not observe joint effects between OSA risk and insomnia symptoms for neuroendocrine hormones and coagulation factors. However, concurring with a high prevalence of OSA among insomnia patients and vice versa [32], we found a significant association between OSA risk and insomnia symptoms with frequent awakenings and non-restorative sleep driving this association. As we adjusted for an overlap between OSA risk and insomnia symptoms, we may interpret that in the setting of acute MI, neuroendocrine and coagulation abnormalities differ substantially between high OSA risk and insomnia symptoms

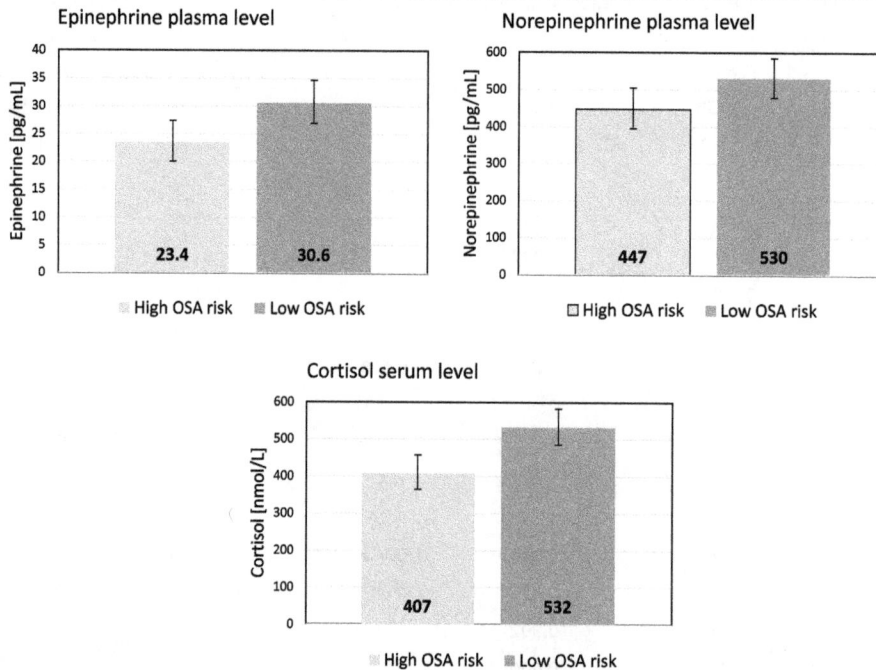

Fig. 1 Risk of obstructive sleep apnea and mean values of neuroendocrine measures. The bar graphs illustrate the significant differences in epinephrine ($p = 0.015$), norepinephrine ($p = 0.049$) and cortisol ($p = 0.001$) levels between subjects with high ($n = 77$) vs. low ($n = 113$) risk of obstructive sleep apnea (OSA), expressed as geometric mean values with 95% confidence interval. Adjustments were made for age, sex, education, Charlson comorbidity index, positive history of hypertension/high cholesterol/depression, body mass index, smoking, alcohol consumption, physical activity, previous myocardial infarction (MI), ST-segment MI, number of stenotic coronary arteries, Global Registry of Acute Coronary Events risk score, acute distress, and sleep difficulties

and even between individual insomnia symptoms. We particularly found difficulties in initiating sleep to be significantly associated with NEPI and fibrinogen, and difficulties maintaining sleep also with NEPI, whereas waking up during the night and nonrestorative sleep showed no association with neuroendocrine hormones and coagulation factors whatsoever.

Increased fibrinogen levels in acute MI patients with more severe insomnia symptoms is compatible with a prothrombotic state, one mechanism that may possibly increase the risk of recurrent atherothrombotic events [21]. In addition to having rheological and hemostatic properties, fibrinogen is also an inflammatory molecule (i.e., an acute phase reactant), and inflammation and sleep disturbances are reciprocally linked with each other [57]. However, as we measured fibrinogen only once, but inquired about insomnia symptoms covering the preceding 4 weeks, we are unable to make any causal inferences. For instance, it is possible that insomnia symptoms were already associated with elevated fibrinogen before MI and/or even a contributing factor to MI onset, although exaggerated fibrinogen production during the acute phase could also have occurred in those with more severe insomnia symptoms. Clearly, our finding in fibrinogen needs replication, as we did not observe a relation

between insomnia symptoms and the other two prothrombotic markers. Future studies should also include measures of impaired fibrinolysis, particularly plasminogen activator inhibitor-1 [16, 19].

Regarding neuroendocrine dysregulation, low endogenous COR levels in CHD patients with high OSA risk could result in less curtailing of vascular inflammation and atherosclerosis progression, respectively [58]. Indeed, low cortisol levels at admission were previously shown to predict early death in patients with acute MI [59]. Likewise, low catecholamine levels, found in those with high OSA risk and more sleep difficulties in our study, are implied in increased systemic inflammation [60]. Moreover, in OSA, due to the accompanying SNS hyperactivity, beta-2-adrenergic receptors are desensitized [61], a mechanism that may result in blunted beta-2-adrenergic receptor-mediated anti-inflammatory effects of catecholamines [60]. As coagulation activation relates to catecholamine and cortisol activity [30, 31], comparably low SNS and HPA activation in relation to sleep problems may help to explain why neuroendocrine dysregulation was no associated with coagulation factors in patients with high OSA risk and insomnia symptoms, respectively.

That patients with OSA might not mount an appropriate stress response to ACS could not only have

Norepinephrine plasma level

Fibrinogen plasma level

Fig. 2 Sleep difficulties and mean values of neuroendocrine and coagulation measures. The bar graphs illustrate the significant differences in norepinephrine ($p = 0.010$) and fibrinogen ($p = 0.003$) levels between subjects with poor sleep (i.e., sleep difficulties on more than 7 days in the previous 4 weeks; $n = 52$) and those with good sleep ($n = 138$), expressed as geometric mean values with 95% confidence interval. Adjustments were made for age, sex, education, Charlson comorbidity index, positive history of hypertension/high cholesterol/depression, body mass index, smoking, alcohol consumption, physical activity, previous myocardial infarction (MI), ST-segment MI, number of stenotic coronary arteries, Global Registry of Acute Coronary Events risk score, acute distress, and risk of obstructive sleep apnea

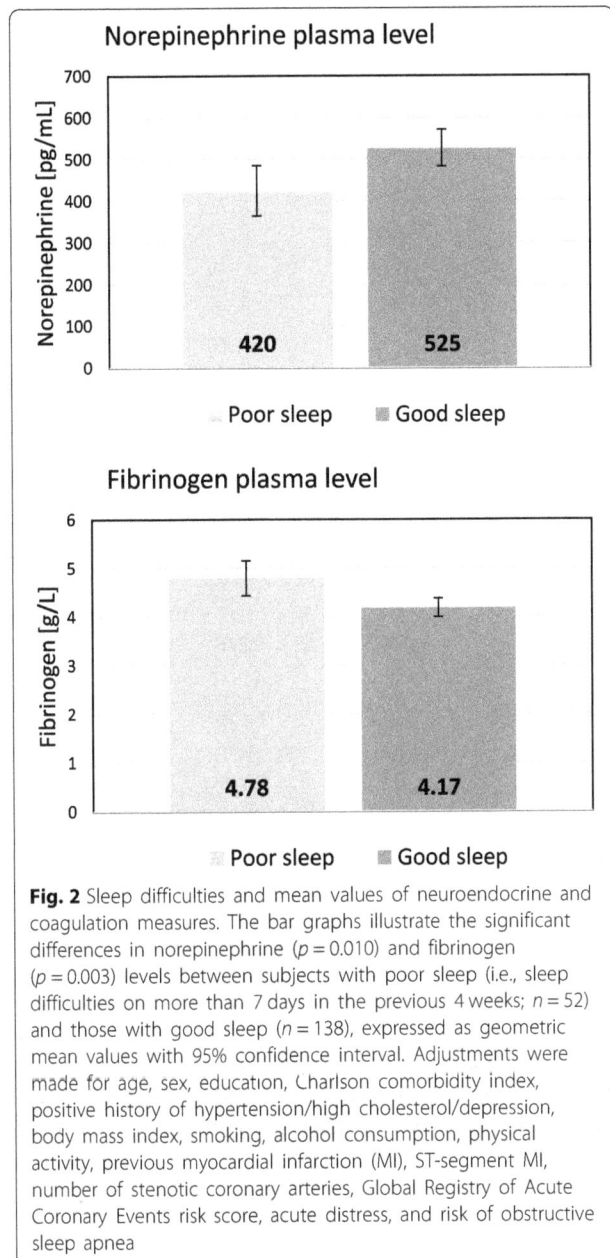

production [64]. A lower sympathoadrenal response in the setting of ACS might result in less oxidative stress and myocardial damage, respectively.

Our study has several limitations worth mentioning. Most importantly, the lack of objective measures of sleep architecture, sleep duration and sleep apnea testing does not allow us to draw firm conclusions. To better differentiate between effects of OSA risk and insomnia symptoms, polysomnography or the additional inclusion of validated screening tools, such as the Berlin questionnaire and the Epworth Sleepiness Scale would have yielded data that are more reliable. We were particularly unable to tease apart influences of obstructive versus central sleep apnea that is prevalent in ACS. Moreover, objective short sleep duration is an important factor driving activation of the stress system and cardiometabolic morbidity in patients with insomnia [65]. However, it should also be mentioned that the acute cardiac situation influences sleep macro- and microarchitecture [66], which can complicate the diagnostic process. The STOP screening questionnaire is not very sensitive and specific for moderate-to-severe sleep-disordered breathing in CHD [42], but also in other disorders [42, 67] and in population-based studies [45]. A high sensitivity to detect more severe forms of OSA in patients with coronary artery bypass surgery was associated with low specificity [42], which increases the risk of false positives. The STOP questionnaire does not allow a firm assessment of OSA severity. Follow-up sleep studies would have been necessary for this purpose. It is not clear how the modified STOP questionnaire influenced its sensitivity and specificity. The omission of loudness of snoring may have overestimated the prevalence of patients classified with high OSA risk. Nonetheless, the majority of patients who reported a history of sleep apnea were in this group, suggesting our slightly modified STOP tool showed clinically useful sensitivity. Although time of blood collection did not significantly relate to coagulation and neuroendocrine measures, given their circadian variation, the difference in the time of assessment is a limitation. Although we applied an established method to replace missing data, the fact that 24% of patients missed catecholamine measures is a further limitation. We controlled for a range of important covariates, but residual confounding through for instance combined effects of emergency medications remains a possibility. This weakens the interpretation of the relationships which only emerged as significant in the covariate-adjusted analyses. In turn, non-significant results must be interpreted with caution, as we did not perform a power calculation for this ancillary sleep study. Body mass index, a driver of neuroendocrine and coagulation measures, was self-reported. Although we controlled for acute distress during MI, the

deleterious consequences for cardiac prognosis, as there is data from animal models to suggest that chronic intermittent hypoxia is a potentially adaptive stimulus for the myocardium in OSA [62]. One study in humans found more severe OSA to be associated with less cardiac injury during non-fatal ACS, proposing that ischemic preconditioning due to chronic intermittent hypoxia could be a possible explanation [63]. Although the involved physiological mechanisms are still elusive, there may be pro-angiogenic and anti-oxidant effects of intermittent hypoxia [62, 63]. For instance, as increased sympathetic tone and elevated catecholamine levels in OSA might be associated with increased reactive oxygen species

Table 3 Multivariate relationship between sleep problems and coagulation factors

Entered variables	Fibrinogen		D-dimer		VWF	
	Partial corr.	P	Partial corr.	P	Partial corr.	P
Age	−0.059	0.439	−0.125	0.102	−0.006	0.942
Male sex	−0.073	0.343	−0.083	0.278	−0.114	0.137
Education	**−0.190**	**0.012**	−0.096	0.208	−0.018	0.810
Charlson index	0.115	0.133	**0.177**	**0.020**	0.021	0.779
Hypertension history	0.078	0.309	0.037	0.628	−0.034	0.654
High cholesterol history	0.041	0.591	−0.063	0.409	−0.049	0.522
Depression history	**−0.178**	**0.019**	0.037	0.627	−0.060	0.432
Body mass index	0.133	0.081	−0.011	0.890	0.136	0.075
Smoking	0.032	0.678	−0.061	0.426	0.003	0.973
Alcohol consumption	−0.054	0.477	0.087	0.253	0.032	0.674
Physical activity	−0.090	0.238	0.069	0.367	−0.012	0.877
Previous MI	0.047	0.538	**0.155**	**0.042**	0.082	0.286
ST-elevation MI	**0.158**	**0.038**	0.019	0.800	0.010	0.898
Stenotic coronary arteries	0.074	0.331	−0.083	0.280	0.003	0.972
GRACE risk score	0.102	0.180	**0.279**	**< 0.001**	**0.276**	**< 0.001**
Acute distress	0.033	0.668	0.060	0.430	0.126	0.097
Sleep difficulties	**0.158**	**0.037**	0.040	0.600	0.079	0.299
High risk of OSA	−0.038	0.618	−0.082	0.283	0.017	0.828
Model statistic	$R^2 = 0.216$ $F_{18,171} = 2.61$ $P = 0.001$		$R^2 = 0.245$ $F_{18,171} = 3.08$ $P < 0.001$		$R^2 = 0.236$ $F_{18,171} = 2.93$ $P < 0.001$	

Linear regression model with all variables entered in one block. Significant partial correlation coefficients (Partial corr.) and P-values are given in bold
GRACE Global Registry of Acute Cardiac Events, MI myocardial infarction, OSA obstructive sleep apnea, VWF von Willebrand factor

specifics of our sample with substantially distressed patients need to be considered when generalizing the findings to other cohorts of ACS patients. Distressed patients may have over-reported sleep difficulties in their effort to make sense of the situation. However, about 70% of patients experience at least moderate distress and fear of dying during ACS [68]. As is common in ACS studies, less than 20% of our patients were women, which precluded sex-stratified analyses, which might result in different findings for women and men [10, 11].

Conclusions

In patients admitted with acute MI, high OSA risk and insomnia symptoms might differently affect neuroendocrine and coagulation activity. While a high OSA risk was associated with neuroendocrine dysregulation, indicating SNS and HPA axis hypoactivity, insomnia symptoms, particularly problems initiating or maintaining sleep, showed a relation with reduced SNS activity and a prothrombotic state. Low cortisol and catecholamine levels might result in less curtailing of vascular inflammation, and elevated fibrinogen levels might evoke a prothrombotic state, with such pathophysiology helping to explain adverse outcome of MI patients with sleep problems. In turn, the finding of lower neuroendocrine hormones in patients with acute MI and a high OSA risk may also inform further studies to better understand potentially cardioprotective mechanisms of chronic intermittent hypoxia.

Abbreviations
ACS: Acute coronary syndrome; CHD: Coronary heart disease; COR: Cortisol; CVD: Cardiovascular disease; EPI: Epinephrine; GRACE: Global Registry of Acute Cardiac Events; HPA: Hypothalamic-pituitary adrenal; MI: Myocardial infarction; NEPI: Norepinephrine; OSA: Obstructive sleep apnea; SNS: Sympathetic nervous system; STEMI: ST-elevation myocardial infarction; VWF: Von Willebrand factor

Acknowledgements
Not applicable.

Funding
This study was financially supported by grant No. 140960 from the Swiss National Science Foundation to RvK (PI), JPS, US, HZ and JB. Additional support came from the Teaching and Research Directorate, Bern University Hospital, Switzerland.

Authors' contributions

RvK had full access to all data in the study and takes responsibility for the integrity of the data and the accuracy of the data analysis. RvK was responsible for statistical analysis and writing of the first draft of the manuscript. MP and REML were responsible for the acquisition of the data. RvK, MP, JPS, JB, HZ, US, and REML were responsible for the study concept and design, interpretation of data, critical revision of the manuscript for intellectual content, and approval of the manuscript for submission.

Competing interests

The authors declare that they have no competing interests.

Author details

[1]Department of Consultation-Liaison Psychiatry and Psychosomatic Medicine, University Hospital Zurich, Culmannstrasse 8, CH-8091 Zurich, Switzerland. [2]Department of Cardiology, Clinic Barmelweid, Barmelweid, Switzerland. [3]Complementary and Integrative Medicine, University of Zurich, Zurich, Switzerland. [4]Department of Clinical Psychology and Psychotherapy, University of Bern, Bern, Switzerland. [5]Medical Faculty, University of Zurich, Zurich, Switzerland. [6]Department of Psychiatry, Clienia Schlössli AG, Oetwil am See, Switzerland.

References

1. Jordan AS, McSharry DG, Malhotra A. Adult obstructive sleep apnoea. Lancet. 2014;383(9918):736–47.
2. Sateia MJ. International classification of sleep disorders-third edition: highlights and modifications. Chest. 2014;146(5):1387–94.
3. Fu Y, Xia Y, Yi H, Xu H, Guan J, Yin S. Meta-analysis of all-cause and cardiovascular mortality in obstructive sleep apnea with or without continuous positive airway pressure treatment. Sleep Breath. 2017;21(1):181–9.
4. Wang X, Ouyang Y, Wang Z, Zhao G, Liu L, Bi Y. Obstructive sleep apnea and risk of cardiovascular disease and all-cause mortality: a meta-analysis of prospective cohort studies. Int J Cardiol. 2013;169(3):207–14.
5. He Q, Zhang P, Li G, Dai H, Shi J. The association between insomnia symptoms and risk of cardio-cerebral vascular events: a meta-analysis of prospective cohort studies. Eur J Prev Cardiol. 2017;24(10):1071–82.
6. Li M, Zhang XW, Hou WS, Tang ZY. Insomnia and risk of cardiovascular disease: a meta-analysis of cohort studies. Int J Cardiol. 2014;176(3):1044–7.
7. Sofi F, Cesari F, Casini A, Macchi C, Abbate R, Gensini GF. Insomnia and risk of cardiovascular disease: a meta-analysis. Eur J Prev Cardiol. 2014;21(1):57–64.
8. Xie W, Zheng F, Song X. Obstructive sleep apnea and serious adverse outcomes in patients with cardiovascular or cerebrovascular disease: a PRISMA-compliant systematic review and meta-analysis. Medicine (Baltimore). 2014;93(29):e336.
9. Zhao Y, Yu BY, Liu Y, Liu Y. Meta-analysis of the effect of obstructive sleep apnea on cardiovascular events after percutaneous coronary intervention. Am J Cardiol. 2017;120(6):1026–30.
10. Clark A, Lange T, Hallqvist J, Jennum P, Rod NH. Sleep impairment and prognosis of acute myocardial infarction: a prospective cohort study. Sleep. 2014;37(5):851–8.
11. Leineweber C, Kecklund G, Janszky I, Akerstedt T, Orth-Gomér K. Poor sleep increases the prospective risk for recurrent events in middle-aged women with coronary disease. The Stockholm female coronary risk study. J Psychosom Res. 2003;54(2):121–7.
12. Appels A, Kop W, Bär F, de Swart H, Mendes de Leon C. Vital exhaustion, extent of atherosclerosis, and the clinical course after successful percutaneous transluminal coronary angioplasty. Eur Heart J. 1995;16(12):1880–5.
13. Lévy P, Kohler M, McNicholas WT, Barbé F, McEvoy RD, Somers VK, Lavie L, Pépin JL. Obstructive sleep apnoea syndrome. Nat Rev Dis Primers. 2015;1:15015.
14. Baltzis D, Bakker JP, Patel SR, Veves A. Obstructive sleep apnea and vascular diseases. Compr Physiol. 2016;6(3):1519–28.
15. Motivala SJ. Sleep and inflammation: psychoneuroimmunology in the context of cardiovascular disease. Ann Behav Med. 2011;42(2):141–52.
16. von Känel R, Loredo JS, Ancoli-Israel S, Mills PJ, Natarajan L, Dimsdale JE. Association between polysomnographic measures of disrupted sleep and prothrombotic factors. Chest. 2007;131(3):733–9.
17. Mausbach BT, Ancoli-Israel S, von Känel R, et al. Sleep disturbance, norepinephrine, and D-dimer are all related in elderly caregivers of people with Alzheimer disease. Sleep. 2006;29(10):1347–52.
18. von Känel R, Ancoli-Israel S, Dimsdale JE, et al. Sleep and biomarkers of atherosclerosis in elderly Alzheimer caregivers and controls. Gerontology. 2010;56(1):41–50.
19. Mehra R, Xu F, Babineau DC, Tracy RP, Jenny NS, Patel SR, Redline S. Sleep-disordered breathing and prothrombotic biomarkers: cross-sectional results of the Cleveland family study. Am J Respir Crit Care Med. 2010;182(6):826–33.
20. Shitrit D, Peled N, Shitrit AB, Meidan S, Bendayan D, Sahar G, Kramer MR. An association between oxygen desaturation and D-dimer in patients with obstructive sleep apnea syndrome. Thromb Haemost. 2005;94(3):544–7.
21. Toss H, Lindahl B, Siegbahn A, Wallentin L. Prognostic influence of increased fibrinogen and C-reactive protein levels in unstable coronary artery disease. FRISC study group. Fragmin during instability in coronary artery disease. Circulation. 1997;96(12):4204–10.
22. Lee KW, Lip GY, Tayebjee M, Foster W, Blann AD. Circulating endothelial cells, von Willebrand factor, interleukin-6, and prognosis in patients with acute coronary syndromes. Blood. 2005;105(2):526–32.
23. Oldgren J, Linder R, Grip L, Siegbahn A, Wallentin L. Coagulation activity and clinical outcome in unstable coronary artery disease. Arterioscler Thromb Vasc Biol. 2001;21(6):1059–64.
24. Brügger-Andersen T, Pönitz V, Staines H, Grundt H, Hetland Ø, Nilsen DW. The prognostic utility of D-dimer and fibrin monomer at long-term follow-up after hospitalization with coronary chest pain. Blood Coagul Fibrinolysis. 2008;19(7):701–7.
25. Dimsdale JE, Coy T, Ziegler MG, Ancoli-Israel S, Clausen J. The effect of sleep apnea on plasma and urinary catecholamines. Sleep. 1995;18(5):377–81.
26. Balbo M, Leproult R, Van Cauter E. Impact of sleep and its disturbances on hypothalamo-pituitary-adrenal axis activity. Int J Endocrinol. 2010;2010:759234.
27. Rodenbeck A, Huether G, Rüther E, Hajak G. Interactions between evening and nocturnal cortisol secretion and sleep parameters in patients with severe chronic primary insomnia. Neurosci Lett 2002;324(2):159–163.
28. Backhaus J, Junghanns K, Hohagen F. Sleep disturbances are correlated with decreased morning awakening salivary cortisol. Psychoneuroendocrinology. 2004;29(9):1184–91.
29. Kong AP, Chan NN, Chan JC. The role of adipocytokines and neurohormonal dysregulation in metabolic syndrome. Curr Diabetes Rev. 2006;2(4):397–407.
30. von Känel R, Dimsdale JE. Effects of sympathetic activation by adrenergic infusions on hemostasis in vivo. Eur J Haematol. 2000;65(6):357–69.
31. von Känel R, Kudielka BM, Abd-el-Razik A, Gander ML, Frey K, Fischer JE. Relationship between overnight neuroendocrine activity and morning haemostasis in working men. Clin Sci (Lond). 2004;107(1):89–95.
32. Luyster FS, Buysse DJ, Strollo PJ Jr. Comorbid insomnia and obstructive sleep apnea: challenges for clinical practice and research. J Clin Sleep Med. 2010;6(2):196–204.
33. Gupta MA, Knapp K. Cardiovascular and psychiatric morbidity in obstructive sleep apnea (OSA) with insomnia (sleep apnea plus) versus obstructive sleep apnea without insomnia: a case-control study from a nationally representative US sample. PLoS One. 2014;9(3):e90021.
34. Luyster FS, Kip KE, Buysse DJ, Aiyer AN, Reis SE, Strollo PJ Jr. Traditional and nontraditional cardiovascular risk factors in comorbid insomnia and sleep apnea. Sleep. 2014;37(3):593–600.
35. Zhang J, Ma RC, Kong AP, et al. Relationship of sleep quantity and quality with 24-hour urinary catecholamines and salivary awakening cortisol in healthy middle-aged adults. Sleep. 2011;34(2):225–33.
36. Jackowska M, Ronaldson A, Brown J, Steptoe A. Biological and psychological correlates of self-reported and objective sleep measures. J Psychosom Res. 2016;84:52–5.
37. Meister R, Princip M, Schmid JP, Schnyder U, Barth J, Znoj H, Herbert C, von Känel R. Myocardial Infarction – Stress Prevention INTervention (MI-SPRINT) to reduce the incidence of posttraumatic stress after acute myocardial infarction through trauma-focused psychological counseling: study protocol for a randomized controlled trial. Trials. 2013;14:329.
38. Edmondson D, Richardson S, Falzon L, Davidson KW, Mills MA, Neria Y. Posttraumatic stress disorder prevalence and risk of recurrence in acute coronary syndrome patients: a meta-analytic review. PLoS One. 2012;7:e38915.
39. Edmondson D, von Känel R. Post-traumatic stress disorder and cardiovascular disease. Lancet Psychiatry. 2017;4(4):320–9.

40. Windecker S, Kolh P, Alfonso F, et al. 2014 ESC/EACTS Guidelines on myocardial revascularization: The Task Force on Myocardial Revascularization of the European Society of Cardiology (ESC) and the European Association for Cardio-Thoracic Surgery (EACTS)Developed with the special contribution of the European Association of Percutaneous Cardiovascular Interventions (EAPCI). Eur Heart J. 2014;35(37):2541–619.

41. Roffi M, Patrono C, Collet JP, et al. 2015 ESC Guidelines for the management of acute coronary syndromes in patients presenting without persistent ST-segment elevation: Task Force for the Management of Acute Coronary Syndromes in Patients Presenting without Persistent ST-Segment Elevation of the European Society of Cardiology (ESC). Eur Heart J. 2016;37(3):267–315.

42. Chung F, Yegneswaran B, Liao P, et al. STOP questionnaire: a tool to screen patients for obstructive sleep apnea. Anesthesiology. 2008;108(5):812–21.

43. Nunes FS, Danzi-Soares NJ, Genta PR, Drager LF, Cesar LA, Lorenzi-Filho G. Critical evaluation of screening questionnaires for obstructive sleep apnea in patients undergoing coronary artery bypass grafting and abdominal surgery. Sleep Breath. 2015;19(1):115–22.

44. Haddad A. Validierung eines miniaturisierten Gerätes zum präoperativen Screening bei Patienten mit gesichertem oder mutmaßlichem obstruktiven Schlafapnoesyndrom und Validierung des sogenannten STOP-Fragebogens. Dissertation Medizinische Fakultät, Universität Duisburg-Essen, 2015.

45. Silva GE, Vana KD, Goodwin JL, Sherrill DL, Quan SF. Identification of patients with sleep disordered breathing: comparing the four-variable screening tool, STOP, STOP-Bang, and Epworth Sleepiness Scales. J Clin Sleep Med. 2011;7(5):467–72.

46. Jenkins CD, Stanton BA, Niemcryk SJ, Rose RM. A scale for the estimation of sleep problems in clinical research. J Clin Epidemiol. 1988;41(4):313–21.

47. Ehrenreich H, Schuck J, Stender N, et al. Endocrine and hemodynamic effects of stress versus systemic CRF in alcoholics during early and medium term abstinence. Alcohol Clin Exp Res. 1997;21(7):1285–93.

48. Coen Herak D, Milos M, Zadro R. Evaluation of the Innovance D-DIMER analytical performance. Clin Chem Lab Med. 2009;47(8):945–51.

49. Bopp M, Minder CE. Swiss National Cohort. Mortality by education in German speaking Switzerland, 1990-1997: results from the Swiss National Cohort. Int J Epidemiol. 2003;32(3):346–54.

50. Charlson ME, Pompei P, Ales KL, CR MK. A new method of classifying prognostic comorbidity in longitudinal studies: development and validation. J Chronic Dis. 1987;40(5):373–83.

51. Fox KA, Dabbous OH, Goldberg RJ, et al. Prediction of risk of death and myocardial infarction in the six months after presentation with acute coronary syndrome: prospective multinational observational study (GRACE). BMJ. 2006;333(7578):1091.

52. von Känel R, Hari R, Schmid JP, Saner H, Begré S. Distress related to myocardial infarction and cardiovascular outcome: a retrospective observational study. BMC Psychiatry. 2011;11:98.

53. Perneger TV. What's wrong with Bonferroni adjustments? BMJ. 1998;316:1236–8.

54. Cohen J. Statistical power for the behavioral sciences, ed 3. New York: Academic Press; 1988.

55. Le Grande MR, Neubeck L, Murphy BM, McIvor D, Lynch D, McLean H, Jackson AC. Screening for obstructive sleep apnoea in cardiac rehabilitation: a position statement from the Australian Centre for Heart Health and the Australian cardiovascular health and rehabilitation association. Eur J Prev Cardiol. 2016;23(14):1466–75.

56. Coryell VT, Ziegelstein RC, Hirt K, Quain A, Marine JE, Smith MT. Clinical correlates of insomnia in patients with acute coronary syndrome. Int Heart J. 2013;54(5):258–65.

57. Irwin MR, Opp MR. Sleep Health: Reciprocal regulation of sleep and innate immunity. Neuropsychopharmacology. 2017;42(1):129–55.

58. Waller C, Bauersachs J, Hoppmann U, et al. Blunted cortisol stress response and depression-induced hypocortisolism is related to inflammation in patients with CAD. J Am Coll Cardiol. 2016;67(9):1124–6.

59. Reynolds RM, Walker BR, Haw S, et al. Low serum cortisol predicts early death after acute myocardial infarction. Crit Care Med. 2010;38(3):973–5.

60. Elenkov IJ. Neurohormonal-cytokine interactions: implications for inflammation, common human diseases and well-being. Neurochem Int. 2008;52(1–2):40–51.

61. Mills PJ, Dimsdale JE, Coy TV, Ancoli-Israel S, Clausen JL, Nelesen RA. Beta 2-adrenergic receptor characteristics in sleep apnea patients. Sleep. 1995;18(1):39–42.

62. Yin X, Zheng Y, Liu Q, Cai J, Cai L. Cardiac response to chronic intermittent hypoxia with a transition from adaptation to maladaptation: the role of hydrogen peroxide. Oxidative Med Cell Longev. 2012;2012:569520.

63. Shah N, Redline S, Yaggi HK, et al. Obstructive sleep apnea and acute myocardial infarction severity: ischemic preconditioning? Sleep Breath. 2013;17(2):819–26.

64. Khayat R, Patt B, Hayes D Jr. Obstructive sleep apnea: the new cardiovascular disease. Part I: obstructive sleep apnea and the pathogenesis of vascular disease. Heart Fail Rev. 2009;14(3):143–53.

65. Vgontzas AN, Fernandez-Mendoza J, Liao D, Bixler EO. Insomnia with objective short sleep duration: the most biologically severe phenotype of the disorder. Sleep Med Rev. 2013;17(4):241–54.

66. Schiza SE, Simantirakis E, Bouloukaki I, et al. Sleep patterns in patients with acute coronary syndromes. Sleep Med. 2010;11(2):149–53.

67. Westlake K, Plihalova A, Pretl M, Lattova Z, Polak J. Screening for obstructive sleep apnea syndrome in patients with type 2 diabetes mellitus: a prospective study on sensitivity of Berlin and STOP-bang questionnaires. Sleep Med. 2016;26:71–6.

68. Whitehead DL, Strike P, Perkins-Porras L, Steptoe A. Frequency of distress and fear of dying during acute coronary syndromes and consequences for adaptation. Am J Cardiol. 2005;96(11):1512–6.

Effect of Erythropoietin in patients with acute myocardial infarction: five-year results of the REVIVAL-3 trial

Birgit Steppich[1]* ⓘ, Philip Groha[1], Tareq Ibrahim[2], Heribert Schunkert[2], Karl-Ludwig Laugwitz[2], Martin Hadamitzky[1], Adnan Kastrati[1], Ilka Ott[1] and for the Regeneration of Vital Myocardium in ST-Segment Elevation Myocardial Infarction by Erythropoietin (REVIVAL-3) Study Investigators

Abstract

Background: Erythropoietin (EPO) has been suggested to promote cardiac repair after MI. However, the randomized, double-blind, placebo controlled REVIVAL-3 trial showed that short term high dose EPO in timely reperfused myocardium does not improve left ventricular ejection fraction after 6 months. Moreover, the study raised safety concerns due to a trend towards a higher incidence of adverse clinical events as well as a increase in neointima formation after treatment with EPO. The present study therefore aimed to assess the 5-year clinical outcomes.

Methods: After successful reperfusion 138 patients with STEMI were randomly assigned to receive epoetin beta (3.33×10^4 U, $n = 68$) or placebo ($n = 70$) immediately, 24 and 48 h after percutaneous coronary intervention. The primary outcome of the present study- the combined incidence of MACE 5 years after randomization - occurred in 25% of the patients assigned to epoetin beta and 17% of the patients assigned to placebo (RR 1.5; 95% CI 0.8-3.5; $p = 0.26$). Target lesion revascularization was required in 15 patients (22.1%) treated with epoetin-ß and 9 patients (12.9%) treated with placebo ($p = 0.15$). Analysis of patients in the upper and lower quartile of baseline hemoglobin as an indirect estimate of endogenous erythropoietin levels revealed no significant impact of endogenous erythropoietin on efficiency of exogen administered epoetin-ß in terms of death and MACE.

Conclusion: These long-term follow-up data show that epoetin beta does not improve clinical outcomes of patients with acute myocardial infarction.

Keywords: Erythropoietin, Acute myocardial infarction, REVIVAL-3 trial

Background

Despite continually improved treatment regimens the rate of death and heart failure is still substantially high after ST-elevation myocardial infarction (STEMI) [1–3].

The extent of myocardial necrosis is a main predictor of mortality and morbidity after STEMI. Cardiac necrosis is not only determined by the myocardial ischemia itself, but also driven by secondary damage upon reperfusion, the ischemia-reperfusion-injury. While the ischemia-induced necrosis can effectively be treated by timely myocardial reperfusion using percutaneous coronary intervention (PCI), reperfusion-induced necrosis is still barely preventable [4].

Erythropoietin (Epo), a hypoxia induced hormone, has been shown to play a cardioprotective role in various experimental models of myocardial ischemia and ischemia-reperfusion via pleiotropic actions [5]. Besides stimulation of haematopoesis, Epo induces mobilization of endothelial progenitor cells and promotes neovascularization and angiogenesis [6, 7]. It also exhibits anti-apoptotic, anti-inflammatory and anti-oxidative properties

* Correspondence: bigitsteppich@yahoo.de
[1]Deutsches Herzzentrum der Technischen Universität München, Lazarettstr. 36, 80636 Munich, Germany
Full list of author information is available at the end of the article

in the heart [5], where cardiomyocytes and endothelial cells express functional Epo receptors [8, 9].

However, despite promising results of experimental and preclinical studies, we -like most other clinical trials- showed in the randomized, double-blind, placebo controlled REVIVAL-3 trial, that short-term, high dose epoetin beta in addition to successful PCI in STEMI does neither reduce infarct size nor improve left ventricular function at 6 months [10–12]. On the contrary we observed a trend towards a higher incidence of adverse clinical events 6 month after epoetin beta treatment as well as a significant increase in neointima formation in the erythropoietin group [13]. This raises safety concerns about the use of erythropoietin in patients with acute MI. By promoting neointima formation and imparing arterial healing, erythropoietin might affect clinical outcomes of STEMI patients over the longer term. Moreover legacy or memory effects can influence clinical prognosis even long after cessation of drug administration [14]. However clinical outcome data more than 12 month after erythropoietin therapy have never been reported in patients treated for myocardial infarction. Thus, the aim of the present trial was to assess the impact of high-dose, short term erythropoietin on long-term clinical outcomes in STEMI patients. For this purpose we extended the follow up of the REVIVAL-3 trial, which compared 3 daily IV doses of 33,000 I.U. of rhEpoetin beta administered immediately, 24 and 48 h after PCI in STEMI to placebo treatment, up to 5 years.

Methods

Patients and protocol

The detailed study design and main results from the REVIVAL-3 trial have been published previously [10]. In brief, the REVIVAL-3 study was a prospective, randomized, double-blind, placebo-controlled trial allocating patients with acute STEMI in a 1:1 ratio after successful primary PCI to medical treatment with either epoetin beta or placebo as a supplement to treatment according to guidelines.

To be included patients had to present with a first STEMI within 24 h of symptom onset and had to have an angiographic left ventricular ejection fraction (LVEF) of less than 50% by visual estimation in the angiogramm. The study drug was given immediately after successful PCI in the catheterization laboratory as well as 24 and 48 h after randomization. Each time, patients received either 3.33×10^4 IU of recombinant human epoetin-β (NeoRecormon; F. Hoffmann-La Roche, Basel, Switzerland) or a matching placebo intravenously for 30 min. The periprocedural antithrombotic therapy consisted of 600 mg of clopidogrel orally, 500 mg aspirin, and unfractionated heparin with or without abciximab intravenously. Heparin was given as a bolus of 140 IU or 70 IU in case of additional abciximab

(0.25 mg/kg body weight bolus, followed by an infusion of 0.125 µg/kg per min for 12 h). Postinterventional all patients recieved clopidogrel 75 mg twice a day for 3 days followed by 75 mg/d for at least 6 months. Aspirin 100 mg twice a day was recommended indefinitely.

The study protocol was approved by the institutional ethics committee and all patients gave written informed consent for participation in the study. The study has been registered in clinicaltrials.gov (NCT00390832).

One hundred thirty-eight patients were randomized, from January 2007 to November 2008 at the Deutsches Herzzentrum and 1st Medizinische Klinik rechts der Isar, to epoetin-ß ($n = 68$) or placebo ($n = 70$) and finally included in the present extended follow up study.

Clinical follow-up

The pre-specified primary end point of the main REVIVAL-3 trial was LVEF 6 months after random assignment measured by MRI. Other end points included infarct size at 5 days and 6 months and clinical adverse events (death, recurrent myocardial infarction, stroke, and infarct-related artery revascularization) at 30 days and 6 months.

Epoetin did not improve LVEF or reduce infarct size at 6 months follow up. On the contrary, there was a trend toward a higher adverse event rate with erythropoietin at 6 months.

The primary outcome of interest for the current analysis was the combined incidence of major adverse cardiac events (MACE), including death, recurrent MI, stroke, coronary bypass surgery (ACVB) and target vessel revascularistion, 5 years after randomization. The incidence of the individual components of the primary end point was also assessed. Information on vital status, recurrent MI, target vessel revascularization and stroke was collected by annual telephone interviews and from hospital records. In case the patients reported cardiac symptoms during the interview, complete clinical, electrocardiogram, and laboratory examination was performed in the outpatient clinic or by the referring physician. Reinfarction was defined as the onset of recurrent symptoms of ischemia combined with new ST-segment elevations and/or a second increase of serum CK or CK-MB to at least twice the upper limit of the normal range. Target vessel revascularization was defined as PCI or bypass grafting of the infarct-related coronary artery after primary PCI.

Statistical analysis

All data were analyzed on the basis of the intention-to-treat principle using data from all patients as randomized. Categorical data are presented as counts or proportions (%). Continuous data are presented as mean ± standard deviation. Differences between the groups were assessed using χ^2 or Fisher exact test for categorical data and t test for continuous data. The cumulative incidence of the composite end point during the 5-year–follow up was evaluated with the Kaplan Meier method. Survival free of adverse events was defined as the interval from randomization until the event of interest. Data for patients who did not have an event of interest were censored at the date of the last follow-up. The difference in the composite event rate between the 2 study groups was checked for significance by means of a Cox proportional hazards model, which also allowed the calculation of the respective hazard ratio with its 95% confidence interval. A 2-tailed probability value < 0.05 was considered to indicate statistical significance. All analyses were performed using S-plus statistical package (S-PLUS, In- sightful Corp., Seattle, Washington).

Results

All 138 patients enrolled in the REVIVAL-3 trial were included in the present extend follow up study. All had received the randomly assigned medication: 68 epoetin-ß and 70 placebo. One hundred thirty-four patients (97%) completed the 5-years follow up, while 4 patients were lost to follow up. Detailed baseline characteristics of the patients have been published previously and were similarly distributed in the two treatment groups. Table 1 summarizes some key data of the study population.

The mean age of the patients was 59.1 (±13.0) years in the epoetin-ß group and 62.1 (±12.3) years in the control group, with a proportion of males of 82% versus 74%. The median time from symptom onset to PCI was 252 (interquartile range 175–413) minutes in patients receiving epoetin-ß and 253 (interquartile range 165–457) minutes in patients in the control group. Baseline angiographic LVEF was 46% in both groups, indicating substantial myocardial infarction. The majority of patients presented with multi-vessel-disease (62% versus 71%) and was treated with drug-eluting stents (93% versus 95%). Although epoetin-ß induced an increase in circulating reticulocytes 5 days after random assignment ($11.3 \pm 3.8 \times 10^4/\mu l$ versus $10.9 \pm 4.18 \times 10^4/\mu l$; $p = 0.563$ to $34.2 \pm 9.58 \times 10^4/\mu l$ versus $16.8 \pm 6.58 \times 10^4/\mu l$; $p = 0.001$) and a rise in the maximal platelet count ($265 \pm 70 \times 10^9/l$ versus $232 \pm 74 \times 10^9/l$, $P = 0.011$), it was not associated with a rise in maximal hemoglobin levels (14.8 ± 1.6 mg/dl versus 15 ± 1.3 mg/dl, $P = 0.593$).

Clinical outcome

Table 2 summarizes the major clinical events registered after hospital discharge in both patient groups over the extended follow-up. A total of 14 patients (10%) died during the 5-years study period, 8 (11.8%) in the epoetin-ß and 6 (8.6%) in the control group ($p = 0.53$; Fig. 1a).

Table 1 Key characteristics of the study population

	Epoetin-ß (n = 68)	Placebo (n = 70)
Age, mean y (±SD)	59.1 (13.0)	62.1 (12.3)
Women, n(%)	12 (18)	18 (26)
Body mass index, mean (±SD)	28 (4)	27 (4)
Diabetes, n(%)	11 (16)	10 (14)
Current smoker, n(%)	29 (43)	30 (43)
Multivessel disease, n(%)	42 (62)	50 (71)
Angiographic LVEF, mean % (±SD)	46 (8)	46 (8)
Infarct related coronary artery, n(%)		
LAD	34 (50)	31 (44)
RCA	19 (33.9)	18 (31.0)
LCX	7 (12.5)	12 (20.7)
LMCA	0	1 (1)
Initial TIMI flow grade, n(%)		
0	35 (52)	41 (59)
1	11 (16)	11 (14)
2	20 (29)	15 (21)
3	2 (3)	4 (6)
Final TIMI flow grade, n(%)		
1	0	1 (1)
2	5 (7)	6 (9)
3	63 (93)	63 (90)
Type of intervention, n(%)		
Bare metal stent	3 (4)	3 (4)
Drug-eluting stent	63 (93)	66 (95)
Balloon angioplasty	2 (3)	1 (1)
Creatine kinase-MB max, U/L (range)	201 (121–450)	213 (124–312)
Symtom onset to PCI, min (range)	252 (175–413)	253 (165–457)
Hemoglobin max, mean g/dl (±SD)	14.8 (1.6)	15 (1.3)

Table 2 Summary of major clinical events registered after hospital discharge in both patient groups over the 5-year follow-up

	EPO (n = 68)	Placebo (n = 70)	
Death; n(%)	8 (11.8)	6 (8.6)	p = 0.53
MI; n(%)	4 (5.9)	2 (2.9)	p = 0.38
Death or MI; n(%)	10 (14.7)	7 (10.0)	p = 0.40
Stroke; n(%)	1 (1.5)	0 (0)	p = 0.31
Death or MI or Stroke; n(%)	10 (14.7)	7 (10.0)	p = 0.40
Coronary bypass surgery; n(%)	1 (1.5)	0 (0)	p = 0.31
Target lession revascularization; n(%)	15 (22.1)	9 (12.9)	p = 0.15
MACE; n(%)	17 (25.0)	12 (17.1)	p = 0.26

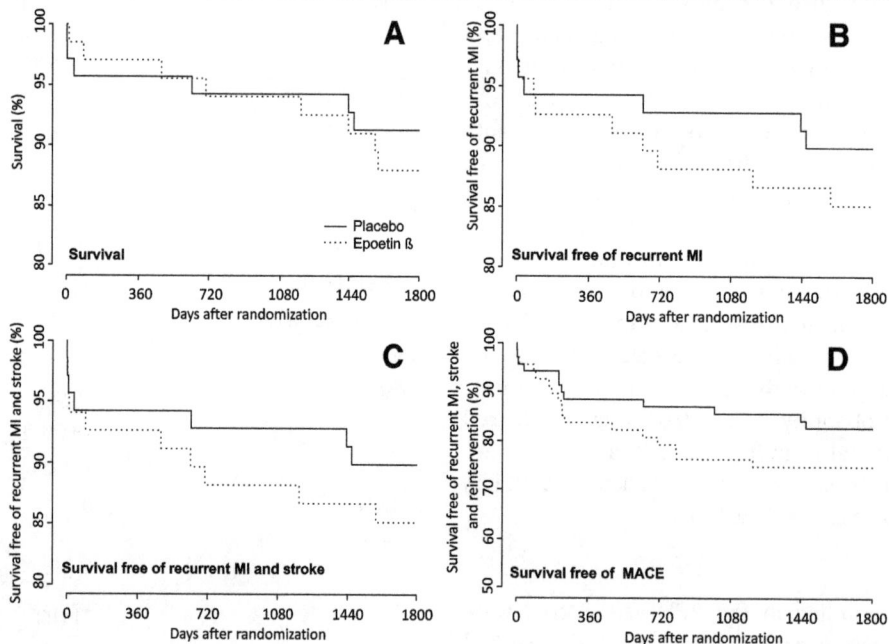

Fig. 1 Kaplan-Meier-Curves showing the cumulative event rates according to Epoetin beta therapy or Placebo. A Analysis of survival. B Analysis of survival free of recurrent myocardial infarction (MI). C Analysis of survival free of recurrent MI and stroke. D Analysis of survival free of MACE (recurrent MI, stroke and reintervention)

While 2 epoetin-ß patients and 3 placebo patients had died during the initial 6 month follow up, 6 patients receiving epoetin-ß and 3 patients receiving placebo died between 6 month and 5 years. Individual causes of death are shown in Table 3.

Six patients (4.3%) experienced MI, 2 (2.9%) in the placebo and 4 (5.9%) in the epoetin-ß group. Only 1 (1.5%)

Table 3 Summary of patients who died during the 5 year follow up period

Patient #	Group	Cause of death
1	Placebo	cardiogenic shock
2	Placebo	cardiogenic shock
3	EPO	lung embolism
4	Placebo	sudden cardiac death
5	EPO	septic shock, stroke
6	EPO	cancer
7	Placebo	after orthopedic surgery
8	EPO	sudden cardiac death
9	EPO	unknown
10	Placebo	cancer
11	EPO	sudden cardiac death
12	Placebo	unknown
13	EPO	unknown
14	EPO	unknown

Patient # 1–5 died 1–186 days after randomization. Patient # 7–14 died 187–1860 days after randomization

patient in the epoetin-ß group suffered a stroke ($p = 0.31$). Coronary bypass surgery was also needed in 1 (1.5%) epoetin-ß patient and none of the control patient ($p = 0.31$). Target lesion revascularization was required in 15 patients (22.1%) treated with epoetin-ß and 9 patients (12.9%) treated with placebo ($p = 0.15$).

Figure 1b and c show the cumulative event rates of survival free of recurrent MI and survival free of recurrent MI and stroke.

The current primary outcome - the cumulative incidence of MACE 5 years after randomization - occurred in 25% ($n = 17$) of the patients assigned to epoetin-ß and 17% ($n = 12$) of the patients assigned to placebo (RR 1.5; 95% CI 0.8-3.5; $p = 0.26$; Fig. 1d).

To analyze if elevated endogenous erythropoietin levels might have interfered with effects of exogenous administered epoetin-ß, we stratified the patients according to their hemoglobin level on admission. Since serum erythropoietin levels rise in an exponential manner with a decrease in hemoglobin levels [15], we analyzed clinical outcome of patients in the lower (Hb < 14,1 g/dl) and the upper (Hb > 15,5 g/dl) quartile of hemoglobin concentration on admission separately. While the lower quartile consisted of 16 control patients and 23 erythropoietin-treated patients, the upper quartile comprised 34 patients, 19 treated by placebo and 15 by erythropoietin. During the 5 years follow up 1 death in the placebo group and 5 deaths in the erythropoietin group occurred in the lower Hb-quartile (Kaplan Meier estimates of death: 6.2% placebo, 21.7% epoetin-ß; $p = 0.19$), whereas 2 control and none of the erythropoietin patients experienced death in the upper Hb-quartile (Kaplan Meier estimates of death: 10.5% placebo, 0% epoetin-ß; $p = 0.20$). The cumulative incidence of MACE 5 years after randomization occurred in 21.7% ($n = 5$) of the patients assigned to epoetin-ß and 18.8% ($n = 3$) of the patients assigned to placebo in the lower hemoglobin quartile ($p = 0.82$) and in 20% ($n = 3$) in epoetin-ß and 21.1% ($n = 4$) in placebo treated patients of the upper quartile ($p = 0.94$).

Discussion

This extended follow-up of the REVIVAL-3 trial revealed that high-dose, short-term epoetin-ß in addition to successful PCI does not improve clinical long-term outcomes of patients with acute myocardial infarction.

To the best of our knowledge, this is currently the study with the longest follow up analyzing erythropoietin effects in STEMI patients up to 5 years. All previous trials focused on the first 6 month and to date only the large HEBE III trial has provided one year follow up results [16].

While most other trials have to deal with the problem of a selective patient inclusion with small infarct sizes the REVIVAL-3 trial only randomized large infarctions affecting approximately 27–28% of the left ventricle with impaired LV-Function [10]. This ensures, that erythropoietin effects have been tested in an adequate ischemic condition.

Prognosis of patients with STEMI remains complicated by a substantial number of death, reinfarction and heart failure. According to real life registries like the REAL register the 3-year cumulative incidence of death is about 17.5% and MACE about 22.9% in STEMI patients treated by timely PCI with DES (drug eluting stents) [3]. Due to closely supervised and optimized therapy in the setting of RCT (randomzied controlled clinical trials) the present study has a somewhat lower however still substantial 5-year cumulative incidence of death (10%) and MACE (21%).

Since the extent of myocardial necrosis is a major determinant of adverse postinfarction-outcome, therapies able to further reduce infarct size are urgently needed. According to experimental in vivo and ex-vivo studies erythropoietin seemed to be such a promising candidate by its angiogenic, anti-inflammatory, anti-hypertrophic and anti-apoptotic properties [17]. It attenuated infarct expansion and detrimental cardiac remodeling, reduced infarct size and improved functional recovery in animal models of ischemic cardiac injury [5]. However our results are in line with the majority of clinical studies and recent meta-analyses, who all failed to demonstrate a benefit for shortterm erythropoetin therapy in PCI-

treated STEMI patients in terms of both cardiac function and clinical prognosis [11, 18, 19]. A lot has been speculated about this erythropoietin paradox - why the overwhelming cardioprotective effects in animal studies could not be translated into humans.

Animal experiments were conducted in two major experimental models, MI induced by permanent ligation of a coronary artery or by temporary occlusion followed by reperfusion. In the model of permanent occlusion animals were mostly treated by a single intraperitoneal dose of 3000–5000 IU/kg of body weight erythropoietin immediately after ligation or even before [20, 21]. The best results were achieved when EPO was applied at the time of occlusion. Dose regimes in cardiac ischemia-reperfusion worked also primarily with high doses of 2500–5000 IU/kg of body weight erythropoietin intraperitoneal or intravenous and most regimes included a dose given even before ischemia was induced. Most effective results were observed when treatment was applied no later than at the time of reperfusion, i.e., 30–90 min from coronary occlusion. In contrast the majority of clinical trials did not adjust the erythropoietin dose to the individual body weight, in fact doses ranged between 30000–60000 IU, which corresponds to 430–860 IU/kg for a 70 kg patient. Drug application was carried out between 6 to 48 h in average after symptom onset [20, 21].

Therefore as a possible explanation of the erythropoietin-paradox, mostly dosing and timing of erythropoietin-administration has been supposed to be inappropriate, especially since experimental studies have shown the existence of a dose-dependent therapeutic window of time subsequent to reperfusion [22]. Beyond this window the erythropoietin induced tissue-protection is reduced or even abolished.

For example, Moon et al. showed in a rat model of permanent coronary ligation, that erythropoietin mediated cardioprotection with 3000 IU/kg of body weight was still effective when administration was delayed up to 12 h after ischemic injury, but not if the treatment was delayed for 24 h. With the lowest effective dose of 150 IU/kg of body weight beneficial effects were only observed when administered within 4 h. This efficacy was already lost when the administration was delayed by 8 h [23].

Our trial is among the studies with the highest erythropoietin doses used, nevertheless still substantial lower than those used in animal studies, and increasing the dosage further would mean increasing the risk of thromboembolic events due to elevated heamatocrit levels [24]. On the other hand, we administered erythropoietin as soon as possible in our clinical setting, namely immediately with PCI. However the average time from symptom-onset to PCI was about 250 min, exceeding the above mentioned critical time window limit of 4 h according to animal studies. Therefore, application of erythropoietin even in advance to PCI or intracoronary might be necessary to be protective and beneficial. The recently published Intra-Co-EpoMI trial however failed to demonstrate reduction of infarct size 3 months after randomized intracoronary administration of a single dose darbepoetin-alpha in STEMI patients [25]. Another novel, promising approach to increase erythropoietin doses and thereby prolong the therapeutic window without increasing the thromboembolic risk, might be the new erythropoietin derivates, which display no haematopoietic effects by preserved cardioprotection [26].

A central issue of the erythropoietin paradox however might lay in the difference between animal models and the real human world [27].

Erythropoietin mediated cardioprotective effects seem to differ across species. While cardioprotection has been clearly shown in ischemia-reperfusion models in small rodents including mouse and rabbit, experiments in larger animals such as sheep and pig were either negative or controversial [20, 21]. As mentioned above experimental studies testing erythropoietin effects in myocardial infarction mostly used healthy animals and mimicked myocardial ischemia by mechanical injury of the coronary artery. This basically contrasts the process of MI in humans. Although MI is an acute phenomenon it develops on the basis of atherosclerosis and is the final stage of this chronic complex disease. STEMI patients often experience periods of stable or unstable angina with hypoxia and/or hypoperfusion and suffer from different degrees of congestive heart failure. Therefore, they can exhibit pathologically elevated erythropoietin levels leading to erythropoietin resistance. It has been shown, that raised endogenous plasma erythropoietin concentrations in patients with congestive heart failure are associated with increased cardiovascular mortality [28]. This might also explain why we not only found no improvement of clinical outcome, but observed a trend towards an increase in MACE following epoetin beta - a trend we had already seen in the original REVIVAL 3 trial after 6 months of follow up. While 62–71% of our study patients presented with multivessel disease, in the current metaanalysis on patient level by Fokkema et al. only 36% of the patients included had multivessel disease indicating a less advanced, pronounced and preceded disease process [11]. Therefore, Epoetin-ß therapy might have encountered different endogenous erythropoietin levels, resulting in the observed adverse outcome.

Separate analysis of patients in the upper and lower quartile of baseline hemoglobin as an indirect estimate of endogenous erythropoietin levels revealed no significant impact of endogenous erythropoietin on efficiency of exogen administered epoetin-ß in terms of death and MACE - although a definitive conclusion can´t be drawn, since the event numbers are too small. However endogenous erythropoietin might not be the only confounder present. Hypertension, diabetes, aging and concomitant medication can also interfere with erythropoietin-mediated cardioprotection in clinical settings. Morphine, statins, ACE-inhibitors, angiotensin II receptor blockers, antidiabetics and clopidogrel are known to influence conditioning-induced cardioprotection and might overdrive or damp beneficial erythropoietin effects [20].

The REVEAL study by Najjar et al. on 222 patients with STEMI showed a higher incidence of death, MI, stroke and stent thrombosis upon erythropoietin use during the first 12 weeks. A subgroup analysis even revealed increased infarct size among erythropoietin patients 70 years or older [29]. Although other studies on erythropoietin in STEMI patients did not find an increased risk of adverse events over the short term, side effects of erythropoietin therapy are evident for other indications like heart failure, renal disease, anemia or cancer [30, 31]. In patients with systolic heart failure and anemia darbopoetin was accompanied by a significant increase in thrombembolic events and septic shock [32]. Side effects have been linked to erythropoietin induced increases in haematocrit, blood viscosity, blood pressure, vasoconstriction or platelet function [33]. In the present study the non-significant rise in adverse clinical events after 5 years was mainly driven by more frequent target vessel revascularization in response to epoetin beta. Corresponding quantitative coronary angiography after six months revealed an increase in segment diameter stenosis in the epoetin beta group ($32 \pm 19\%$ vs. $26 \pm 14\%$, p = 0.046). Despite a subtle induction of circulating progenitor cells by erythropoietin, the observed increase in neointima formation was not associated with progenitor cell mobilization [13]. In a rat carotid artery model of vascular injury erythropoietin induced excessive neointima formation [34]. Experimental studies in vascular lesions in mice are less clear: one study reported inhibition of neointima hyperplasia due to enhanced reendothelialisation by mobilized endothelial progenitor cells and resident endothelial cells [35], while another study described increased neointima formation upon erythropoietin treatment due to enhanced smooth muscle cell proliferation by paracrine effects of the endothelium [36]. A clinical trial, designed to analyze the effect of erythropoietin on restenosis, failed to demonstrate, that short-term 'low-dose' epoetin beta prevented neointimal hyperplasia in PCI-treated AMI patients [37].

Our study is limited by the fact, that the REVIVAL-3 trial was powered to detect differences in left ventricular ejection fraction and was not designed to evaluate effects on long-term clinical outcomes. Although the relatively low number of patients enrolled precludes definitive conclusions about clinical prognosis, we believe that the herein presented data can provide nevertheless valuable insights, since 97% of the study patients completed the 5-year clinical follow-up and it´s to date the only study providing clinical outcome data more than 12 month after epoetin treatment in AMI.

Conclusion

These 5 years follow-up data show that short-term use of 3 IV doses epoetin beta in PCI-treated STEMI patients does not improve clinical long-term prognosis. Our results further support the erythropoietin paradox and advise caution regarding the application of erythropoietin in patients with STEMI.

Abbreviations
REVIVAL: Regenerate Vital Myocardium by Vigorous Activation of Bone Marrow Stem cells; STEMI: ST-elevation myocardial infarction; MI: Myocardial infarction; PCI: Percutaneous coronary intervention; EPO: Erythropoietin; LVEF: Left ventricular ejection fraction; MACE: Major adverse cardiac events; MRI: Magnetic resonance imaging; ACVB: Coronary bypass surgery

Acknowledgments
We appreciate the invaluable contribution of the medical and technical staffs operating in the coronary care units, nuclear medicine, and catheterization laboratories of the participating institutions.

Funding
There is no external or commercial funding to be reported. The REVIVAL-3 trial was solely sponsored by the German Heart Center.

Authors'contributions
Design, conception and conduction of the study: IO, AK; coordination of the study and data collection: PG, TI, HS, K-LL, MH,, AK, IO, BS; statistical analysis and data interpretation: IO, AK, MH, BS; manuscript writing: BS. All authors read and approved the final manuscript.

Competing interest
The authors declare that they have no competing interests.

Author details
[1]Deutsches Herzzentrum der Technischen Universität München, Lazarettstr. 36, 80636 Munich, Germany. [2]Medizinische Klinik Klinikum rechts der Isar der Technischen Universität München, Ismaningerstr. 22, 81675 Munich, Germany.

References
1. Campo G, Guastaroba P, Marzocchi A, Santarelli A, Varani E, Vignali L, Sangiorgio P, Tondi S, Serenelli C, De Palma R, Saia F. Impact of COPD on long-term outcome after ST-segment elevation myocardial infarction receiving primary percutaneous coronary intervention. Chest. 2013;144(3):750–7.
2. Campo G, Saia F, Guastaroba P, Marchesini J, Varani E, Manari A, Ottani F, Tondi S, De Palma R, Marzocchi A. Prognostic impact of hospital readmissions after primary percutaneous coronary intervention. Arch Intern Med. 2011;171(21):1948–9.
3. Campo G, Saia F, Percoco G, Manari A, Santarelli A, Vignali L, Varani E, Benassi A, Sangiorgio P, Tarantino F, Magnavacchi P, De Palma R, Guastaroba P, Marzocchi A. Long-term outcome after drug eluting stenting in patients with ST-segment elevation myocardial infarction: data from the REAL registry. Int J Cardiol. 2010;140(2):154–60.
4. Dominguez-Rodriguez A, Abreu-Gonzalez P, Reiter RJ. Cardioprotection and pharmacological therapies in acute myocardial infarction: Challenges in the current era. World J Cardiol. 2014;6(3):100–6.
5. Sanchis-Gomar F, Garcia-Gimenez JL, Pareja-Galeano H, Romagnoli M, Perez-Quilis C, Lippi G. Erythropoietin and the heart: physiological effects and the therapeutic perspective. Int J Cardiol. 2014;171(2):16–125.
6. Heeschen C, Aicher A, Lehmann R, Fichtlscherer S, Vasa M, Urbich C, Mildner-Rihm C, Martin H, Zeiher AM, Dimmeler S. Erythropoietin is a potent physiologic stimulus for endothelial progenitor cell mobilization. Blood. 2003;102(4):1340–6.
7. van der Meer P, Lipsic E, Henning RH, Boddeus K, van der Velden J, Voors AA, van Veldhuisen DJ, van Gilst WH, Schoemaker RG. Erythropoietin induces neovascularization and improves cardiac function in rats with heart failure after myocardial infarction. J Am Coll Cardiol. 2005;46(1):125–33.
8. Anagnostou A, Liu Z, Steiner M, Chin K, Lee ES, Kessimian N, Noguchi CT. Erythropoietin receptor mRNA expression in human endothelial cells. Proc Natl Acad Sci U S A. 1994;91(9):3974–8.
9. Wright GL, Hanlon P, Amin K, Steenbergen C, Murphy E, Arcasoy MO. Erythropoietin receptor expression in adult rat cardiomyocytes is associated with an acute cardioprotective effect for recombinant erythropoietin during ischemia-reperfusion injury. FASEB J. 2004;18(9):1031–3.
10. Ott I, Schulz S, Mehilli J, Fichtner S, Hadamitzky M, Hoppe K, Ibrahim T, Martinoff S, Massberg S, Laugwitz KL, Dirschinger J, Schwaiger M, Kastrati A, Schömig A, REVIVAL-3 Study Investigators. Erythropoietin in patients with acute ST-segment elevation myocardial infarction undergoing primary percutaneous coronary intervention: a randomized, double-blind trial. Circ Cardiovasc Interv. 2010;3(5):408–13.
11. Fokkema M, van der Meer LP, Rao SV, Belonje AM, Ferrario M, Hillege HL, Katz SD, Lipšic E, Ludman AJ, Ott I, Prunier F, Choi DJ, Toba K, van Veldhuisen DJ, Voors AA. Safety and clinical outcome of erythropoiesis-stimulating agents in patients with ST-elevation myocardial infarction: A meta-analysis of individual patient data. Am Heart J. 2014;168(3):354–62. e352.
12. Ali-Hassan-Sayegh S, Mirhosseini SJ, Tahernejad M, Mahdavi P, Haddad F, Shahidzadeh A, Lotfaliani MR, Sedaghat-Hamedani F, Kayvanpour E, Weymann A, Sabashnikov A, Popov AF. Administration of erythropoietin in patients with myocardial infarction: does it make sense? An updated and comprehensive meta-analysis and systematic review. Cardiovasc Revasc Med. 2015;16(3):179–89.
13. Stein A, Mohr F, Laux M, Thieme S, Lorenz B, Cetindis M, Hackl J, Groha P, Demetz G, Schulz S, Mehilli J, Schömig A, Kastrati A, Ott I. Erythropoietin-induced progenitor cell mobilisation in patients with acute ST-segment-elevation myocardial infarction and restenosis. Thromb Haemost. 2012; 107(4):769–74.
14. Chalmers J, Cooper ME. UKPDS and the legacy effect. N Engl J Med. 2008; 359(15):1618–20.
15. Mastromarino V, Volpe M, Musumeci MB, Autore C, Conti E. Erythropoietin and the heart: facts and perspectives. Clin Sci. 2011;120(2):51–63.
16. Fokkema ML, Kleijn L, Van der Meer P, Belonje AM, Achterhof SK, Hillege HL, Van 't Hof A, Jukema JW, Peels HO, Henriques JP, ten Berg JM, Vos J, van Gilst WH, van Veldhuisen DJ, Voors AA. Long term effects of epoetin alfa in patients with ST- elevation myocardial infarction. Cardiovasc Drugs Ther. 2013;27(5):433–9.
17. Wen Y, Zhang XJ, Ma YX, Xu XJ, Hong LF, Lu ZH. Erythropoietin attenuates hypertrophy of neonatal rat cardiac myocytes induced by angiotensin-II in vitro. Scand J Clin Lab Invest. 2009;69(4):518–25.
18. Gao D, Ning N, Niu X, Dang Y, Dong X, Wei J, Zhu C. Erythropoietin treatment in patients with acute myocardial infarction: a meta-analysis of randomized controlled trials. Am Heart J. 2012;164(5):715–27. e711.
19. Wen Y, Xu J, Ma X, Gao Q. High-dose erythropoietin in acute ST-segment elevation myocardial infarction: a meta-analysis of randomized controlled trials. Am J Cardiovasc Drugs. 2013;13(6):435–42.
20. Roubille F, Prunier F, Barrère-Lemaire S, Leclercq F, Piot C, Kritikou EA, Rhéaume E, Busseuil D, Tardif JC. What is the role of erythropoietin in acute myocardial infarct? Bridging the gap between experimental models and clinical trials. Cardiovasc Drugs Ther. 2013;27(4):315–31.

21. Talan MI, Latini R. Myocardial infarction: cardioprotection by erythropoietin. Methods Mol Biol. 2013;982:265–302.

22. Talan MI, Ahmet I, Lakatta EG. Did clinical trials in which erythropoietin failed to reduce acute myocardial infarct size miss a narrow therapeutic window? PLoS One. 2012;7(4):e34819.

23. Moon C, Krawczyk M, Lakatta EG, Talan MI. Therapeutic effectiveness of a single vs multiple doses of erythropoietin after experimental myocardial infarction in rats. Cardiovasc Drugs Ther. 2006;20(4):245–51.

24. Greenberg G, Assali A, Vaknin-Assa H, Brosh D, Teplitsky I, Fuchs S, Battler A, Kornowski R, Lev EI. Hematocrit level as a marker of outcome in ST-segment elevation myocardial infarction. Am J Cardiol. 2010;105(4):435–40.

25. Roubille F, Micheau A, Combes S, Thibaut S, Souteyrand G, Cayla G, Bonello L, Lesavre N, Sportouch-Dukhan C, Klein F, Berboucha S, Cade S, Cung TT, Raczka F, Macia JC, Gervasoni R, Cransac F, Leclercq F, Barrère-Lemaire S, Paganelli F, Mottref P, Vernhet Kovacsik H, Ovize M, Piot C. Intracoronary administration of darbepoetin-alpha at onset of reperfusion in acute myocardial infarction: results of the randomized Intra-Co-EpoMI trial. Arch Cardiovasc Dis. 2013;106(3):135–45.

26. Sanchis-Gomar F, Perez-Quilis C, Lippi G. Erythropoietin receptor (EpoR) agonism is used to treat a wide range of disease. Mol Med. 2013;19:62–4.

27. Seifirad S. An emerging need for developing new models for myocardial infarction as a chronic complex disease: lessons learnt from animal vs. human studies on cardioprotective effects of Erythropoietin in reperfused myocardium. Front Physiol. 2014;5:44.

28. van der Meer P, Voors AA, Lipsic E, Smilde TD, van Gilst WH, van Veldhuisen DJ. Prognostic value of plasma erythropoietin on mortality in patients with chronic heart failure. J Am Coll Cardiol. 2004;44(1):63–7.

29. Najjar SS, Rao SV, Melloni C, Raman SV, Povsic TJ, Melton L, Barsness GW, Prather K, Heitner JF, Kilaru R, Gruberg L, Hasselblad V, Greenbaum AB, Patel M, Kim RJ, Talan M, Ferrucci L, Longo DL, Lakatta EG, Harrington RA, REVEAL Investigators. Intravenous erythropoietin in patients with ST-segment elevation myocardial infarction: REVEAL: a randomized controlled trial. JAMA. 2011;305(18):1863–72.

30. Pfeffer MA, Burdmann EA, Chen CY, Cooper ME, de Zeeuw D, Eckardt KU, Feyzi JM, Ivanovich P, Kewalramani R, Levey AS, Lewis EF, McGill JB, McMurray JJ, Parfrey P, Parving HH, Remuzzi G, Singh AK, Solomon SD, Toto R, TREAT Investigators. A trial of darbepoetin alfa in type 2 diabetes and chronic kidney disease. N Engl J Med. 2009;361(21):2019–32.

31. Macdougall IC, Roger SD, de Francisco A, Goldsmith DJ, Schellekens H, Ebbers H, Jelkmann W, London G, Casadevall N, Hörl WH, Kemeny DM, Pollock C. Antibody-mediated pure red cell aplasia in chronic kidney disease patients receiving erythropoiesis-stimulating agents: new insights. Kidney Int. 2012;81(8):727–32.

32. Swedberg K, Young JB, Anand IS, Cheng S, Desai AS, Diaz R, Maggioni AP, McMurray JJ, O'Connor C, Pfeffer MA, Solomon SD, Sun Y, Tendera M, VanVeldhuisen DJ, RED-HF Committees; RED-HF Investigators. Treatment of anemia with darbepoetin alfa in systolic heart failure. N Engl J Med. 2013; 368(13):1210–9.

33. Fishbane S, Besarab A. Mechanism of increased mortality risk with erythropoietin treatment to higher hemoglobin targets. Clin J Am Soc Nephrol. 2007;2(6):1274–82.

34. Reddy MK, Vasir JK, Hegde GV, Joshi SS, Labhasetwar V. Erythropoietin induces excessive neointima formation: a study in a rat carotid artery model of vascular injury. J Cardiovasc Pharmacol Ther. 2007;12(3):237–47.

35. Janmaat ML, Heerkens JL, de Bruin AM, Klous A, de Waard V, de Vries CJ. Erythropoietin accelerates smooth muscle cell-rich vascular lesion formation in mice through endothelial cell activation involving enhanced PDGF-BB release. Blood. 2010;115(7):1453–60.

36. Urao N, Okigaki M, Yamada H, Aadachi Y, Matsuno K, Matsui A, Matsunaga S, Tateishi K, Nomura T, Takahashi T, Tatsumi T, Matsubara H. Erythropoietin-mobilized endothelial progenitors enhance reendothelialization via Akt-endothelial nitric oxide synthase activation and prevent neointimal hyperplasia. Circ Res. 2006;98(11):1405–13.

37. Taniguchi N, Nakamura T, Sawada T, Matsubara K, Furukawa K, Hadase M, Nakahara Y, Nakamura T, Matsubara H. Erythropoietin prevention trial of coronary restenosis and cardiac remodeling after ST-elevated acute myocardial infarction (EPOC-AMI): a pilot, randomized, placebo-controlled study. Circ J. 2010;74(11):2365–71.

22

Post-cardiac injury syndrome in acute myocardial infarction patients undergoing PCI

Yan Gao[1]*[iD], Nanette H. Bishopric[2], Hong-wei Chen[3], Jiang-tao Li[1], Yu-lang Huang[1] and He-xun Huang[1]

Abstract

Background: In the era of primary percutaneous coronary intervention (PPCI), the incidence of post-cardiac injury syndrome (PCIS) in patients with acute myocardial infarction (AMI) following PPCI has become less common. However, the intrinsic pathogenesis of this medical condition remains largely uncertain. Unlike the prior reports, the present paper provides new mechanistic clues concerning the pathogenesis of PCI-related PCIS.

Case presentation: A 45-year-old male with AMI had developed an early onset of PCIS at 3 h after PPCI. A significantly slower TIMI flow (grade ≤ 2) for the culprit arteries was observed through follow-up coronary angiography (CAG); no stent thrombosis or any significant evidence of iatrogenic trauma due the intervention procedures was found. Nevertheless, the the serum level of HsCRP showed similar variation trend as the neutrophil count and troponin T in continuous blood monitoring, which suggested a potential association between PPCI-related coronary microvascular dysfunction (CMD) and pathogenesis of PCIS.

Conclusions: The reported case had excessive inflammatory reaction and CMD resulting from cardiac ischemia-reperfusion injury in an AMI patient with risk factors of endothelial dysfunction. There exists a potential reciprocal causation between PCIS and performance of PPCI in the AMI patient who was susceptible to endothelial damage.

Keywords: Post-cardiac injury syndrome, Acute myocardial infarction, Primary percutaneous coronary intervention, Coronary microvascular dysfunction

Background

Post-cardiac injury syndrome (PCIS) is referred to as an autoimmune reaction resulting from a variety of cardiac insults, including myocardial necrosis, cardiac trauma and surgery. In the era of primary percutaneous coronary intervention (PPCI), the incidence of PCI-related PCIS has been reported as lower than 0.5%, while its intrinsic pathogenesis remains completely uncertain [1]. Here we report an unusual case of early-onset PCIS after PPCI for acute myocardial infarction (AMI) plus post-operative coronary microvascular dysfunction (CMD). We further discuss the possible pathogenesis and risk alleviation of PCI-related PCIS.

Case presentation

A 45-year-old male with known risk factors of endothelial dysfunction (including smoking and hyperlipidemia) had typical episodes of angina for 3 days. Characteristic dynamic changes of electrocardiogram (ECG) and cardiac marker of myocardial necrosis troponinT (cTnT) suggested posterior STEMI. Emergency coronary angiography (CAG) revealed complete proximal occlusion of the circumflex artery (Fig. 1a). A drug eluting stent was deployed to the proximal left circumflex artery (p-LCX). Final angiogram revealed that the PPCI was successful (Fig. 1b). Three hours later, the patient developed dyspnea and persistent pleural chest pain, and the ECG showed widespread concave ST segment elevations and PR segment depression (Fig. 2a). A follow-up CAG was performed 33 h after PPCI, and no stent thrombosis or any significant evidence of iatrogenic trauma due to the intervention procedures was found. But a significant slower TIMI flow (grade ≤ 2 grade) (Fig. 1c) and abnormal TIMI myocardial

---
* Correspondence: gaoyan_0222@163.com
[1]Department of Cardiovascular Medicine, Shenzhen Shekou People's Hospital, Shenzhen 518067, Guangdong, China
Full list of author information is available at the end of the article

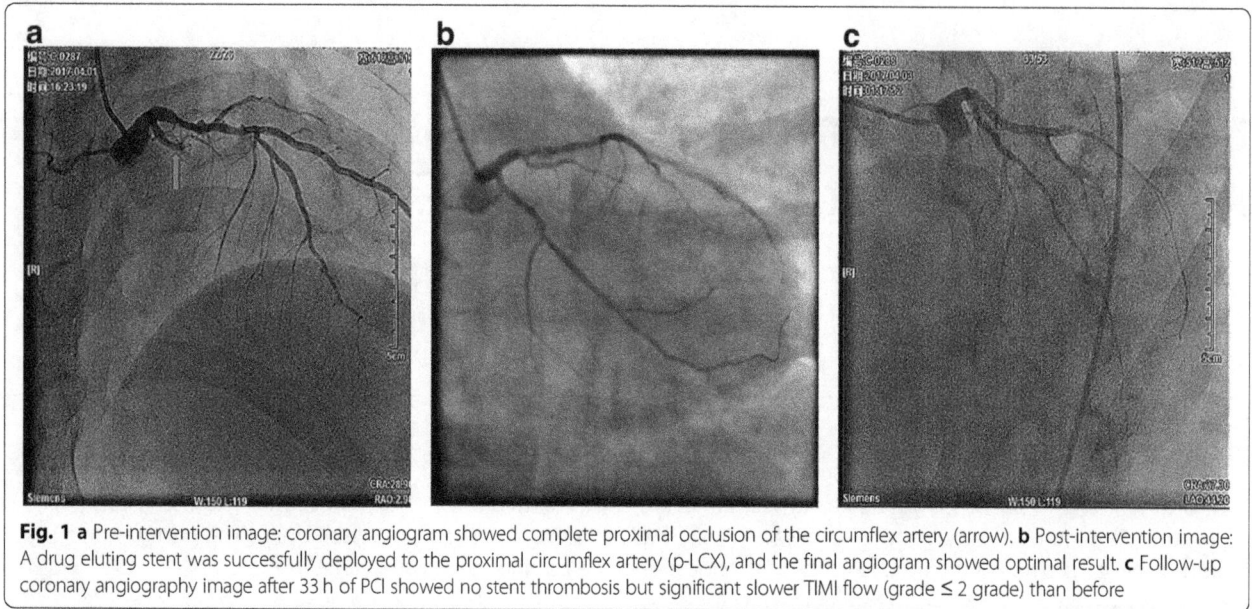

Fig. 1 a Pre-intervention image: coronary angiogram showed complete proximal occlusion of the circumflex artery (arrow). **b** Post-intervention image: A drug eluting stent was successfully deployed to the proximal circumflex artery (p-LCX), and the final angiogram showed optimal result. **c** Follow-up coronary angiography image after 33 h of PCI showed no stent thrombosis but significant slower TIMI flow (grade ≤ 2 grade) than before

perfusion frame count (TMPFC = 140 frames, at a filming rate of 30 frames/sec.) in the culprit arteries were seen through CAG. Consistent ST segment elevation on ECG with an increase in cTnT, but no recurrent CK-MB peak, seemed to suggest that the persistent focal myocardial injury might possibly involve coronary microvascular dysfunction (CMD). In recent years, assessing coronary flow reserve (CFR) by intracoronary Doppler guide wire and positron emission tomography (PET) is considered the gold standard for quantitative assessment of coronary microcirculation disorder. But this method is technically complex and very expensive, and therefore not applicable to the present case based on the patient's condition and intention. Chest CT scan showed mild pleural effusion and interstitial infiltration in both lungs (Fig. 2b, c), and UCG revealed mild pericardial effusion with posterior wall motion disappearance (Fig. 2d, e). Blood test showed that the serum concentration of HsCRP was persistently increasing; neutrophil count and the level of cTnT were elevated in parallel with HsCRP increase in the early and later stage of PCIS, respectively (Fig. 3). The erythrocyte sedimentation rate (ESR) (83 m/s) was also significantly elevated as another inflammatory marker, while the concentration of Anti-Streptolysin O (ASO) and Antinuclear Antibody (ANA) associated with rheumatic and tuberculosis disease and B-type natriuretic peptide (BNP 107 pg/ml) was still in the normal range. So we concluded that the patient had developed PCIS. After receiving full anti-ischemic drug treatment and aspirin at an anti-inflammatory dose, the patient was symptom-free during hospitalization. The pericardial effusion was gradually resolved along with the recovery of serum concentration of HsCRP and cTnT to the normal levels at 3 weeks after PPCI.

Discussion and conclusions

PICS has been used to describe early-onset pleuropericarditis after AMI and coronary catheterization. The former is also called Dressler syndrome, the onset of which usually occurs 3–4 weeks after AMI. A widely accepted hypothesis about this syndrome is that an autoimmune response against heart antigens leads to generalized pericardial inflammation and pericarditis [2]. In the era of PPCI, the incidence of Dressler syndrome and PCI-related PCIS has been decreasing. Although the pathogenesis remains generally uncertain, there has been some presumption that an autoimmune pathogenesis triggered by myocardial necrosis already exists before PPCI [3] and that iatrogenic trauma may be done to the pericardial and/or pleural mesothelial cells [4]. Here we report a rare case of PCIS with CMD following PPCI. Similar to the case reported by Jin-Seok Park in 2010 [5], the PCIS occurring in our case after PCI also had an atypical early onset, and the clinical features included pleuritic chest pain, low fever, pericardial and/or pleural effusions.

Furthermore, the present case seemed to suggest that the increase of inflammatory marker in AMI patients with PCIS had potential association with PCI-related CMD and the subsequent persistent focal myocardial injury. According to the evidences from animal models [6] and clinical study [7], cardiac neutrophil activation along with the release of proinflammatory cytokines will cause damage to the microvascular endothelial and pericardial/pleural mesothelial cells. And this may finally result in CMD and pleural pericarditis along with myocardial ischemia and reperfusion. In addition, Frohlich GM et al. [8] and Robbers LF et al. [9] have also demonstrated recently that inflammatory responses due to perfusion

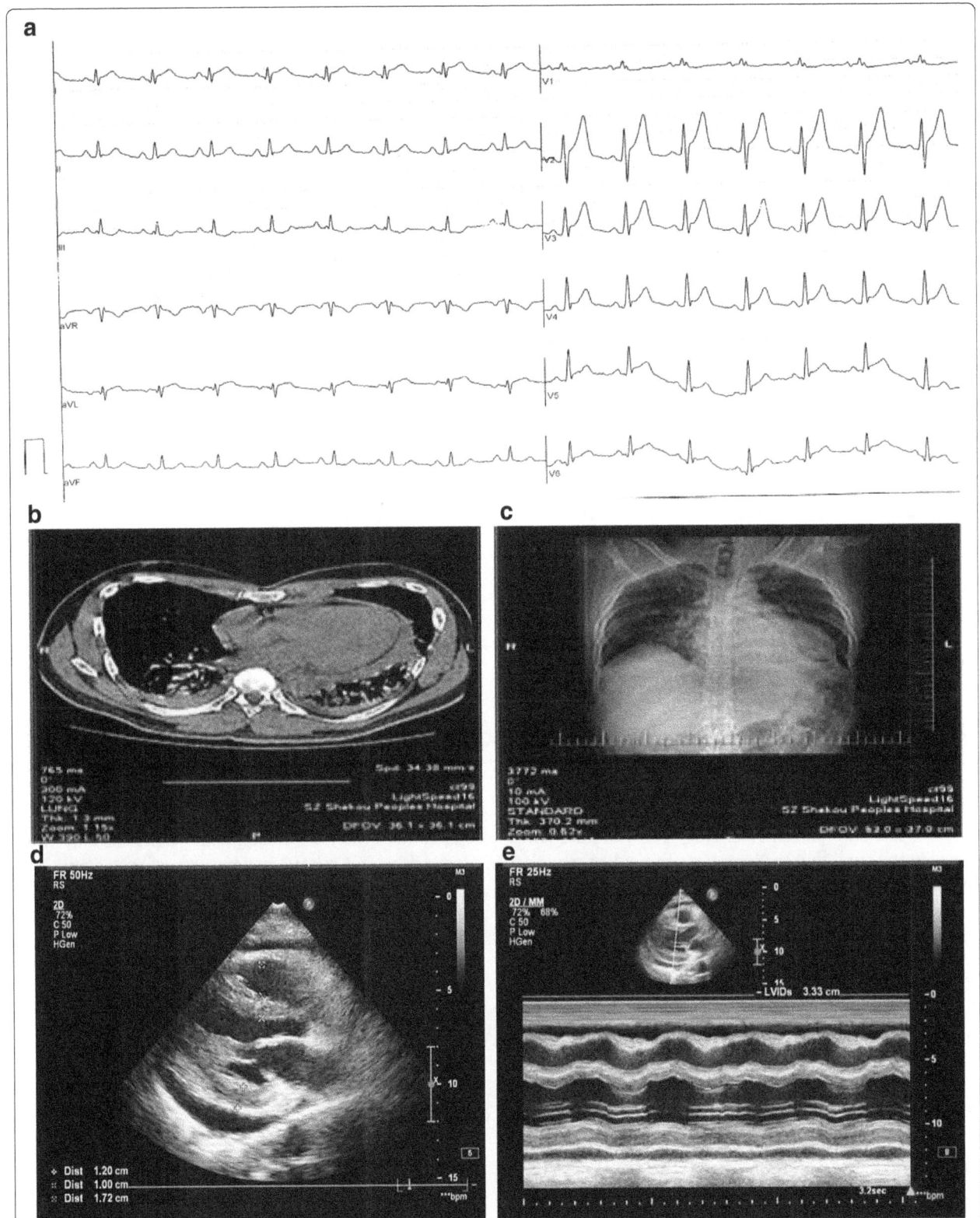

Fig. 2 a After 24 h of PCI, the twelve-lead ECG showed wide spread concave ST segment elevations. **b** and **c** Chest CT scan showed mild pleural effusion and interstitial infiltration in both lungs. **d** and **e** UCG revealed mild pericardial effusion with posterior wall motion disappearance

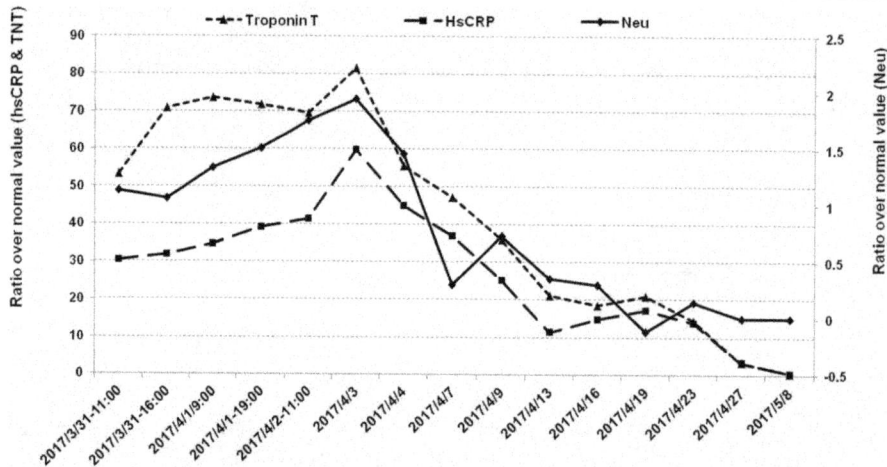

Fig. 3 Blood test showed Neutrophil count and the serum concentration of cTnT were elevated in parallel with HsCRP increase in the early and later stage of PCIS, respectively

injury stimulates the production of chemokines, cytokines, and adhesion molecules, which is probably associated with CMD and coronary microvascular obstruction. This further contributes to the development of myocardial no-reflow and myocardial hematoma. According to the report of Jin-Seok Park et al. [5], in a patient with PCIS after a successful PCI, there were some red blood cells present in the drained pericardial effusion. This suggested that the myocardial hematoma due to PCI-related CMD is likely to cause leakage of the blood into the pericardial space and thus plays an important role in the pathogenesis of PCIS.

The risk factors of microcirculatory dysfunction included smoking, obesity, hyperlipidemia, hyperuricemia, diabetes and chronic kidney disease (CKD) besides AMI. It has been found that the long-term present of stimulating signals which can induce endothelial injury may mediate the DNA methylation of chromosomes, leading to changes in chromosomal structure and function and enhancing the regulatory effect of stress signals on the signaling pathways related to endothelial injury [10]. Chromosome remodeling of endothelial cells may be caused by long-term smoking of this patient, who was thus susceptible to endothelial damage with a "metabolic memory effect". The above situation can enhance the I/R-related endothelial damage after PCI, resulting in severe impairment of coronary microcirculatory structure and coronary flow reserve/diastolic function. It has been reported by Matteo et al. [11] that CKD can promote microcirculatory dysfunction and lead to a decrease in diastolic dysfunction and cardiac reserve function impairment. Our patient showed a persistent increase of cTnT even after the infarct-related artery (IRA) was opened by PCI. This possibly resulted from myocardial focal necrosis caused by cigarette smoking-aggravated microcirculatory dysfunction and a decrease in myocardial blood flow perfusion.

Besides, in the present case, the level of inflammatory marker also matched up with the consistent elevation of cTnT, which was probably associated with the persistent focal myocardial injury due to CMD. This agrees with the recent studies reported by Vilahur G et al. [12], who showed that extensive necrosis of ischemic cardiomyocytes in hypoperfused myocardium might activate the innate immune response, triggering an increase of compensatory inflammation. At present,the correlation between perioperative PCIS and CMD in AMI needs to be further explored.

In conclusions, findings in the present case seemed to suggest that excessive inflammatory reaction and CMD triggered by PCI-related ischemia-reperfusion injury may be the potential reciprocal causation of PCIS. So we should pay more attention to the severe inflammatory reaction and CMD resulting from cardiac ischemia-reperfusion injury in an AMI patient with risk factors of endothelial dysfunction, although this condition poses a real challenge, especially in the PCIS-predisposed individuals.

Abbreviations
ANA: Antinuclear Antibody; ASO: Anti-Streptolysin O; BNP: Natriuretic peptide; CAG: Coronary angiography; CFR: Coronary flow reserve; CMD: Coronary microvascular dysfunction; ESR: Erythrocyte sedimentation rate; hs-CRP: Hypersensitive C-reactive protein; PCIS: Post-cardiac injury syndrome; PET: Positron emission tomography; p-LCX: Proximal of left circumflex artery; PPCI: Primary percutaneous coronary intervention; TIMI: Thrombolysis in myocardial infarction; TNT: Troponin T

Acknowledgements
Not applicable.

Funding
Not applicable.

Authors' contributions
GY analyzed and interpreted the patient data and wrote the manuscript. NHB reviewed the patient data and revised the manuscript. CHW participated discussion of patients data. LJT, HYL, HHX were responsible for patient treatment and nursing and data collection. All authors read and approved the final manuscript.

Competing interests
The authors declare that they have no competing interests.

Author details
[1]Department of Cardiovascular Medicine, Shenzhen Shekou People's Hospital, Shenzhen 518067, Guangdong, China. [2]Departments of Medicine, Molecular and Cellular Pharmacology and Pediatrics, University of Miami Miller School of Medicine, Miami, FL, USA. [3]Department of Interventional Diagnosis and Treatment, Shenzhen Longhua Central Hospital, Shenzhen 518067, Guangdong, China.

References
1. Jaworska-Wilczynska M, Abramczuk E, Hryniewiecki T. Postcardiac injury syndrome. Med Sci Monit. 2011;17:13–4.
2. Dressler W. The postmyocardial infarction syndrome. AMA Arch Int Med. 1959;103:28–42.
3. Setoyama T, Furukawa Y, Abe M, Nakagawa Y, Kita T, Kimura. Acute pleuropericarditis after coronary stenting: a case report. Circ J. 2006;70:358–61.
4. Imazio M, Brucato A, Rovere ME, Adler Y. Contemporary features, risk factors, and prognosis of the postpericardiotomy syndrome. Am J Cardiol. 2011;108:1183–7.
5. Park JS, Kim DH, Choi WG, Woo SI, Kwan J, Park KS, Lee WH, Lee JJ, Choi YJ. Postcardiac injury syndrome after percutaneous coronary intervention. Yonsei Med J. 2010;51:284–6.
6. Neumann FJ, Ott I, Gawaz M, Richardt G, Holzapfel H, Jochum M, Schömig A. Cardiac release of cytokines and inflammatory responses in acute myocardial infarction. Circulation. 1995;92:748–55.
7. Carbone F, Nencioni A, Mach F, Vuilleumier N, Montecucco F. Pathophysiological role of neutrophils in acute myocardial infarction. Thromb Haemost. 2013;110:501–14.
8. Frohlich GM, Meier P, White SK, Yellon DM, Hausenloy DJ. Myocardial reperfusion injury: looking beyond primary PCI. Eur Heart J. 2013;34:1714–22.
9. Robbers LF, Eerenberg ES, Teunissen PF, Jansen MF, Hollander MR, Horrevoets AJ, Knaapen P, Nijveldt R, Heymans MW, Levi MM, van Rossum AC, Niessen HW, Marcu CB, Beek AM, van Royen N. Magnetic resonance imaging-defined areas of microvascular obstruction after acute myocardial infarction represent microvascular destruction and haemorrhage. Eur Heart J. 2013;34:2346–53.
10. Roberts AC, Porter KE. Cellular and molecular mechanisms of endothelial dysfunction in diabetes. Diab Vasc Dis Res. 2013;10(6):472–82.
11. Tebaldi M, Biscaglia S, Fineschi M, Manari A, Menozzi M, Secco GG, Di Lorenzo E, D'Ascenzo F, Fabbian F, Tumscitz C, Ferrari R, Campo G, Vilahur G, Badimon L. Fractional flow reserve evaluation and chronic kidney disease: analysis from a multicenter Italian registry (the FREAK study). Catheter Cardiovasc Interv. 2016;88(4):555–62.
12. Vilahur G, Badimon L. Ischemia/reperfusion activates myocardial innate mmune response: the key role of the toll-like receptor. Front Physiol. 2014;5:496.

23

Association between admission anemia and long-term mortality in patients with acute myocardial infarction: results from the MONICA/KORA myocardial infarction registry

Miriam Giovanna Colombo[1,2*] (iD), Inge Kirchberger[1,2,3], Ute Amann[1,2,3], Margit Heier[1,2], Christian Thilo[4], Bernhard Kuch[4,5], Annette Peters[2] and Christa Meisinger[1,2,3]

Abstract

Background: Previous studies have shown that the presence of anemia is associated with increased short- and long-term outcomes in patients with acute myocardial infarction (AMI). This study aims at examining the impact of admission anemia on long-term, all-cause mortality following AMI in patients recruited from a population-based registry. Contrary to most prior studies, we distinguished between patients with mild and moderate to severe anemia.

Methods: This prospective study was conducted in 2011 patients consecutively hospitalized for AMI that occurred between January 2005 and December 2008. Patients who survived more than 28 days after AMI were followed up until December 2011. Hemoglobin (Hb) concentration was measured at hospital admission and classified according to the World Health Organization (WHO). Mild anemia was defined as Hb concentration of 11 to < 12 g/dL in women and 11 to < 13 g/dL in men; moderate to severe anemia as Hb concentration of < 11 g/dL. Adjusted Cox regression models were calculated to compare survival in patients with and without anemia.

Results: Mild anemia and moderate to severe anemia was found in 183 (9.1%) and 100 (5%) patients, respectively. All-cause mortality after a median follow-up time of 4.2 years was 11.9%. The Cox regression analysis showed significantly increased mortality risks in both patients with mild (HR 1.74, 95% CI 1.23–2.45) and moderate to severe anemia (HR 2.05, 95% CI 1.37–3.05) compared to patients without anemia.

Conclusion: This study shows that anemia adversely affects long-term survival following AMI. However, further studies are needed to confirm that anemia can solely explain worse long-term outcomes after AMI.

Keywords: Myocardial infarction, Anemia, Hemoglobin, Mortality

Background

Anemia found in patients with acute myocardial infarction (AMI) and measured at hospital admission has been identified as an independent predictor of adverse outcomes such as cardiac events, major bleeding as well as short- and long-term mortality [1–5]. Defined according to the World Health Organization (WHO), anemia is present in women and men if hemoglobin (Hb) concentration falls below 12 g/dL and 13 g/dL, respectively [6]. Compared with the prevalence in the general population (3.8%) [7], anemia is more frequently encountered in patients hospitalized for cardiac events [8, 9]. Ranging from 11% to 38% the presence of anemia varied widely across prior studies in patients with AMI [10, 11].

The majority of previous studies in patients with AMI focused on comparing those with and without anemia

* Correspondence: miriam.colombo@helmholtz-muenchen.de
[1]MONICA/KORA Myocardial Infarction Registry, Central Hospital of Augsburg, Augsburg, Germany
[2]Institute of Epidemiology, Helmholtz Zentrum München, German Research Center for Environmental Health (GmbH), Neuherberg, Germany
Full list of author information is available at the end of the article

neglecting severity of anemia. However, since it is a common condition found in hospitalized patients, severity of anemia might be important to consider [11]. In addition, results from long-term studies covering observation periods beyond 5 years are scarce. Therefore, the aim of this study was to examine the association between admission anemia and long-term, all-cause mortality in patients with AMI recruited from the MONICA/KORA myocardial infarction registry and to incorporate severity of anemia into the analysis.

Methods

The data for this study were derived from the Myocardial Infarction Registry that was established in Augsburg as part of the WHO project MONICA (Monitoring Trends and Determinants in Cardiovascular disease) in 1984. All coronary deaths and cases of non-fatal AMI occurring among the inhabitants of the city of Augsburg and the 2 adjacent counties (600,000 inhabitants) have been continuously registered since then. The population-based registry was included into the KORA (Cooperative Health Research in the Region of Augsburg) framework when the MONICA project ended in 1995.

Patients aged between 25 and 74 years, who were admitted to one out of 8 hospitals in the study area were included. Written informed consent had to be obtained before patients were included into the cohort. More detailed information on case identification, diagnostic classification of events and quality control of the data can be found in previous publications [12, 13]. Trained study nurses interviewed the participants during hospital stay using a standardized questionnaire. In order to confirm the information provided by the patients and to collect additional information, the patients' medical chart was reviewed. Both methods of data collection and questionnaires have been approved by the ethics committee of the Bavarian Medical Association (Bayerische Landesärztekammer) and the study was performed in accordance with the Declaration of Helsinki.

We conducted this prospective study in consecutive patients hospitalized for AMI between January 1, 2005 and December 31, 2008. Patients were followed up for all-cause mortality, the outcome of this study, until December 31, 2011. The vital status of study participants after hospital discharge was determined through population registries located in- and outside the study region. Patients were included in this study if they survived longer than 28 days after AMI had occurred. Those with missing information on both admission Hb concentration ($n = 68$) as well as relevant covariates ($n = 176$) were excluded. The final study population consisted of 2011 patients with AMI.

Presence of anemia was defined based on Hb concentration (g/dL) measured at hospital admission and patients were categorized according to WHO classification

of anemia [6]. Mild anemia was defined as Hb concentration of 11 to < 12 g/dL in women and 11 to < 13 g/dL in men. Moderate to severe anemia was present when Hb concentration was below 11 g/dL. Since only thirteen patients had severe anemia (Hb < 8 g/dL), no further subdivisions were made.

In order to examine whether an impaired renal function was present, we used the estimated glomerular filtration rate (eGFR) and applied the Modification of Diet in Renal Disease (MDRD) study equation (eGFR (ml/min/1.73 m^2) = 186.3 × (serum creatinine$^{-1.154}$) x (age$^{-0.203}$) × 0.742 (if female) × 1.212 (if black)) [14] to calculate it. Risk factors such as history of angina pectoris, prior myocardial infarction, hypertension, hyperlipidemia, diabetes mellitus, stroke as well as patients' smoking habits were covered during the interview conducted by the study nurses and confirmed by chart review (except for history of stroke and smoking habits). Body mass index (BMI; kg/m^2), systolic and diastolic blood pressure as well as heart rate and AMI classification (ST-segment elevation myocardial infarction (STEMI), non-ST-segment elevation myocardial infarction (NSTEMI) or bundle branch block) were derived from chart review only. Echocardiography, ventriculography and radionuclide ventriculography were used to determine whether patients had a reduced left ventricular ejection fraction (LVEF < 30%). Furthermore, medications administered at discharge were documented. The majority of patients received antiplatelet agents, angiotensin-converting enzyme inhibitors (ACEI) or angiotensin-receptor-blockers (ARB), beta-blockers and statins at discharge and therefore, we included these medications as one covariate (4 evidence-based medications (EBM); yes/no). In-hospital procedures such as percutaneous coronary intervention (PCI) and coronary artery bypass graft (CABG) were determined by chart review. Since in-hospital complications rarely occurred, a single covariate was generated including the occurrence of cardiac arrest, pulmonary edema, bradycardia, re-infarction, ventricular tachycardia, ventricular fibrillation or cardiogenic shock.

Possible differences in survival were tested using Kaplan-Meyer plots as well as log-rank tests. Hazard ratios (HR) for all-cause mortality according to anemia status were calculated using Cox regression models. Three different models were calculated: 1) an unadjusted model, 2) a model adjusted for age and sex, and 3) a model adjusted for age, sex, previous MI, angina pectoris, hyperlipidemia, diabetes, stroke, eGFR, heart rate, AMI type, LVEF, discharge medications, PCI and in-hospital complications. Covariates made it into the latter model if the corresponding log-rank-test was statistically significant ($p < 0.05$) and if they proved to make a statistically significant contribution to predicting all-cause mortality in a model together with anemia status. We graphically tested whether the assumption of proportional hazards (parallel lines of log (–log (event)) versus log of event times) was valid for each covariate. Time-dependent interaction terms were included if the assumption was rejected. The covariates age and sex were included into each model independent of statistical significance. Due to frequently missing data, LVEF was entered into the regression model as a dummy coded variable (LVEF < 30%; yes/no/missing). The variance inflation factor (VIF) was used to detect multicollinearity among covariates [15]. Furthermore, we calculated adjusted Cox regression models for increasing observation periods ranging from one to 6 years.

As a sensitivity analysis, we calculated a Cox regression model including all patients who were originally excluded from our study population due to missing information on any covariate ($n = 176$). We adjusted this model for sex and age. Patients without anemia served as the reference category for all analyses. P-values of < 0.05 were considered statistically significant. The analyses were performed using statistical software package SAS version 9.2 (SAS Institute Inc., Cary, NC).

Results

In total, 283 AMI patients (14.1%) were considered anemic based on admission Hb concentration. Of those patients, 183 (64.7%) were mildly anemic, whereas 100 (35.3%) had moderate to severe anemia. Male patients accounted for 75.6% of the total study population and the mean age was 60.9 ± 9.6 years. Further patient characteristics are summarized in Table 1.

Patients without anemia differed from the group with anemia concerning a majority of patient characteristics: they were significantly younger, had a higher BMI and were more likely to smoke (see Table 1). In terms of known comorbidities and other risk factors, the non-anemia group was overall healthier. They were less likely to have diabetes and to have suffered from prior myocardial infarction, angina pectoris and stroke. Additionally, they had a significantly higher eGFR on admission. Patients with anemia were less likely to receive antiplatelet agents, ACEIs/ARBs and statins, but more often received diuretics and insulin at hospital discharge. Patients with anemia more often had a LVEF < 30% and information on LVEF was more frequently missing than in patients without anemia.

During a median follow-up time of 4.2 years (IQR 3.1–5.4), 241 (12.0%) patients with AMI died. Patients with anemia had a significantly higher long-term mortality ($n = 85$, 30.0%) compared to patients without anemia ($n = 156$, 9.0%). A higher percentage of patients died in the group with moderate to severe anemia ($n = 37$, 37.0%) than in the group with mild anemia ($n = 48$, 26.2%). Kaplan-Meier plots showing survival curves stratified by anemia status and the corresponding log-rank p-value are provided in Fig. 1. Patients who died during follow-up were significantly older, had a lower eGFR and were more likely to have an impaired LVEF compared to those without an event during follow-up

(data not shown). Furthermore, they received four EBM at discharge significantly less often (data not shown).

Results of the Cox regression analyses are shown in Table 2.

In the unadjusted model, patients with mild anemia and patients with moderate to severe anemia had significantly increased mortality risks compared to the non-anemia group by factor of 3.35 and 5.22, respectively. With increasing adjustment, HRs decreased but still remained statistically significant. Interaction terms were each included in a regression model together with anemia status due to a rejected proportionality assumption for sex, age, BMI, smoking habits, history of angina pectoris, history of diabetes, AMI type, LVEF, eGFR and heart rate. None of the interaction terms made a statistically significant contribution to the models. Despite the adjustment, patients with moderate to severe anemia still had a 2 times higher mortality risk (HR 2.05, 95% CI 1.37–3.05) compared to the reference group. In patients with mild anemia, the risk of dying was increased by 74% in the final model (HR 1.74, 95% CI 1.23–2.45). Possible multicollinearity among covariates was rejected since the VIF did not exceed the threshold value of 2.5.

Cox regression models for increasing observation periods showed decreasing HRs in both groups with anemia (see Additional file 1: Figure S1). After 1 year, both anemia groups had a 2.4-times increased risk of dying. The risk decreased to HRs of 1.7 and 2.1 in patients with mild anemia and moderate to severe anemia 6 years after AMI, respectively. Estimates drifted apart starting at 3 years of observation period.

The sensitivity analysis showed increased HRs in patients with moderate to severe anemia (HR 4.19 vs. 3.94) and attenuated HRs in patients with mild anemia (HR 2.46 vs. 2.71) compared to the results from our actual study population (see Additional file 2: Table S1). The estimates remained statistically significant.

Discussion

In the present analysis, we demonstrated that anemia on admission both the mild and moderate to severe type was associated with higher long-term all-cause mortality in patients hospitalized for AMI. HRs attenuated after multivariate adjustment, but a considerable and statistically significant difference in mortality risk persisted. Similar risks for patients in both anemia groups were found 1 year after AMI before they decreased and drifted apart with increasing observation periods.

In patients with coronary artery disease, the prevalence of anemia on admission varied widely across previous studies and ranged from 11% [10] to up to 38% [11]. Compared to most previous studies, the prevalence of anemia in our population (14.1%) was low [1, 8, 10, 11, 16–21]. Those studies focused either only on patients with STEMI or

Table 1 Baseline characteristics and long-term mortality of patients with AMI by anemia status ($n = 2011$)

	Anemia[a] ($n = 283$)			Non-anemia[d] ($n = 1728$)	p Value
	Total	Mild anemia[b] ($n = 183$)	Moderate to severe anemia[c] ($n = 100$)		
Socio-demographic characteristics					
Age (years)	64.8 ± 8.5	64.5 ± 8.5	65.4 ± 8.4	60.1 ± 9.6	< 0.0001
Female	70 (24.7)	43 (23.5)	27 (27.0)	440 (25.5)	0.7838
Living alone, ($n = 1939$)	54 (20.7)	35 (20.2)	19 (21.6)	291 (17.34)	0.4057
Risk factors and medical history					
BMI (kg/m^2), ($n = 1934$)	27.2 ± 4.8	27.4 ± 4.8	26.8 ± 4.9	28.0 ± 4.5	0.0272
Smoking status, ($n = 1886$)					< 0.0001
Smoker	55 (22.7)	36 (22.5)	19 (23.2)	661 (40.2)	
Ex-smoker	102 (41.2)	70 (43.8)	32 (39.0)	515 (31.3)	
Never smoker	85 (35.1)	54 (33.8)	31 (37.8)	468 (28.5)	
Prior myocardial infarction	41 (14.5)	24 (13.2)	17 (17.0)	165 (9.6)	0.0228
Angina pectoris	71 (25.1)	51 (27.9)	20 (20.0)	282 (16.3)	0.0004
Hypertension	230 (81.3)	142 (77.6)	88 (88.0)	1367 (79.1)	0.0830
Hyperlipidemia	164 (58.0)	107 (58.5)	57 (57.0)	1118 (64.7)	0.0884
Diabetes	123 (43.5)	68 (37.2)	55 (55.0)	488 (28.2)	< 0.0001
Stroke	38 (13.4)	21 (11.5)	17 (17.0)	85 (4.9)	< 0.0001
Laboratory markers					
Hemoglobin (g/dL)	11.2 ± 1.6	12.1 ± 0.6	9.5 ± 1.3	14.8 ± 1.3	< 0.0001
eGFR (ml/min/1.73m^2)	63.9 (43.4–85.5)	65.9 (47.4–83.4)	60.3 (35.9–88.4)	78.3 (64.4–92.3)	< 0.0001
eGFR < 60 ml/min/1.73m^2	122 (43.1)	73 (39.9)	49 (49.0)	329 (19.0)	< 0.0001
Clinical characteristics					
Systolic blood pressure (mmHg)	120 ± 17	120 ± 16	121 ± 19	118 ± 15	0.0746
Diastolic blood pressure (mmHg)	68 ± 10	68 ± 10	67 ± 11	69 ± 10	0.1236
Heart rate (bpm)	73 ± 11	73 ± 11	73 ± 10	71 ± 10	0.0004
AMI type					< 0.0001
STEMI	63 (22.3)	46 (25.14)	17 (17.0)	616 (35.6)	
NSTEMI	194 (68.6)	120 (65.6)	74 (74.0)	1019 (59.0)	
Bundle branch block	26 (9.2)	17 (9.3)	9 (9.0)	93 (5.4)	
LVEF ($n = 1188$)					0.0021
LVEF < 30%	4 (2.9)	3 (1.6)	1 (1.0)	38 (2.2)	
LVEF ≥30%	132 (46.6)	87 (47.5)	45 (45.0)	1014 (58.7)	
Missing	147 (51.9)	93 (50.8)	54 (54.0)	676 (39.1)	
Medication at discharge					
Antiplatelet agents	263 (92.9)	172 (94.0)	91 (91.0)	1686 (97.6)	< 0.0001
ACEIs/ARBs	225 (79.5)	149 (81.4)	76 (76.0)	1493 (86.4)	0.0045
Beta-blocker	271 (95.8)	175 (95.6)	96 (96.0)	1728 (96.1)	0.9595
Statins	239 (84.5)	161 (88.0)	78 (78.0)	1636 (94.7)	< 0.0001
4 EBM	178 (62.9)	125 (68.3)	53 (53.0)	1358 (78.6)	< 0.0001
Calcium channel blocker	49 (17.3)	33 (18.0)	16 (16.0)	216 (12.5)	0.0758
Diuretics	184 (65.0)	115 (62.8)	69 (69.0)	877 (50.8)	< 0.0001
Insulin	57 (20.1)	30 (16.4)	27 (27.0)	147 (8.5)	< 0.0001
Other antidiabetic agents	51 (18.0)	31 (16.9)	20 (20.0)	225 (13.0)	0.0594

Table 1 Baseline characteristics and long-term mortality of patients with AMI by anemia status ($n = 2011$) *(Continued)*

	Anemia[a] ($n = 283$)			Non-anemia[d] ($n = 1728$)	p Value
	Total	Mild anemia[b] ($n = 183$)	Moderate to severe anemia[c] ($n = 100$)		
In-hospital treatment					
PCI	139 (49.1)	102 (55.7)	37 (37.0)	1335 (77.3)	< 0.0001
CABG	66 (23.3)	39 (21.3)	27 (27.0)	235 (13.6)	< 0.0001
Any in-hospital complication[e]	51 (18.0)	31 (16.9)	20 (20.0)	229 (13.3)	0.0773
Outcome					
All-cause mortality	85 (30.0)	48 (26.2)	37 (37.0)	156 (9.0)	< 0.0001

AMI acute myocardial infarction, *ACEI* angiotensin-converting enzyme inhibitor, *ARB* angiotensin-receptor blocker, *BMI* body mass index, *CABG* coronary artery bypass graft, *EBM* evidence-based medications (antiplatelet agents, ACEIs/ARBs, beta-blockers, statins), *eGFR* estimated glomerular filtration rate, *LVEF* left ventricular ejection fraction, *PCI* percutaneous coronary intervention

Data are presented as n (%), mean ± standard deviation or median (interquartile range (25%-quartile – 75%-quartile))

[a] Anemia: Hemoglobin (Hb) concentration of < 12 g/dL in women, Hb concentration of < 13 g/dL in men

[b] Mild anemia: Hb concentration of 11 g/dL to < 12 g/dL in women, Hb concentration of 11 g/dL to < 13 g/dL in men

[c] Moderate to severe anemia: Hb concentration of < 11 g/dL in men and women

[d] Non-anemia: Hb concentration of ≥12 g/dL in women, Hb concentration of ≥13 g/dL in men

[e] Any in-hospital complication includes at least one of the following: cardiac arrest, pulmonary edema, bradycardia, re-infarction, ventricular tachycardia, ventricular fibrillation, cardiogenic shock

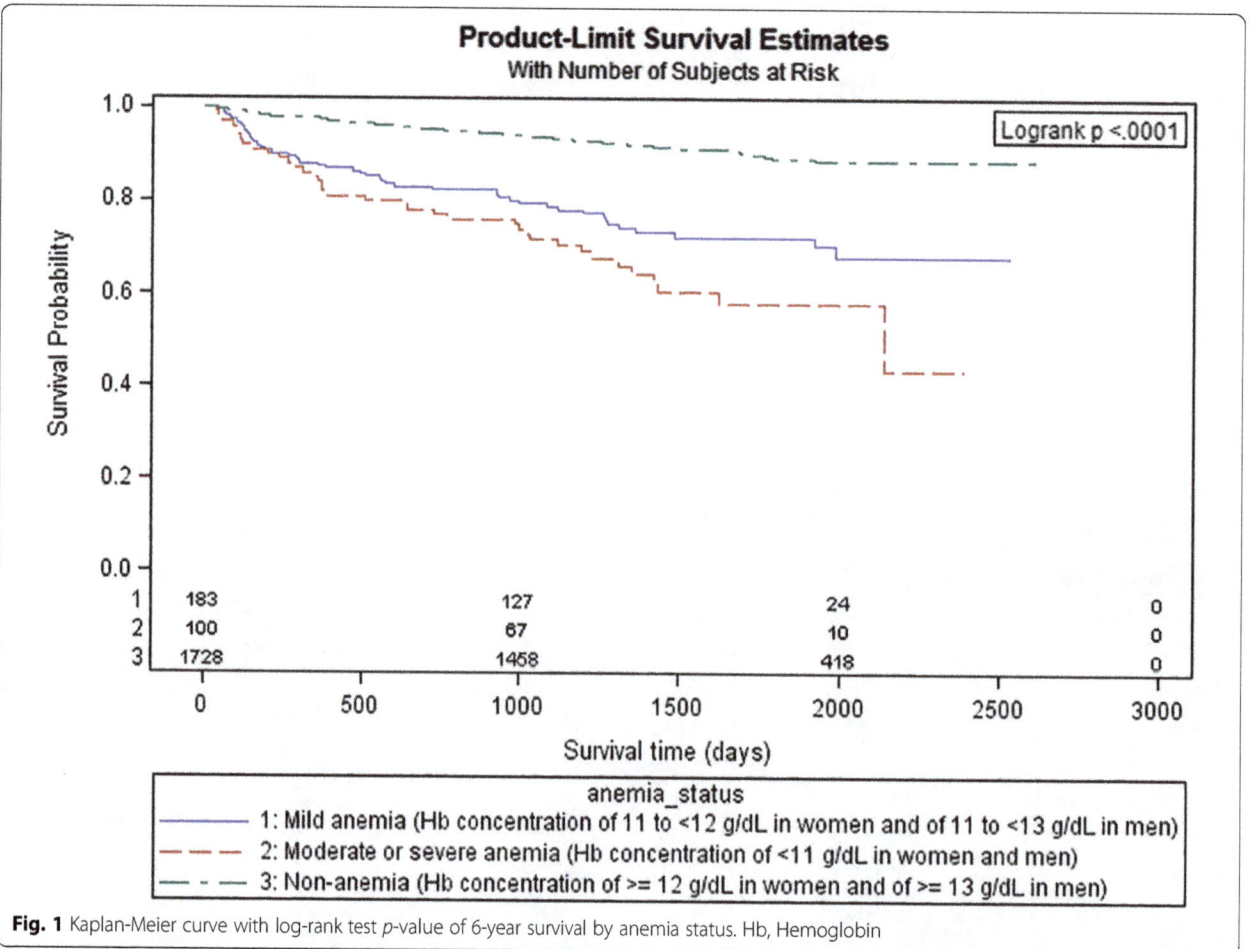

Fig. 1 Kaplan-Meier curve with log-rank test *p*-value of 6-year survival by anemia status. Hb, Hemoglobin

Table 2 Cox regression models for long-term mortality following AMI by anemia status ($n = 2011$)

	Anemia[a] ($n = 283$)								Non-anemia[d] ($n = 1728$)
	Total			Mild anemia[b] ($n = 183$)			Moderate to severe anemia[c] ($n = 100$)		
	HR [95% CI]	p Value		HR [95% CI]	p Value		HR [95% CI]	p Value	HR [95% CI]
Unadjusted model	3.99 [3.07–5.20]	< 0.0001		3.35 [2.45–4.68]	<.00001		5.22 [3.64–7.48]	< 0.0001	Ref.
Model 1[e]	3.13 [2.39–4.11]	< 0.0001		2.71 [1.95–3.77]	< 0.0001		3.94 [3.73–5.68]	< 0.0001	Ref.
Model 2[f]	1.85 [1.37–2.49]	< 0.0001		1.74 [1.23–2.45]	0.0017		2.05 [1.37–3.05]	0.0004	Ref.

AMI acute myocardial infarction, *CI* confidence interval, *HR* hazard ratio, *Ref* reference category

[a] Anemia: Hemoglobin (Hb) concentration of < 12 g/dL in women, Hb concentration of < 13 g/dL in men

[b] Mild anemia: Hb concentration of 11 g/dL to < 12 g/dL in women, Hb concentration of 11 g/dL to < 13 g/dL in men

[c] Moderate to severe anemia: Hb concentration of < 11 g/dL in men and women

[d] Non-anemia: Hb concentration of ≥12 g/dL in women, Hb concentration of ≥13 g/dL in men

[e] Model 1: Adjusted for age and sex

[f] Model 2: Model 1 + previous myocardial infarction, angina pectoris, hyperlipidemia, diabetes, stroke, eGFR, heart rate, AMI type (STEMI, NSTEMI, Bundle branch block), left-ventricular ejection fraction (LVEF) < 30%, medications at discharge (evidence-based medications (antiplatelet agents, angiotensin-converting-enzyme inhibitor (ACEI), angiotensin-receptor blocker (ARB), beta-blocker, statins), calcium channel blockers, diuretics), percutaneous coronary intervention (PCI) and any in-hospital complication

included all patients with acute coronary syndrome (ACS), which might explain the disparities. A higher prevalence of anemia was found in previous studies in patients with AMI [1, 5, 11]. This could derive from the fact that we excluded patients who survived for 28 days or less, which reduced the prevalence of anemia in our study population.

In line, studies with observation periods of at least 1 year found significant associations between admission anemia and long-term mortality [1, 16, 18, 22–24]. Anemia predicted 1-year survival in ACS patients [18] and 2-year survival or AMI in men with ACS [22]. In patients with STEMI, anemia was significantly associated with an increased cardiovascular mortality risk after 21 months [23], major cardiovascular events (MACE) after 5-years [16] and all-cause mortality after 6-years of follow-up [24]. Ducrocq et al. examined 3541 patients with AMI and found a 5-year mortality risk increased by 40% in patients with anemia (HR 1.4, 95% CI 1.2–1.6) [1]. In comparison, the mortality risk found in patients with anemia from our study population was increased by 80%. Among other known risk factors, Ducrocq et al. adjusted their regression analysis for in-hospital bleeding and transfusion [1]. Studies have shown that patients with anemia are more susceptible to experience major bleeding after cardiac events and revascularization [3, 25], which might also affect their long-term mortality risk [1, 25]. Apart from advising to use certain antiplatelet agents with care to avoid bleeding in patients with anemia after AMI [26], current clinical practice guidelines do not provide specific recommendations for the management of anemia in those patients [27]. In terms of AMI treatment using PCI, a study showed that radial instead of femoral access might reduce the risk of bleeding in patients with AMI [28]. Due to the lower risk of bleeding, the radial access might also be preferable when performing PCI in patients with anemia. Furthermore, assuming that patients with anemia are more likely to receive blood transfusion than patients

without anemia, an increased risk of "transfusion-associated mortality" [29] might exist. Clinical practice guidelines regarding blood transfusion recommend a Hb threshold of 7–8 g/dL in hospitalized patients [30]. However, transfusion should be taken into consideration in patients with acute coronary syndrome and a Hb concentration of 8–10 g/dL [30]. Data on both in-hospital bleeding and transfusion were not collected in the framework of the registry and, therefore, the possibility exists that we overestimated the mortality risk in patients with anemia. Given the prognostic importance, future studies should include data on bleeding as well as blood transfusions and a Hb threshold for blood transfusion in patients with AMI should be determined.

Furthermore, we subdivided patients with anemia and found increased mortality risks already in patients with mildly reduced Hb concentration. This could have been concealed in previous studies only distinguishing between patients with anemia and those without. Younge et al. examined patients with ACS (defined as STEMI or NSTEMI) who were followed up for over 20 years and found significantly increased mortality risks in those with moderate (HR 1.13) and severe anemia (HR 1.39), but not in those with mild anemia [11]. In their study, patients with anemia were subdivided by tertiles, which deviated from the WHO classification. The cut-off points, especially those for men with mild anemia (12.2–13.0 g/dL vs. 11–13 g/dL in our study) might be responsible for different survival estimates found in their study [11]. Nonetheless, both our and their results stress the need to account for severity of anemia in future studies. Furthermore, our analysis of increasing observation periods showed that severity of anemia might not be important in the first 2 years after AMI but might become more relevant in subsequent years.

Inconsistent with our results, a study in patients with STEMI treated with primary PCI did not confirm an association after 3 years of follow-up [19]. Besides it being a single center study, differences in study population could explain the inconsistency with our results. Furthermore, the authors argue that not anemia itself might negatively impact long-term survival, but rather other comorbidities could explain the worse prognosis [19]. In our study and most previous studies [1, 10, 11, 23], patients with anemia were more likely to be older, were affected by more comorbidities, had an impaired eGFR as well as a lower LVEF. Even though important comorbidities were included in our analysis, data on other measures of overall health status were not available. Additionally, patients with anemia differed from those without anemia regarding in-hospital treatment. They were less often treated with PCI, but more frequently with CABG, which might be an indicator of more advanced coronary artery disease. In line, previous studies demonstrated that anemic patients were less often treated with PCI [18, 21] and experienced worse outcomes after PCI, e.g. increased risks for stent thrombosis, long-term mortality, MACE and bleeding [3, 4, 23, 31]. Furthermore, patients with anemia were less likely to receive 4 EBM at hospital discharge, which is considered the standard of care in patients after AMI and has been shown to significantly reduce long-term mortality [32]. Out of the 4 EBM, both patients with mild and moderate to severe anemia were less likely to receive antiplatelet agents, ACEIs/ARBs and statins compared to patients without anemia. In line, a study in STEMI patients showed that those with anemia were less frequently treated according to guidelines in terms of pharmacological treatment compared to those without anemia [20]. However, less often receiving 4 EBM could also be a consequence of other pre-existing diseases apart from anemia such as impaired renal function [33].

Multiple factors might influence long-term mortality after AMI in patients with anemia. When anemia is present, the amount of oxygen delivered to the heart during AMI is further decreased, myocardial tissue oxygenation is likely to be insufficient and cardiac output is increased [31, 34]. Possibly entailing an impaired recovery after AMI [16], anemia might affect mortality, but cannot solely explain the significantly worse long-term outcomes in patients with AMI. Even though both mild and moderate to severe anemia did predict an increased risk for long-term mortality independent of a number of confounders in our study population, treatment strategies that aim at increasing Hb concentration in patients with AMI and anemia might not significantly benefit long-term survival. In line, a recent randomized controlled trial demonstrated that administering erythropoietin after PCI, a hypoxia-induced hormone that also regulates Hb concentration, did not have beneficial effects on long-term outcomes [35].

Our study is characterized by several strengths. Data was collected in the framework of a population-based registry and patients with AMI were consecutively enrolled. Important risk factors such as comorbidities, in-hospital treatment and complications, relevant laboratory values as well as medications received at hospital discharge were included in our analysis. A longer follow-up than most previous studies and the analysis of increasing observation periods add valuable information to existing research.

This study has limitations. First, even though several risk factors potentially affecting survival after AMI were included, data on cancer, gastro-intestinal or other chronic diseases was not collected. Second, we had no information on the etiology of anemia and how it was treated (e.g. using iron therapy). Knowing the cause of abnormal Hb concentrations would considerably contribute to the understanding of the association between anemia and long-term mortality. Third, any other events occurring after hospital-discharge apart from all-cause mortality and possibly affecting survival could not be monitored. Fourth, a reduced LVEF is a marker for heart failure and data on LVEF was not available in all patients in our study population. Since we included those patients with missing values for left-ventricular ejection fraction we cannot rule out potential bias. Finally, due to the methodological limitations of an observational study, a causal relationship between admission anemia and long-term mortality cannot be established with absolute certainty and the possibility of reverse causation exists.

Conclusion

Both mild and moderate to severe anemia were associated with significantly increased long-term, all-cause mortality risks in our study population and low admission Hb concentration needs to be considered as a risk factor in patients with AMI. However, even though our results confirm what most other studies have found in patients with AMI before, it remains unclear if anemia alone can predict long-term mortality after AMI or if it is merely a proxy for worse overall health. Future studies need to take severity of anemia, bleeding events and blood transfusion as well as overall health status into account.

Additional files

Additional file 1: Figure S1. Hazard ratios for long-term mortality in patients with AMI and anemia covering increasing observation periods. Reference: Non-anemia: Hemoglobin (Hb) concentration of ≥12 g/dL in women, Hb concentration of ≥13 g/dL in men. Mild anemia: Hb concentration of 11 g/dL to < 12 g/dL in women, Hb concentration of 11 g/dL to < 13 g/dL in men. Moderate to severe anemia: Moderate to severe anemia: Hb concentration of < 11 g/dL in women and men. 95% Confidence intervals (CI) are represented by vertical lines above and below the HR estimates; 95% CI for mild anemia: dashed line; 95% CI for moderate to severe anemia: continuous line. AMI, Acute myocardial infarction; CI, Confidence interval; Hb, Hemoglobin; HR, Hazard ratio. (PDF 49 kb)

Additional file 2: Table S1. Results of the sensitivity analysis (n = 2187). (DOCX 16 kb)

Abbreviations

ACEI: Angiotensin-converting enzyme inhibitor; ACS: Acute coronary disease; AMI: Acute myocardial infarction; ARB: Angiotensin-receptor blockers; BMI: Body mass index; CABG: Coronary artery bypass graft; EBM: Evidence-based medication; eGFR: Estimated glomerular filtration rate; Hb: Hemoglobin; HR: Hazard ratio; IQR: Interquartile range; KORA: Cooperative Health Research in the Region of Augsburg; LVEF: Left ventricular ejection fraction; MACE: Major cardiovascular event; MDRD: Modification of Diet in Renal Disease; MI: Myocardial infarction; MONICA: Monitoring Trends and Determinants in Cardiovascular disease; NSTEMI: Non-ST-segment elevation myocardial infarction; PCI: Percutaneous coronary intervention; SD: Standard deviation; SPC: Serum potassium concentration; STEMI: ST-elevation myocardial infarction; VIF: Variance inflation factor; WHO: World Health Organization

Acknowledgements

We thank all members of the Helmholtz Zentrum München, Institute of Epidemiology and the field staff in Augsburg who were involved in the planning and conduct of the study. We wish to thank the local health departments, the office-based physicians and the clinicians of the hospitals within the study area for their support. Finally, we express our appreciation to all study participants.

Funding

The KORA research platform and the MONICA Augsburg studies were initiated and financed by the Helmholtz Zentrum München, German Research Center for Environmental Health, which is funded by the German Federal Ministry of Education, Science, Research and Technology and by the State of Bavaria. Since the year 2000, the collection of MI data has been co-financed by the German Federal Ministry of Health to provide population-based MI morbidity data for the official German Health Report (see www.gbe-bund.de). Steering partners of the MONICA/KORA Infarction Registry, Augsburg, include the KORA research platform, Helmholtz Zentrum München and the Department of Internal Medicine I, Cardiology, Central Hospital of Augsburg.

Authors' contributions

MGC, IK and CM conceived the study. MGC performed the statistical analyses and drafted the manuscript. CM, UA, MH, BK, CT and AP contributed to the interpretation of data. CM, MH, BK and CT contributed to data acquisition. IK, UA, MH, CT, BK, AP and CM read, critically revised and approved the final manuscript.

Competing interests

The authors declare that they have no competing interests.

Author details

[1]MONICA/KORA Myocardial Infarction Registry, Central Hospital of Augsburg, Augsburg, Germany. [2]Institute of Epidemiology, Helmholtz Zentrum München, German Research Center for Environmental Health (GmbH), Neuherberg, Germany. [3]Chair of Epidemiology, Ludwig-Maximilians-Universität München, UNIKA-T, Augsburg, Germany. [4]Department of Internal Medicine I – Cardiology, Central Hospital of Augsburg, Augsburg, Germany. [5]Department of Internal Medicine/ Cardiology, Hospital of Nördlingen, Nördlingen, Germany.

References

1. Ducrocq G, Puymirat E, Steg PG, Henry P, Martelet M, Karam C, Schiele F, Simon T, Danchin N. Blood transfusion, bleeding, anemia, and survival in patients with acute myocardial infarction: FAST-MI registry. Am Heart J. 2015;170(4):726–34. e722
2. Leibundgut G, Gick M, Morel O, Ferenc M, Werner KD, Comberg T, Kienzle RP, Buettner HJ, Neumann FJ. Discordant cardiac biomarker levels independently predict outcome in ST-segment elevation myocardial infarction. Clin Res Cardiol. 2016;105(5):432–40.
3. Wang X, Qiu M, Qi J, Li J, Wang H, Li Y, Han Y. Impact of anemia on long-term ischemic events and bleeding events in patients undergoing percutaneous coronary intervention: a system review and meta-analysis. J Thorac Dis. 2015;7(11):2041–52.
4. Nikolsky E, Mehran R, Aymong ED, Mintz GS, Lansky AJ, Lasic Z, Negoita M, Fahy M, Pocock SJ, Na Y, et al. Impact of anemia on outcomes of patients undergoing percutaneous coronary interventions. Am J Cardiol. 2004;94(8):1023–7.
5. Aronson D, Suleiman M, Agmon Y, Suleiman A, Blich M, Kapeliovich M, Beyar R, Markiewicz W, Hammerman H. Changes in haemoglobin levels during hospital course and long-term outcome after acute myocardial infarction. Eur Heart J. 2007;28(11):1289–96.
6. Haemoglobin concentrations for the diagnosis of anaemia and assessment of severity. Vitamin and Mineral Nutrition Information System [http://www.who.int/vmnis/indicators/haemoglobin.pdf].
7. Martinsson A, Andersson C, Andell P, Koul S, Engstrom G, Smith JG. Anemia in the general population: prevalence, clinical correlates and prognostic impact. Eur J Epidemiol. 2014;29(7):489–98.
8. Ang DS, Kao MP, Noman A, Lang CC, Struthers AD. The prognostic significance of early and late anaemia in acute coronary syndrome. QJM. 2012;105(5):445–54.
9. Jonsson A, Hallberg AC, Edner M, Lund LH, Dahlstrom U. A comprehensive assessment of the association between anemia, clinical covariates and outcomes in a population-wide heart failure registry. Int J Cardiol. 2016;211:124–31.
10. Bolinska S, Sobkowicz B, Zaniewska J, Chlebinska I, Bolinski J, Milewski R, Tycinska A, Musial W. The significance of anaemia in patients with acute ST-elevation myocardial infarction undergoing primary percutaneous coronary intervention. Kardiol Pol. 2011;69(1):33–9.
11. Younge JO, Nauta ST, Akkerhuis KM, Deckers JW, van Domburg RT. Effect of anemia on short- and long-term outcome in patients hospitalized for acute coronary syndromes. Am J Cardiol. 2012;109(4):506–10.
12. Meisinger C, Hormann A, Heier M, Kuch B, Lowel H. Admission blood glucose and adverse outcomes in non-diabetic patients with myocardial infarction in the reperfusion era. Int J Cardiol. 2006;113(2):229–35.
13. Kuch B, Heier M, von Scheidt W, Kling B, Hoermann A, Meisinger C. 20-year trends in clinical characteristics, therapy and short-term prognosis in acute myocardial infarction according to presenting electrocardiogram: the MONICA/KORA AMI registry (1985-2004). J Intern Med. 2008;264(3):254–64.
14. Levey AS, Bosch JP, Lewis JB, Greene T, Rogers N, Roth D. A more accurate method to estimate glomerular filtration rate from serum creatinine: a new prediction equation. Modification of diet in renal disease study group. Ann Intern Med. 1999;130(6):461–70.
15. When can you safely ignore multicollinearity? [http://statisticalhorizons.com/multicollinearity].
16. Uchida Y, Ichimiya S, Ishii H, Kanashiro M, Watanabe J, Hayano S, Suzuki S, Takeshita K, Sakai S, Amano T, et al. Impact of admission anemia on coronary microcirculation and clinical outcomes in patients with ST-segment elevation myocardial infarction undergoing primary percutaneous coronary intervention. Int Heart J. 2015;56(4):381–8.
17. Barbarova I, Klempfner R, Rapoport A, Wasserstrum Y, Goren I, Kats A, Segal G. Avoidance of blood transfusion to patients suffering from myocardial injury and severe anemia is associated with increased long-term mortality: a retrospective cohort analysis. Medicine (Baltimore). 2015;94(38):e1635.
18. Kunadian V, Mehran R, Lincoff AM, Feit F, Manoukian SV, Hamon M, Cox DA, Dangas GD, Stone GW. Effect of anemia on frequency of short- and long-term clinical events in acute coronary syndromes (from the acute catheterization and urgent intervention triage strategy trial). Am J Cardiol. 2014;114(12):1823–9.
19. Rathod KS, Jones DA, Rathod VS, Bromage D, Guttmann O, Gallagher SM, Mohiddin S, Rothman MT, Knight C, Jain AK, et al. Prognostic impact of anaemia on patients with ST-elevation myocardial infarction treated by primary PCI. Coron Artery Dis. 2014;25(1):52–9.
20. Riley RF, Newby LK, Don CW, Alexander KP, Peterson ED, Peng SA, Gandhi SK, Kutcher MA, Amsterdam EA, Herrington DM. Guidelines-based treatment of anaemic STEMI patients: practice patterns and effects on in-hospital mortality: a retrospective analysis from the NCDR. Eur Heart J Acute Cardiovasc Care. 2013;2(1):35–43.
21. Sulaiman K, Prashanth P, Al-Zakwani I, Al-Mahmeed W, Al-Motarreb A, Al Suwaidi J, Amin H, Asaad N, Hersi A, Al Faleh H, et al. Impact of anemia on in-hospital, one-month and one-year mortality in patients with acute coronary syndrome from the Middle East. Clin Med Res. 2012;10(2):65–71.

22. Cavusoglu E, Chopra V, Gupta A, Clark LT, Eng C, Marmur JD. Usefulness of anemia in men as an independent predictor of two-year cardiovascular outcome in patients presenting with acute coronary syndrome. Am J Cardiol. 2006;98(5):580–4.

23. Ayhan E, Aycicek F, Uyarel H, Ergelen M, Cicek G, Gul M, Osmonov D, Yildirim E, Bozbay M, Ugur M, et al. Patients with anemia on admission who have undergone primary angioplasty for ST elevation myocardial infarction: in-hospital and long-term clinical outcomes. Coron Artery Dis. 2011;22(6):375–9.

24. Tomaszuk-Kazberuk A, Bolinska S, Mlodawska E, Lopatowska P, Sobkowicz B, Musial W. Does admission anaemia still predict mortality six years after myocardial infarction? Kardiol Pol. 2014;72(6):488–93.

25. Tsujita K, Nikolsky E, Lansky AJ, Dangas G, Fahy M, Brodie BR, Dudek D, Mockel M, Ochala A, Mehran R, et al. Impact of anemia on clinical outcomes of patients with ST-segment elevation myocardial infarction in relation to gender and adjunctive antithrombotic therapy (from the HORIZONS-AMI trial). Am J Cardiol. 2010;105(10):1385–94.

26. Ibanez B, James S, Agewall S, Antunes MJ, Bucciarelli-Ducci C, Bueno H, Caforio ALP, Crea F, Goudevenos JA, Halvorsen S, et al. 2017 ESC guidelines for the management of acute myocardial infarction in patients presenting with ST-segment elevation. Rev Esp Cardiol (Engl Ed). 2017;70(12):1082.

27. Kwok CS, Tiong D, Pradhan A, Andreou AY, Nolan J, Bertrand OF, Curzen N, Urban P, Myint PK, Zaman AG, et al. Meta-analysis of the prognostic impact of anemia in patients undergoing percutaneous coronary intervention. Am J Cardiol. 2016;118(4):610–20.

28. Bagai J, Little B, Banerjee S. Association between arterial access site and anticoagulation strategy on major bleeding and mortality: a historical cohort analysis in the veteran population. Cardiovasc Revasc Med. 2018;19(1 Pt B):95–101.

29. Salisbury AC, Reid KJ, Marso SP, Amin AP, Alexander KP, Wang TY, Spertus JA, Kosiborod M. Blood transfusion during acute myocardial infarction: association with mortality and variability across hospitals. J Am Coll Cardiol. 2014;64(8):811–9.

30. Carson JL, Guyatt G, Heddle NM, Grossman BJ, Cohn CS, Fung MK, Gernsheimer T, Holcomb JB, Kaplan LJ, Katz LM, et al. Clinical practice guidelines from the AABB: red blood cell transfusion thresholds and storage. JAMA. 2016;316(19):2025–35.

31. Pilgrim T, Vetterli F, Kalesan B, Stefanini GG, Raber L, Stortecky S, Gloekler S, Binder RK, Wenaweser P, Moschovitis A, et al. The impact of anemia on long-term clinical outcome in patients undergoing revascularization with the unrestricted use of drug-eluting stents. Circ Cardiovasc Interv. 2012;5(2):202–10.

32. Amann U, Kirchberger I, Heier M, Goluke H, von Scheidt W, Kuch B, Peters A, Meisinger C. Long-term survival in patients with different combinations of evidence-based medications after incident acute myocardial infarction: results from the MONICA/KORA myocardial infarction registry. Clin Res Cardiol. 2014;103(8):655–64.

33. Khedri M, Szummer K, Carrero JJ, Jernberg T, Evans M, Jacobson SH, Spaak J. Systematic underutilisation of secondary preventive drugs in patients with acute coronary syndrome and reduced renal function. Eur J Prev Cardiol. 2017;24(7):724–734.

34. Willis P, Voeltz MD. Anemia, hemorrhage, and transfusion in percutaneous coronary intervention, acute coronary syndromes, and ST-segment elevation myocardial infarction. Am J Cardiol. 2009;104(5 Suppl):34C–8C.

35. Steppich B, Groha P, Ibrahim T, Schunkert H, Laugwitz KL, Hadamitzky M, Kastrati A, Ott I, Regeneration of Vital Myocardium in STSEMIbESI. Effect of erythropoietin in patients with acute myocardial infarction: five-year results of the REVIVAL-3 trial. BMC Cardiovasc Disord. 2017;17(1):38.

24

Association of sleep disturbances within 4 weeks prior to incident acute myocardial infarction and long-term survival in male and female patients: an observational study from the MONICA/KORA Myocardial Infarction Registry

Franziska Nairz[1,2,3], Christa Meisinger[1,2,4], Inge Kirchberger[1,2,4], Margit Heier[1,2], Christian Thilo[5], Bernhard Kuch[5,6], Annette Peters[2] and Ute Amann[1,2,4,*] (iD)

Abstract

Background: Sleep-related investigations in acute myocardial infarction (AMI) patients are rare. The aim of this study was to examine sex-specific associations of patient-reported sleep disturbances within 4 weeks before AMI and long-term survival.

Methods: From a German population-based, regional AMI registry, 2511 men and 828 women, aged 28–74 years, hospitalized with a first-time AMI between 2000 and 2008 and still alive after 28 days, were included in the study (end of follow-up: 12/2011). Frequency of any sleep disturbances within 4 weeks before AMI was inquired by a 6-categorical item summarized to 'never', 'sometimes' and 'nightly'. Cox regression models were calculated.

Results: Over the median follow-up time of 6.1 years (IQR: 4.1) sleep disturbances were reported by 32.3% of male and 48.4% of female patients. During the observation period, 318 men (12.7%) and 131 women (15.8%) died. Men who 'sometimes' had sleep disturbances showed a 56% increased mortality risk compared to those without complaints in an age-adjusted model (HR 1.56; 95%-CI 1.21–2.00). Additional adjustment for confounding variables attenuated the effect to 1.40 (95%-CI 1.08–1.81). Corresponding HRs among women were 0.97 (95%-CI 0.65–1.44) and 0.99 (95%-CI 0.66–1.49). HRs for patients with nightly sleep disturbances did not suggest any association for both sexes.

Conclusions: Our study found that nightly sleep disturbances have no influence on long-term survival in male and female AMI patients. Contrary to women, men who reported sometimes sleep disturbances had a higher mortality. Further investigations on this topic taking into account the role of obstructive sleep apnoea are needed.

Keywords: Sleep disturbance, Myocardial infarction, Long-term mortality, Sex differences

* Correspondence: ute.amann@helmholtz-muenchen.de
[1]Central Hospital of Augsburg, MONICA/KORA Myocardial Infarction Registry, Augsburg, Germany
[2]Helmholtz Zentrum München, German Research Center for Environmental Health (GmbH), Institute of Epidemiology II, Neuherberg, Germany
Full list of author information is available at the end of the article

Background

Sleep disturbances rank as a relevant public health problem in modern society and are expected to increase in the future for several reasons, such as rising job demands combined with 24/7 service availability, inappropriate use of internet or mobile phones at night and ageing populations [1]. Already, about one third of the general population is affected by sleep disturbances in terms of difficulties initiating sleep, maintaining sleep or non-restorative sleep [2]. Sex differences regarding the prevalence of reported insomnia symptoms were shown in previous work and resulted in an estimated female/male ratio of 1.4 which further increased with age [2, 3]. Due to its regenerative function, sleep influences both physical and mental health outcomes. Research in the last decades provided increasing evidence for sleep disturbances - with respect to both sleep quality and quantity - as a risk factor for cardiovascular disease (CVD), cardiac death and all-cause mortality [4–7].

While healthy populations were extensively studied in this context, sleep-related investigations in acute myocardial infarction (AMI) patients are rare. However, previous results indicated that sleep complaints might be associated with disease progression and worse survival prognosis after AMI. Heavy snoring, a proxy for obstructive sleep apnea, was shown to precipitate progression of atherosclerosis in women with AMI or unstable angina pectoris [8] and to be associated with an increased case-fatality in AMI patients [9]. The association between obstructive sleep apnea and risk of CV events and death has been well established in earlier studies [7, 10]. However, recent findings question the impact of obstructive sleep apnea on CV outcomes [11]. Shah et al. [11] suggests a potential cardioprotective effect of obstructive sleep apnea in AMI patients due to ischemic preconditioning. Regarding sleep duration, patients with an acute coronary syndrome who slept less than 7 h per night in the month after the event had an 50% elevated 1-year risk of acute coronary syndrome recurrence and mortality compared to acute coronary syndrome patients who reported longer sleep duration [12]. To our knowledge, only two studies [13, 14] investigated the associations between difficulties initiating sleep or disturbed sleep, respectively, and long-term outcomes in AMI patients. While Condén & Rosenblad [13] followed up recent AMI cases for all-cause mortality without distinction between patients' sex for the analyses, Clark et al. [14] investigated a composite outcome of incidence of or death from recurrent cardiovascular events during a 10-year follow-up and additionally used data originated from the early 90s.

Hence, the aim of our study was to examine the association of patient-reported sleep disturbances within 4 weeks before incident myocardial infarction (MI) and long-term survival, separately for men and women, using data from the percutaneous coronary intervention era. Sleep disturbances in this study were not regarded as a proxy for any sleep disorder but as a complaint perceived by patients which may have an indicative value for their long-term prognosis.

Methods

Data for the present observational study stemmed from the population-based MONICA/KORA MI registry in Augsburg (Southern Bavaria, Germany). The study area comprised a total of about 600,000 inhabitants and eight cooperating hospitals. From the beginning in 1984, all cases of coronary deaths and non-fatal MIs of the study population, aged 25–74 years and resident in the study area, have been continuously documented in the registry. Methods of case identification, diagnostic classification of events, and data quality control have been described in detail elsewhere [15, 16]. Briefly, patients hospitalized for AMI and having survived for at least 24 h after hospitalization were interviewed by trained study nurses after transfer from the intensive care unit. They collected information on socio-demographic characteristics, cardiovascular risk factors, medical history of MI, stroke, comorbidities and information on the acute event using a standardized questionnaire. Additional data on AMI characteristics, treatment, in-hospital complications, comorbidities, vital status and discharge medication were provided by medical chart review.

Based on a total sample of 7115 registered patients between January 1, 2000 and December 31, 2008, our study question was confined to those who had first-time AMI and survived for at least 28 days after the event (n = 4423). We further excluded those without information on sleep disturbances (n = 981) as well as patients with missing data on relevant covariables to be included in final regression models (n = 103), leaving 2511 men and 828 women eligible for the analyses of long-term survival (Fig. 1). Patients with missing values on sleep disturbances had a worse prognosis compared to those with available data (crude Hazard Ratio (HR) for long-term mortality 2.72; 95% confidence interval (CI): 2.29–3.22 (men) and HR 2.14; CI 1.62–2.83 (women)). In most cases, sleep information was lacking because no interview was conducted (96.6%).

Information on sleep disturbances was collected by one questionnaire item. 'How often did you suffer from sleep disturbances within the last 4 weeks?' could be answered by the response categories '1: never', '2: less than once per week', '3: once per week', '4: more than once per week', '5: every night', '6: I do not know'. Patients who indicated the latter (n = 42) were treated as cases with missing data. For the 3-categorical primary

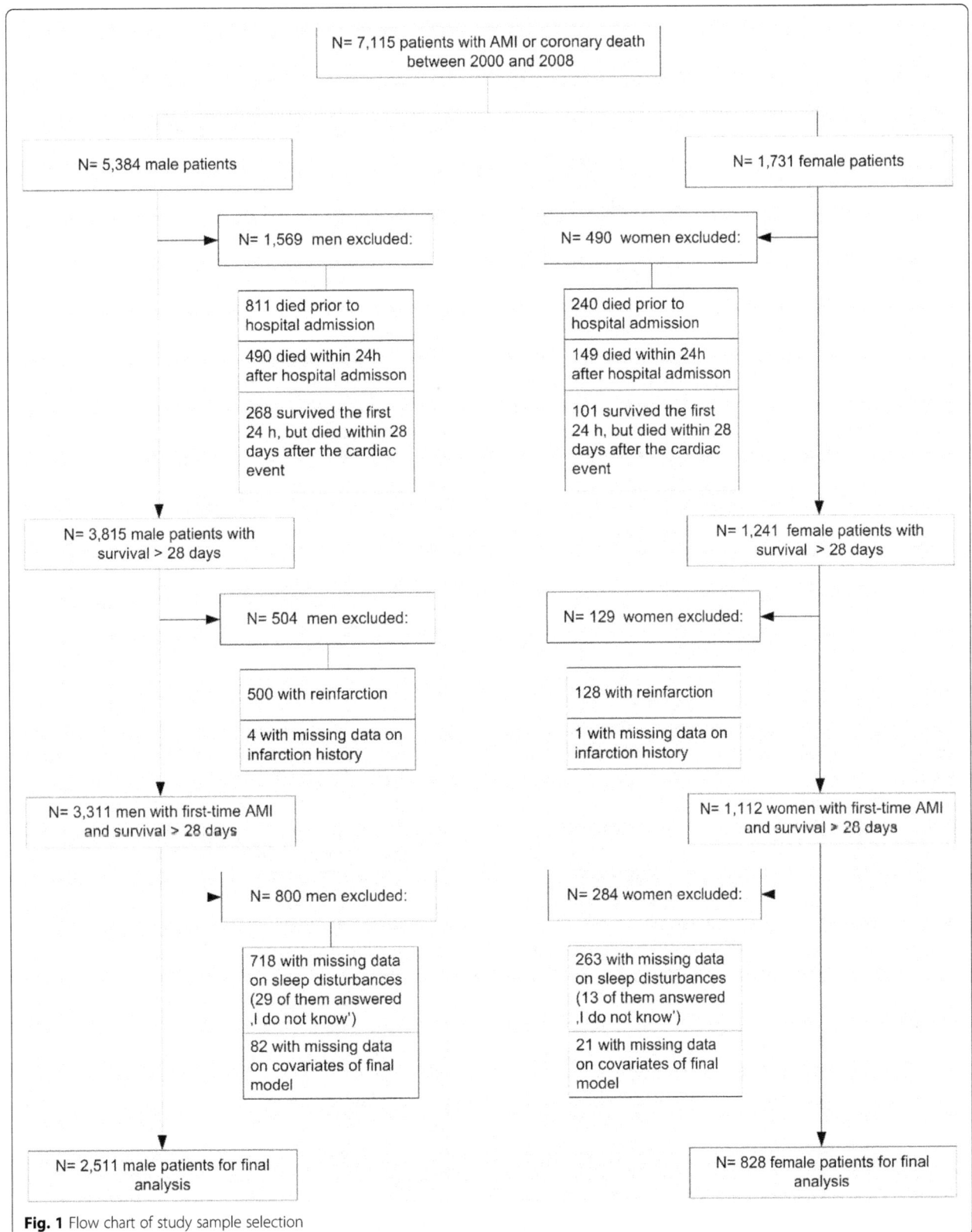

Fig. 1 Flow chart of study sample selection

independent variable 'frequency of sleep disturbances', we summarized answers to 'never' (original category 1), 'sometimes' (original categories 2–4) and 'every night' (original category 5) assuming that patients suffering not at all (1) or nightly (5) would rate themselves rather accurately.

The following covariables were captured and considered for analysis: patients were asked whether they were employed (currently, formerly, never), whether they were married (yes/no) and whether they smoked (currently, formerly, never). The highest acquired school-leaving qualification was captured to evaluate educational level (according to the German school system: 1 = lower secondary school; 2 = secondary school; 3 = high school diploma; 4 = university degree; 5 = other qualification; 6 = refused to reply). This information was dichotomized for analysis as 'low education (< 9 years)' which corresponds to response category 1 (yes/no). Body mass index (BMI) was obtained by assessment of height and weight during the hospital stay and adiposity was defined as $BMI > 30 \, kg/m^2$ (yes/no). While the history of stroke (yes/no) was only determined by self-report, medical history of angina pectoris, hypertension, hyperlipidemia or diabetes (yes/no) was considered if confirmed by chart review. The type of AMI was defined as ST-segment elevation MI (STEMI), Non-ST-segment elevation MI (NSTEMI), bundle branch block, or non-classifiable/ missing. The latter two categories were summarized to 'non-classifiable' for analysis. Regarding primary care, revascularization therapy (yes/no) was defined as having received thrombolysis, percutaneous transluminal coronary angioplasty with or without stenting or coronary artery bypass surgery. A combination of the following four evidence based medications is strongly recommended as standard of care after AMI with reported benefit on long-term survival: anti-platelet agents, beta-blockers, statins and angiotensin-converting enzyme inhibitors or angiotensin-receptor blockers [17]. Thus, we summarized data on medication at hospital discharge to treatment with all 4 evidence based medications (yes/no).

The outcome of interest was all-cause mortality, assessed by checking the vital status of all recorded persons in the MI registry. Local health departments inside and additionally outside the study region were involved in the mortality follow-up assessment, which takes place about every 5 years, in order to ascertain the survival status of all participants including those who had moved out of the study area. Follow-up for this study ended in December 2011. Survival time was measured in days and defined from day of the acute event to the day of death. Patients who were still alive at the end of the follow-up period were censored.

Analyses were done separately for men and women due to differences in CVD risk profile and outcome [18]

and differences in both their reported [3] and objective sleep habits [19, 20], comparable to previous investigations [14]. The primary independent variable was cross-tabulated with potential covariables. Categorical ones were presented as absolute numbers and percentage, and evaluated for differences in frequency distribution with χ^2-test. Continuous data was expressed as median with interquartile range (IQR) and compared using Kruskal-Wallis test as non-parametric equivalent to one-way analysis of variance.

Differences in survival time were determined by Log-Rank test for all categorical variables or simple Cox regression models for continuous age and BMI, respectively.

Except for age, which was a priori determined to be forced in regression models, only those variables were considered for subsequent regression modeling which were significantly associated with either sleep disturbances or long-term survival in sex-specific comparisons.

Kaplan-Meier-curves were generated for the primary independent variable. Differences in survival time between the three strata of the primary independent variable were determined by log rank test. To estimate the magnitude of impact of sleep disturbances on all-cause mortality, several Cox proportional hazard regression models were fitted. Hazard ratios were presented with 95%- confidence intervals and patients never having suffered from sleep disturbances within 4 weeks prior to AMI as reference category. The overall influence of the 3-categorical primary independent variable was evaluated using Likelihood-Ratio tests. First, univariable regression models were calculated for men and women to assess the crude association followed by age-adjusted models. Minimally adjusted models were then individually expanded for covariables sets from the domains socio-demographic/lifestyle, comorbidities and clinical aspects. Finally, a full model - identical for both sexes - was fitted containing all covariables with either significant association in the male or female data set. To control for possible cohort effects, the year of AMI was also included. The potential mediating role of hypertension and diabetes [21, 22] on the association of sleep disturbances and long-time mortality was considered by refitting the full models without these variables.

Proportional hazards assumption was checked graphically (parallel lines of log (−log(survival)) versus log of survival times) for all variables. In case of violating the proportional hazards requirement, a time-dependent variable was created for the respective variable and tested in a bivariate cox regression model for statistical significance. Solely the interaction terms for age and BMI with log (survival) in the female group were statistically significant. Since HRs for the primary independent variable hardly changed when time-dependent variables were included, we decided to report the results for the simple models without interaction terms.

Interaction effects of age with sleep disturbances were tested in bivariate and full models, but failed to reach statistical significance.

To account for the arbitrary categorization of the primary independent variable, sensitivity analyses were performed with the following two alternative categorizations in age-adjusted and full models: 1) another 3-categorical allocation (never [original category 1], occasionally [original categories 2, 3], frequently [original categories 4, 5]) and 2) a binary classification (any sleep disturbances in the prior 4 weeks yes [1]/ no [2–5]). In further sensitivity analyses, we restricted the male study population to those patients with normal weight (BMI ≥ 18.5 and $< 25\,\mathrm{kg/m^2}$), in order to consider potential confounding through obstructive sleep apnea, which occurs more often in overweight men [23]. Finally, crude and age-adjusted models were refitted including also patients with missing data on any of the covariates of the full model.

For all investigations, a significance level of 5% was applied. Data management and analysis were performed using SAS version 9.2 (SAS Institute Inc., Cary, North Carolina).

Results

The study sample consisted of 2511 male and 828 female patients. With a median age of 65 years (IQR: 12) women were older than men (60 (IQR: 15)) and more often diagnosed with hypertension and diabetes.

Baseline socio-demographic data, lifestyle factors, comorbidities, AMI and treatment characteristics of male and female patients stratified by frequency of sleep disturbances are presented in Table 1. Almost 50% of female patients indicated having been affected by sleep disturbances anytime (30.3% sometimes and 18.1% nightly) whereas about 30% of the male sample reported sleep disturbances preceding AMI (22.7 and 9.6%, respectively). These numbers changed in the course of the study period starting with a proportion of 35% of women in the year 2000 up to almost 60% 8 years later. An even stronger increase from early 18% to later 48% reporting any sleep disturbance was observed for men. Median age did not significantly vary across categories of sleep disturbances for both sexes. Overall, none of the analyzed variables were significantly associated with frequency of sleep disturbances in female patients, but for men some differences were detected. Among others, BMI of men was slightly, but significantly, different in the sleep categories with the highest median value in the 'nightly' group (27.7, IQR: 5.3). The proportion of male hypertensive patients increased with frequency of sleep

complaints from 71.8 to 80.1%. The same trend applied to patients diagnosed with angina pectoris. Regarding revascularization therapy, male patients in the bottom as well as in the upper sleep category more often received any of the mentioned treatments.

Median follow-up time was 6.1 years in men and women (IQR: 4.1). Overall, women had a greater long-term mortality rate than men (26 vs. 21 deaths per 1000 person years, respectively). For men, the highest mortality rate was observed for patients who sometimes suffered from sleep disturbances (28 deaths per 1000 person years vs. 19 and 18 deaths per 1000 person years for the bottom and upper category, respectively) while the mortality rate for females did not differ between categories. Kaplan-Meier survival curves visualizing these tendencies in Fig. 2 demonstrated significant differences in survival according to frequency of sleep disturbances for men (Log-Rank, $p = 0.0014$), but not for women (Log-Rank, $p = 0.9690$).

Results from Cox regression analyses are presented in Table 2. The age-adjusted model for men revealed a 56% increased all-cause mortality risk for patients who sometimes suffered from sleep disturbances compared to those reporting no sleep disturbances (HR 1.56; 95%-CI 1.21–2.00) whereas male patients who indicated having had disturbed sleep every night did not show an elevated relative risk (HR 1.00; 95%-CI 0.66–1.51). By separately adding covariables sets from the domains 'socio-demographic/lifestyle', 'comorbidities', and 'clinical aspects' to the age-adjusted model, HRs hardly changed. The decrease of HR [sometimes vs. never] by 5.8% was greatest for the model 'Clinical' and mainly explained by revascularization treatment. The full model finally attenuated the long term mortality risk for the second category to 1.40 (HR, 95%-CI 1.08–1.81). However, the increase remained significant as well as the overall impact of sleep disturbances (Likelihood-Ratio Test $p = 0.0370$).

For women, a relation between sleep disturbances prior to AMI and long-term mortality was detected neither in the age-adjusted or subset models nor in the full model controlled for the same confounders as used in the male model.

When the potential mediator variables hypertension and diabetes were removed individually and together from the full model, HR estimates for sleep disturbances did not change remarkably both for men and women (data not shown). Table 3 summarizes the distribution of the study sample depending on the respective categorization of frequency of sleep disturbances. As sensitivity analysis we refitted the age-adjusted and full model for males and females with alternative categorizations of the primary independent variable. Results of the regression models are shown in Table 4. For the other

Table 1 Sample characteristics for male and female AMI patients stratified by frequency of sleep disturbances

	Men (n = 2511)				Women (n = 828)			
	SLEEP DISTURBANCES			p-value[a]	SLEEP DISTURBANCES			p-value[a]
	never n = 1699	sometimes n = 571	nightly n = 241		never n = 427	sometimes n = 251	nightly n = 150	
Socio-demographic Data								
Age, years [median (IQR)]	60 (15)	60 (15)	60 (14)	0.7213	65 (13)	65 (13)	65 (12)	0.8775
Low Education, < 9 years	1186 (69.8)	407 (71.3)	170 (70.5)	0.7958	351 (82.2)	202 (80.8)	113 (75.3)	0.1894
Married	1378 (81.1)	435 (76.2)	190 (78.8)	0.0375	258 (60.42)	147 (58.57)	91 (60.67)	0.8732
Currently employed	788 (46.4)	243 (42.6)	99 (41.1)	0.1236	98 (22.95)	50 (19.92)	26 (17.33)	0.3057
Lifestyle factors								
BMI, kg/m^2 [median (IQR)]	27.1 (4.8)	27.4 (4.7)	27.7 (5.3)	0.0370	26.8 (7.4)	27.5 (7.1)	27.7 (7.0)	0.5334
Adiposity, BMI > 30 kg/m^2	376 (22.1)	141 (24.7)	69 (28.6)	0.0566	134 (31.4)	86 (34.3)	50 (33.3)	0.7258
Ever Smoker	1280 (75.3)	402 (70.4)	187 (77.6)	0.0322	209 (49.0)	112 (44.6)	76 (50.7)	0.4216
Comorbidities								
Angina	190 (11.2)	104 (18.2)	52 (21.6)	< 0.0001	69 (16.16)	30 (11.95)	31 (20.67)	0.0631
Hypertension	1219 (71.8)	438 (76.7)	193 (80.1)	0.0040	350 (82.0)	206 (82.1)	129 (86.0)	0.5034
Dyslipidemia	1220 (71.8)	394 (69.0)	172 (71.4)	0.4393	310 (72.6)	187 (74.5)	119 (79.3)	0.2665
Diabetes	443 (26.1)	143 (25.0)	59 (24.5)	0.8022	137 (32.1)	82 (32.7)	53 (35.3)	0.7647
Stroke	75 (4.4)	29 (5.1)	15 (6.2)	0.4232	28 (6.6)	15 (6.0)	14 (9.3)	0.4070
Clinical aspects								
Type of Infarction								
STEMI	710 (41.8)	204 (35.7)	86 (35.7)	0.0756	180 (42.2)	87 (34.7)	64 (42.7)	0.2622
NSTEMI	872 (51.3)	323 (56.6)	137 (56.9)		229 (53.6)	149 (59.4)	81 (54.0)	
Bundle Branch Block/non-classifiable	117 (6.9)	44 (7.7)	18 (7.5)		18 (4.2)	15 (6.0)	5 (3.3)	
Revascularization therapy	1521 (89.5)	490 (85.8)	221 (91.7)	0.0175	338 (79.2)	195 (77.7)	111 (74.0)	0.4254
4 EBM at discharge	1221 (71.9)	418 (73.2)	183 (75.9)	0.3852	285 (66.7)	180 (71.7)	111 (74.0)	0.1699
Mortality								
Deceased during follow-up	206 (12.1)	87 (15.2)	25 (10.4)	0.0818	71 (16.6)	37 (14.7)	23 (15.3)	0.7964

Data is presented as absolute number (%) unless otherwise indicated.

AMI acute myocardial infarction, *BMI* Body Mass Index, *EBM* evidence based medication, *IQR* interquartile range, *NSTEMI* Non-ST-segment elevation myocardial infarction, *STEMI* ST-segment elevation myocardial infarction

[a] p-values are obtained from χ^2-tests for categorical data or from Kruksal-Wallis test for continuous data (age and BMI)

3-level variable (categorization 2), the influence of sleep disturbances on long-term mortality in male AMI patients lost overall significance (Likelihood-Ratio Test p = 0.1254). Likewise, the binary comparison failed to reach statistical significance (HR 1.26; 95% CI 1.00–1.60, p = 0.0543). Again, for women no associations were observed.

The association of sleep disturbances and all-cause mortality was not seen any more in the full model restricted to the 629 male patients with normal weight (HR [sometimes vs. never] 1.16, 95%-CI 0.72–1.88 and HR [nightly vs. never] 1.48, 95%-CI 0.76–2.88).

In a final sensitivity analysis, adding the patients with missing data on any covariables of the full model (additionally 82 males and 21 females), no notable changes

regarding the unadjusted and age-adjusted HRs resulted (data not shown).

Discussion

In our study, we found a 40% increased long-term mortality risk in the fully adjusted model for male AMI patients who sometimes, i.e. up to several times a week, suffered from sleep disturbances within 4 weeks before the acute event. For men with nightly sleep disturbances and for women, however, no associations between sleep disturbances and long-term mortality were seen in our data.

Overall, sleep disturbances were reported by 36.3% of our total sample of AMI patients, which is somewhat higher than referred for the general population [2]. The proportion was considerably larger in women than in

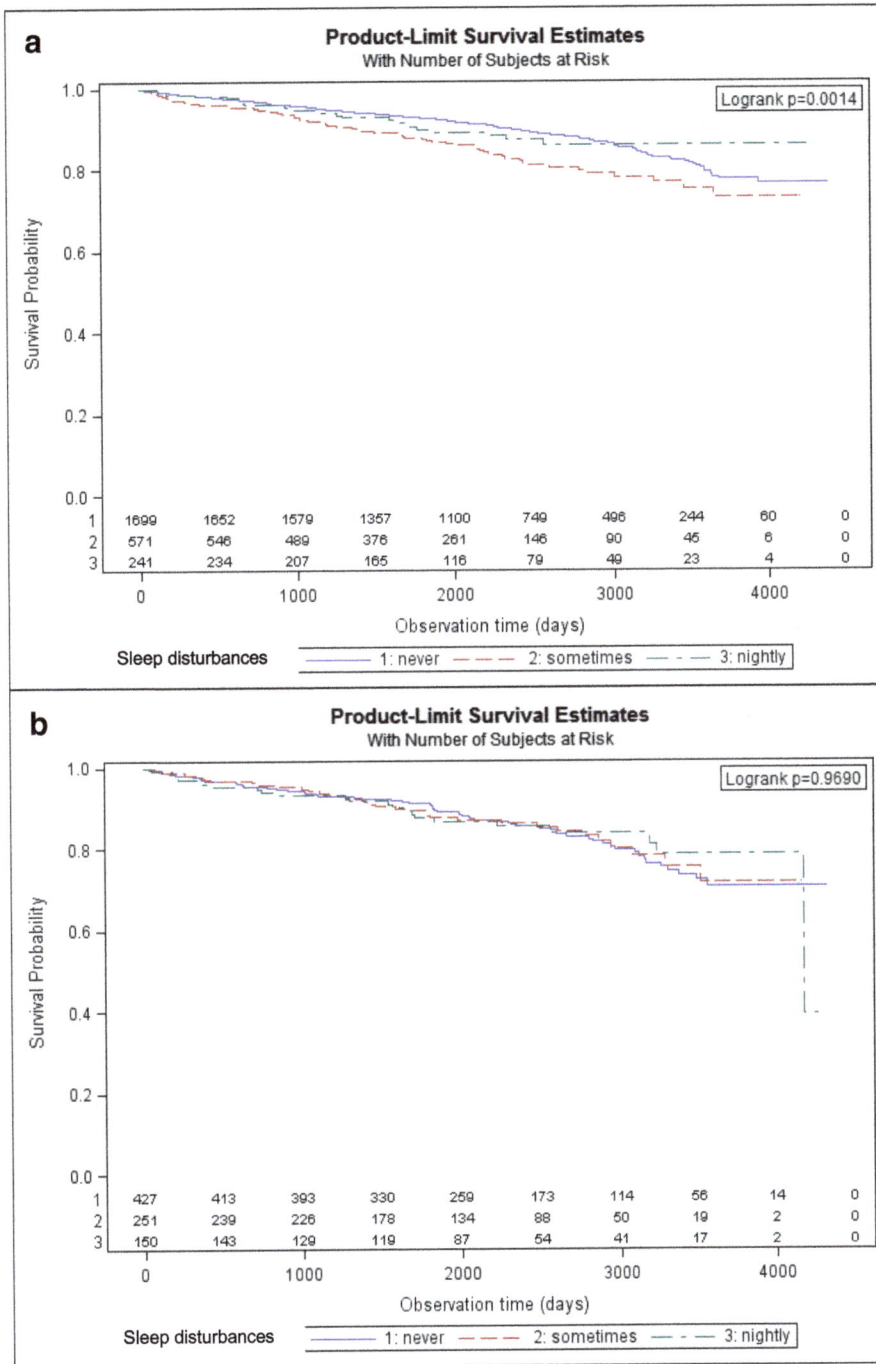

Fig. 2 12-year survival curves for male (**a**) and female (**b**) AMI patients stratified by frequency of sleep disturbances. Footnote: "Differences in survival time between the three strata of the primary independent variable were determined by log rank test."

men (48.4% vs. 32.3%). This was not surprising since women are known to be more frequently affected by insomnia symptoms due to hormonal and physiological differences as well as psychosocial factors [24]. Depression and anxiety disorders which are almost twice as prevalent in women compared to men [25] and are associated with sleep disturbances [26], represent a relevant factor regarding the female predominance in insomnia symptoms [20]. Moreover, prevalence of insomnia was shown to increase in postmenopausal women compared to premenopausal women [27]. With a median age of 65 years in our female study sample, the majority of women could be assumed to be in postmenopausal phase. Finally, sleep disturbances increase with age [2]. This

Table 2 Association of frequency of sleep disturbances within 4 weeks prior to AMI (categorization 1) and long-term mortality in male and female patients

	Frequency of sleep disturbances	Men (n = 2511; 318 deaths)			Women (n = 828; 131 deaths)		
		HR	[95% CI]	p-value[a]	HR	[95% CI]	p-value[a]
Unadjusted model	never	1	Ref.	0.0024	1	Ref.	0.9686
	sometimes	1.58	[1.23–2.03]		1.00	[0.67–1.49]	
	nightly	1.00	[0.66–1.52]		0.94	[0.59–1.51]	
Age-adjusted model	never	1	Ref.	0.0032	1	Ref.	0.9773
	sometimes	1.56	[1.21–2.00]		0.97	[0.65–1.44]	
	nightly	1.00	[0.66–1.51]		0.96	[0.60–1.53]	
Model Lifestyle[b]	never	1	Ref.	0.0038	1	Ref.	0.9665
	sometimes	1.55	[1.20–1.99]		0.96	[0.64–1.43]	
	nightly	0.99	[0.65–1.50]		0.95	[0.59–1.52]	
Model Comorbidities[c]	never	1	Ref.	0.0060	1	Ref.	0.9556
	sometimes	1.50	[1.16–1.93]		0.98	[0.66–1.47]	
	nightly	0.92	[0.60–1.39]		0.93	[0.58–1.49]	
Model Clinical[d]	never	1	Ref.	0.0150	1	Ref.	0.9899
	sometimes	1.47	[1.14–1.89]		0.97	[0.65–1.46]	
	nightly	1.02	[0.67–1.54]		0.97	[0.61–1.57]	
Full model[e]	never	1	Ref.	0.0370	1	Ref.	0.9055
	sometimes	1.40	[1.08–1.81]		0.99	[0.66–1.49]	
	nightly	0.95	[0.62–1.45]		0.90	[0.55–1.46]	

AMI = acute myocardial infarction, CI = confidence interval, HR = Hazard Ratio
[a]p-value obtained from Likelihood-Ratio test for overall significance of 3-categorical variable 'frequency of sleep disturbances' in the respective model
[b]MEN: adjusted for age (cont.), married, low education (< 9 years), employment status, smoking ever and BMI (cont)
WOMEN: adjusted for age (cont.), married and employment status
[c]MEN: adjusted for age (cont.), hypertension, angina, diabetes, dyslipidemia and stroke
WOMEN: adjusted for age, diabetes and stroke
[d]MEN: adjusted for age (cont.), type of infarction, any revascularization treatment (coronary artery bypass surgery, percutaneous coronary intervention (PCI) with/without stenting, or thrombolysis), all four evidence based medications at discharge (antiplatelet agents, beta-blockers, ACEIs/ARBs (Angiotensin-converting enzyme inhibitors/Angiotensin receptor blockers), statins) and year of MI
WOMEN: adjusted for age (cont.), type of infarction, any revascularization treatment and all four evidence based medications at discharge
[e]MEN AND WOMEN: adjusted for age (cont.), low education (< 9 years), married, employment status, ever smoking, BMI (cont.), hypertension, angina, diabetes, dyslipidemia, stroke, type of infarction, any revascularization treatment, all four evidence based medications at discharge and year of MI

Table 3 Distribution of patients and events according to different categorizations of the primary independent variable

Frequency of sleep disturbances within 4 weeks prior to AMI		Men (n = 2511)		Women (n = 828)	
		No. per category (%)	No. of deaths	No. per category (%)	No. of deaths
Original response	never	1699 (67.7)	206	427 (51.6)	71
	< 1 per week	247 (9.8)	40	82 (9.9)	14
	once per week	67 (2.7)	10	31 (3.7)	7
	> 1 per week	257 (10.2)	37	138 (16.7)	16
	nightly	241 (9.6)	25	150 (18.1)	23
Categorization 1	never	1699 (67.7)	206	427 (516)	71
	sometimes	571 (22.7)	87	251 (30.3)	37
	nightly	241 (9.6)	25	150 (18.1)	23
Categorization 2	never	1699 (67.7)	206	427 (51.6)	71
	occasionally	314 (12.5)	50	113 (13.7)	21
	frequently	498 (19.8)	62	288 (34.8)	39
Binary (any time)	no	1699 (67.7)	206	427 (51.6)	71
	yes	812 (32.3)	112	401 (48.4)	60

AMI acute myocardial infarction

Table 4 Association of frequency of sleep disturbances within 4 weeks prior to AMI (categorization 2 and binary split) and long-term mortality in male and female patients

		Men (n = 2511; 318 deaths)			Women (n = 828; 131 deaths)		
		HR	[95% CI]	p-value[a]	HR	[95% CI]	p-value[a]
	Frequency of sleep disturbances						
Age-adjusted model	never	1	Ref.	0.0183	1	Ref.	0.7162
	occasionally	1.52	[1.11–2.07]		1.12	[0.68–1.82]	
	frequently	1.29	[0.97–1.72]		0.90	[0.61–1.33]	
Full model[b]	never	1	Ref.	0.1256	1	Ref.	0.7163
	occasionally	1.37	[1.00–1.87]		1.10	[0.67–1.82]	
	frequently	1.19	[0.89–1.59]		0.89	[0.59–1.33]	
	Sleep disturbances at any time						
Age-adjusted model	no	1	Ref.		1	Ref.	
	yes	1.38	[1.10–1.74]	0.0070	0.96	[0.68–1.36]	0.8330
Full model[b]	no	1	Ref.		1	Ref.	
	yes	1.26	[1.00–1.60]	0.0571	0.95	[0.67–1.36]	0.7854

AMI acute myocardial infarction, *CI* confidence interval, *HR* Hazard Ratio

[a]p-value obtained from Likelihood Ratio test for overall significance of 'frequency of sleep disturbances' in the respective model

[b]adjusted for age (cont.), low education (< 9 years), married, employment status, ever smoking, BMI (cont.), hypertension, angina, diabetes, dyslipidemia, stroke, type of infarction, any revascularization treatment (coronary artery bypass surgery, percutaneous coronary intervention (PCI) with/without stenting, or thrombolysis), all four evidence based medications at discharge (antiplatelet agents, beta-blockers, ACEIs/ARBs (Angiotensin-converting enzyme inhibitors/ Angiotensin receptor blockers), statins) and year of MI

trend might also contribute to the difference in proportions of reported sleep disturbances in our study, as women were significantly older in the analyzed data.

Overall, unadjusted percentages of both men and women who reported sleep disturbances in our study clearly increased within the study period from the year 2000 to 2008 by factor 2.7 and 1.7 respectively. Previous epidemiological studies in several countries presented increasing prevalence of sleep complaints on population-level in the last decades [28]. Among others, the demographic change and growing health problems such as the obesity epidemic were considered as reasons for this development as well as altering occupational requirements such as shift-work and increased work-load [1, 28]. Nevertheless, this trend might be at least in part influenced by a sort of reporting bias due to growing awareness for sleep problems.

Referring to the International Classification of Sleep Disorders – 3rd edition [29] (ICSD-3) and the Diagnostic and Statistical Manual of Mental Disorders – 5th edition [30] (DSM-5) criteria for insomnia disorder, many studies applied a frequency of at least three times per week to rate sleep disturbances as symptomatic [2]. Transferred to our data, 23.5% reported to have suffered from sleep disturbances several times a week or nightly, which corresponds to category 'frequently' in categorization 2 (19.8% of men and 34.8% of women, respectively). These numbers were similar to those stated in two previous studies on the association of sleep disturbances prior to AMI with long-term

outcomes of patients [13, 14], but the assessment and definition of sleep disturbances varied.

In the cohort study by Condén & Rosenblad [13] 23.9% of 732 Swedish AMI patients, recruited between 2006 and 2011, were classified as having insomnia, which was defined in the study as difficulty falling asleep without considering the frequency of occurrence (19.7% of men and 32.7% of women, respectively). Further, the corresponding question was not limited to the period prior to the cardiovascular event and hence might also have captured cases which had problems with initiating sleep as a result of the MI. This could have influenced the survival prognosis in the group of insomnia patients who had an almost 60% elevated, multivariable adjusted, all cause-mortality risk in the period after the first 2 years of follow-up (mean follow-up time 6.0 years) compared to patients not having suffered from difficulties falling asleep. Thus, the relative long-term mortality risk for male and female insomnia patients in Condén & Rosenblad [13] was higher than the fully adjusted HR that we found for men who had sometimes suffered from sleep disturbances (HR 1.40, 95%-CI 1.08–1.81) or men who reported sleep disturbances at any time within 4 weeks prior to AMI (HR 1.26; 95%-CI 1.00–1.60).

In the second previous study investigating long-term outcomes after AMI by Clark et al. [14] based on the Stockholm Heart Epidemiology Program (SHEEP), sleep impairment was assessed in more detail for 1089 male and 499 female patients with first-time AMI between

1992 and 1994. One of four sleep-related aspects was disturbed sleep, which comprised items on general sleep quality, difficulty falling asleep, repeated awakenings, disturbed/uneasy sleep and premature awakenings. More than 20% of the male patients and about one third of the females reported to have experienced disturbed sleep. Unlike in our interrogation, patients were asked for sleep impairment within 1 year prior to initial AMI. Hence, reported sleep disturbances might be more likely associated also with other health problems besides MI. A significantly increased risk for incidence of or death from cardiovascular events (distinguishing AMI [age-adjusted HR 1.73; 95%-CI 1.03–2.91], stroke [multiple adjusted HR 2.61; 95%-CI 1.19–5.76] or heart failure [multiple adjusted HR 2.43, 95%-CI 1.18–4.97]) within a 10-year follow-up was revealed for women but not for men with disturbed sleep at least sometimes a week compared to persons with less frequent or no complaints. As the endpoint of our study was all-cause mortality and we were not able to consider recurrent cardiovascular events after MI and cause-specific mortality, our results were not comparable to the above mentioned study.

Within the framework of topic-related studies, the results of our study therefore had to stand for themselves. We found an association of sometimes experienced sleep disturbances and long-term all-cause mortality in male AMI patients, but not in female patients. Reasons for this sex difference can only be speculative.

Firstly, sex differences in sleep architecture and in implications of sleep disturbances might contribute to the present results. Cross-sectional analyses of healthy participants showed that the percentage of deeper slow wave stage, which is important for regeneration during sleep [31], was significantly lower in men across all age groups and decreased in men getting older but not in women [19, 32]. However, sleep continuity and architecture were shown to change when sleep complaints became pathological. A recent meta-analysis showed a significant reduction of slow wave and rapid eye movement sleep in patients with primary insomnia compared to a good sleeper control group [33]. How far the above-mentioned sex differences hold also for people complaining about sleep disturbances needs to be examined. Secondly, one study found that healthy women were more resilient to the consequences of elevated circulating inflammatory markers induced by sleep disturbances than healthy men [34]. If these observations apply in a similar manner to a MI population, women might cope better with the consequences of sleep disturbances and thus repel a potential adverse impact on long-term survival.

Thirdly, though women across all age strata subjectively reported more sleep complaints than men [3], some studies

revealed no relative differences in polysomnography measurements or even better objective sleep quality for women [20, 24, 32]. Hence, we cannot fully rule out misclassification of female patients as a consequence of misperception of sleep-state to cause sex differences in long-term prognosis in our study and to obscure a potential association in women.

Contrary to what one might expect, we also did not detect an increased mortality risk for patients who suffered nightly from sleep disturbances within 4 weeks preceding the AMI. This may be a result of fewer patients in this category leading to insufficient power to reveal a possible association. Another reason could be a change in individual frequency of sleep disturbances during the follow-up period, particularly as a consequence of the AMI and its severity. As sleep disturbances were assessed only once in our registry, we could not investigate this aspect in our analysis. Adding those patients who suffered more than once per week from disturbed sleep to the nightly group (yielding category 'frequently' of categorization 2), did not reveal a significant increase in mortality risk either. These sensitivity analyses, including the binary comparison, question the robustness of the observed association for male patients found for categorization 1 and stress the need for further investigations. Another reason for our unexpected non-significant result observed in patients who suffered nightly from sleep disturbances might be driven by most resent literature on the role of chronic obstructive sleep apnea as a pre-conditioning stimulus that may have cardioprotective effects in some AMI patients [11]. Shah et al. [11] found a high prevalence (77%) of sleep disordered breathing among patients with AMI and observed that patients with obstructive sleep apnea (35%) develop a less severe cardiac lesion than those without obstructive sleep apnea. These findings question the previous literature that found obstructive sleep apnea to be an independent risk factor for fatal and non-fatal CVD. Nightly sleep disorder caused by non-treated obstructive sleep apnea may have influenced our results and warrants further investigation.

As observational studies still varied widely in the definition of insomnia and other sleep complaints, future research should draw profit from improvements and assimilation of existing diagnostic classification systems of sleep disorders and research diagnostic criteria for insomnia [29, 30]. For this purpose, a harmonization of the assessment of sleep disturbances in epidemiological research would be helpful to yield comparable results and hence to contribute to evident findings. Based on the recently revised ICSD – 3 and DSM-5 criteria for insomnia, a commonly accepted approach to assess sleep disturbances on a population-level should at least specify the kind of symptoms to be captured, their frequency in a defined time period as well as their severity with regard to daytime consequences.

To the best of our knowledge, the present study was the first to examine associations of patient-reported sleep disturbances shortly before AMI and long-term all-cause mortality separately for men and women using data from the percutaneous coronary intervention era.

A further strength of our study is the large sample from a population-based MI registry with high quality and validation standards contributing to the generalizability of our results.

Finally, we were able to adjust for a number of potential confounders, comprising lifestyle factors, comorbidities and clinical aspects.

Nevertheless, some important potential confounders were lacking. First, we were not able to adjust for depressive symptoms though depression is known to be associated with sleep disturbances [26] as well as cardiovascular outcomes and mortality [35].

Likewise, our study did not control for obstructive sleep apnea which may have a confounding influence on the relation between sleep disturbances and long-term mortality after MI [7, 10]. To account for this issue we did a sensitivity analysis in normal weight male patients, as obstructive sleep apnea is more frequent in overweight men [23]. Sleep disturbances were not significant anymore in the full model, but estimates resulted from a markedly smaller patient group with only 11 events in the category of nightly sleep disturbances and have to be treated with caution. However, the aspect of weight was not disregarded in the primary analysis as regression models are adjusted for BMI.

Finally, data on sleep disturbances was based on self report in this study and resulted from only one questionnaire item. However, in clinical practice no objective sleep data will be available either and physicians have to rely on compact patient information. Nevertheless, sleep disturbances in our study were uniquely assessed right after the AMI and we did not know about frequency of sleep disturbances in the follow-up period.

Conclusion

In summary, our data indicate that sleep disturbances were more frequently reported in AMI patients over time with a higher increasing prevalence observed in males. We found an association of sometimes experienced sleep disturbances and long-term all-cause mortality in male but not female AMI patients. In patients who reported nightly sleep disturbances, we did not found a significant association. This unexpected latter result and the sex-differences observed in our study need further investigations considering the diagnosis and treatment of commonly reported obstructive sleep apnea in AMI patients.

Abbreviations
AMI: Acute myocardial infarction; BMI: Body mass index; CI: Confidence interval; CVD: Cardiovascular disease; DSM: Diagnostic and statistical manual of mental disorders; HR: Hazard ratio; ICSD: International classification of sleep disorders; IQR: Interquartile range; KORA: Cooperative health research in the Augsburg region; LR: Likelihood ratio; MI: Myocardial infarction; MONICA: Monitoring trends and determinants in cardiovascular disease; NSTEMI: Non-ST segment elevation myocardial infarction; STEMI: ST-Segment elevation myocardial infarction

Acknowledgements
The KORA research platform and the MONICA Augsburg studies were initiated and financed by the Helmholtz Zentrum München, German Research Center for Environmental Health, which is funded by the German Federal Ministry of Education, Science, Research and Technology and by the State of Bavaria. Since the year 2000, the collection of MI data has been co-financed by the German Federal Ministry of Health to provide population-based MI morbidity data for the official German Health Report (see www.gbe-bund.de). Steering partners of the MONICA/KORA MI Registry, Augsburg, include the KORA research platform, Helmholtz Zentrum München and the Department of Internal Medicine I, Cardiology, Central Hospital of Augsburg.
We thank all members of the Helmholtz Zentrum München, Institute of Epidemiology II and the field staff in Augsburg who were involved in the planning and conduct of the study. We wish to thank the local health departments, the office-based physicians and the clinicians of the hospitals within the study area for their support. Finally, we express our appreciation to all study participants.

Funding
None.

Authors' contributions
FN and UA conceived the study. FN performed the statistical analyses and drafted the manuscript. CM, MH, CT, BK and AP contributed to data acquisition. IK, CM, CT, BK, AP, MP and UA critically revised the manuscript. All authors read and approved the final manuscript.

Competing interests
CT receives personal fees from Novartis, Daiichi Sankyo, Edwards (for lecturing) and from Symetis (for proctoring). Other authors declare that they have no competing interests.

Author details
[1]Central Hospital of Augsburg, MONICA/KORA Myocardial Infarction Registry, Augsburg, Germany. [2]Helmholtz Zentrum München, German Research Center for Environmental Health (GmbH), Institute of Epidemiology II, Neuherberg, Germany. [3]Institute for Medical Informatics, Biometry and Epidemiology (IBE), LMU Munich, Munich, Germany. [4]Ludwig-Maximilians-Universität München, UNIKA-T, Augsburg, Germany. [5]Central Hospital of Augsburg, Department of Internal Medicine I – Cardiology, Augsburg, Germany. [6]Hospital of Nördlingen, Department of Internal Medicine/Cardiology, Nördlingen, Germany. [7]KORA-Herzinfarktregister im Klinikum Augsburg/Helmholtz Zentrum München, Stenglinstr. 2, 86156 Augsburg, Germany.

References
1. Ferrie JE, Kumari M, Salo P, Singh-Manoux A, Kivimaki M. Sleep epidemiology--a rapidly growing field. Int J Epidemiolol. 2011;40:1431–7.
2. Ohayon MM. Epidemiology of insomnia: what we know and what we still need to learn. Sleep Med Rev. 2002;6:97–111.

3. Zhang B, Wing Y. Sex differences in insomnia: a meta-analysis. Sleep. 2006; 29:85–93.

4. Sofi F, Cesari F, Casini A, Macchi C, Abbate R, Gensini GF. Insomnia and risk of cardiovascular disease. A meta-analysis. Eur J Prev Cardiol. 2013;21:57–64.

5. Cappuccio FP, Cooper D, D'Elia L, Strazzullo P, Miller MA. Sleep duration predicts cardiovascular outcomes. A systematic review and meta-analysis of prospective studies. Eur Heart J. 2011;32:1484–92.

6. Fu Y, Xia Y, Yi H, Xu H, Guan J, Yin S. Meta-analysis of all-cause and cardiovascular mortality in obstructive sleep apnea with or without continuous positive airway pressure treatment. Sleep Breath. 2017;21:181–9.

7. Wang X, Zhang Y, Dong Z, Fan J, Nie S, Wei Y. Effect of continuous positive airway pressure on long-term cardiovascular outcomes in patients with coronary artery disease and obstructive sleep apnea: a systematic review and meta-analysis. Respir Res. 2018 Apr 10;19(1):61.

8. Leineweber C, Kecklund G, Janszky I, Åkerstedt T, Orth-Gomér K. Snoring and progression of coronary artery disease: the Stockholm Female Coronary Angiography Study. Sleep. 2004;27:1344–9.

9. Janszky I, Ljung R, Rohani M, Hallqvist J. Heavy snoring is a risk factor for case fatality and poor short-term prognosis after a first acute myocardial infarction. Sleep. 2008;31:801–7.

10. Loke YK, Brown JWL, Kwok CS, Niruban A, Myint PK. Association of obstructive sleep apnea with risk of serious cardiovascular events: a systematic review and meta-analysis. Circ Cardiovasc Qual Outcomes. 2012; 5:720–8.

11. Shah N, Redline S, Yaggi HK, Wu R, Zhao CG, Ostfeld R, et al. Obstructive sleep apnea and acute myocardial infarction severity: ischemic preconditioning? Sleep Breath. 2013;17:819–26.

12. Alcantara C, Peacock J, Davidson KW, Hiti D, Edmondson D. The association of short sleep after acute coronary syndrome with recurrent cardiac events and mortality. Int J Cardiol. 2014;171:e11–2.

13. Conden E, Rosenblad A. Insomnia predicts long-term all-cause mortality after acute myocardial infarction: A prospective cohort study. Int J Cardiol. 2016;215:217–22.

14. Clark A, Lange T, Hallqvist J, Jennum P, Rod NH. Sleep Impairment and prognosis of acute myocardial infarction. A prospective cohort study. Sleep. 2014;37:851–8.

15. Kuch B, Heier M, von Scheidt W, Kling B, Hoermann A, Meisinger C. 20-year trends in clinical characteristics, therapy and short-term prognosis in acute myocardial infarction according to presenting electrocardiogram: the MONICA/KORA AMI Registry (1985-2004). J Intern Med. 2008;264:254–64.

16. Meisinger C, Hörmann A, Heier M, Kuch B, Löwel H. Admission blood glucose and adverse outcomes in non-diabetic patients with myocardial infarction in the reperfusion era. Int J Cardiol. 2006;113:229–35.

17. Amann U, Kirchberger I, Heier M, Goluke H, von Scheidt W, Kuch B, et al. Long-term survival in patients with different combinations of evidence-based medications after incident acute myocardial infarction: results from the MONICA/KORA Myocardial Infarction Registry. Clin Res Cardiol. 2014;103: 655–64.

18. Khamis RY, Ammari T, Mikhail GW. Gender differences in coronary heart disease. Heart. 2016;102:1142–9.

19. Redline S, Kirchner HL, Quan SF, Gottlieb DJ, Kapur V, Newman A. The effects of age, sex, ethnicity, and sleep-disordered breathing on sleep architecture. Arch Intern Med. 2004;164:406–18.

20. Bixler EO, Papaliaga MN, Vgontzas AN, Lin H, Pejovic S, Karataraki M, et al. Women sleep objectively better than men and the sleep of young women is more resilient to external stressors: effects of age and menopause. J Sleep Res. 2009;18:221–8.

21. Gangwisch JE. A review of evidence for the link between sleep duration and hypertension. Am J Hypertens. 2014;27:1235–42.

22. Cappuccio FP, D'Elia L, Strazzullo P, Miller MA. Quantity and quality of sleep and incidence of type 2 diabetes: a systematic review and meta-analysis. Diabetes Care. 2010;33:414–20.

23. Franklin KA, Lindberg E. Obstructive sleep apnea is a common disorder in the population-a review on the epidemiology of sleep apnea. J Thorac Dis. 2015;7:1311–22.

24. Mallampalli MP, Carter CL. Exploring sex and gender differences in sleep health: a Society for Women's Health Research Report. J Women's Health (Larchmt). 2014;23:553–62.

25. Kessler R. Epidemiology of women and depression. J Affect Disord. 2003;74: 5–13.

26. Fava M. Daytime sleepiness and insomnia as correlates of depression. J Clin Psychiatry. 2004;65(Suppl 16):27–32.

27. Moline ML, Broch L, Zak R, Gross V. Sleep in women across the life cycle from adulthood through menopause. Sleep Med Rev. 2003;7:155–77.

28. Ford ES, Cunningham TJ, Giles WH, Croft JB. Trends in insomnia and excessive daytime sleepiness among U.S. adults from 2002 to 2012. Sleep Med. 2015;16:372–8.

29. American Academy of Sleep Medicine International Classification of Sleep Disorders 3rd ed. Darien, IL: American Academy of Sleep Medicine, 2014.

30. American Psychiatric Association. Diagnostic and Statistical Manual of Mental Disorders. 5th ed. Arlington, VA: American Psychiatric Publishing, 2013.

31. Dijk D. Regulation and functional correlates of slow wave sleep. J Clin Sleep Med. 2009;5(Suppl 2):S6–15.

32. Walsleben JA, Kapur VK, Newman AB, Shahar E, Bootzin RR, Rosenberg CE, et al. Sleep and reported daytime sleepiness in normal subjects: The Sleep Heart Health Study. Sleep. 2004;27:293–8.

33. Baglioni C, Regen W, Teghen A, Spiegelhalder K, Feige B, Nissen C, et al. Sleep changes in the disorder of insomnia: a meta-analysis of polysomnographic studies. Sleep Med Rev. 2014;18:195–213.

34. Vgontzas AN, Zoumakis E, Bixler EO, Lin H, Follett H, Kales A, et al. Adverse effects of modest sleep restriction on sleepiness, performance, and inflammatory cytokines. J Clin Endocrinol Metab. 2004;89:2119–26.

35. Hare DL, Toukhsati SR, Johansson P, Jaarsma T. Depression and cardiovascular disease: a clinical review. Eur Heart J. 2014;35:1365–72.

25

Gender differences in all-cause, cardiovascular and cancer mortality during long-term follow-up after acute myocardial infarction

Kristin Marie Kvakkestad[1,2], Morten Wang Fagerland[3], Jan Eritsland[1] and Sigrun Halvorsen[1,2*]

Abstract

Background: Gender differences in short-term mortality in acute myocardial infarction (AMI) have been studied extensively, whereas gender differences in long-term mortality and cause of death largely remain unknown. The aim of this study was to assess the long-term risk of all-cause, cardiovascular and cancer death after AMI in women compared to men.

Methods: Consecutive AMI patients were enrolled in a prospective registry between 2005 and 2011. Date and cause of death were obtained by linkage with the Norwegian Cause of Death Registry, with censoring date 31 December 2012. AMI patients with ST-segment elevation (STEMI, $n = 5159$) and without (NSTEMI, $n = 4899$) were analysed separately.

Results: The 5-years all-cause mortality rates in STEMI were 29% in women vs. 17% in men, and 42% vs. 29% in NSTEMI, respectively. After adjustment for age and other confounders, women with STEMI had similar (HR 1.13 [95% CI: 0.98–1.32]) and women with NSTEMI lower (HR 0.82 [95% CI: 0.73–0.92]) risk of long-term all-cause mortality compared to men. Competing-risks analysis showed no significant gender differences in age-adjusted risk of cardiovascular death nor of cancer death. In both genders, the annual risk of cardiovascular death was low after 1 year, but exceeded annual risk of cancer death throughout follow-up.

Conclusion: During long-term follow-up, women with STEMI had similar and women with NSTEMI lower adjusted risk of all-cause mortality compared to men. Age-adjusted risk of death due to cardiovascular disease was similar in both genders and higher than risk of death due to cancer throughout the follow-up period.

Keywords: Myocardial infarction, Women, Gender, Cardiovascular mortality, Cancer mortality

Background

Several studies have shown a higher risk of short-term mortality after acute myocardial infarction (AMI) in women compared to men [1–4], particularly among younger women with ST-segment elevation myocardial infarction (STEMI) [5–7]. Gender differences in survival are observed also in AMI populations treated with per-cutaneous coronary intervention (PCI) [8, 9]. In other studies, the adjustment for age, cardiovascular (CV) risk factors and treatment have attenuated or eliminated the excess female risk of all-cause mortality [2, 10–13]. Thus, whether or not the underuse of evidence-based treatment can explain the higher mortality in women is an unsettled question.

Little is known about gender differences in all-cause mortality during long-term follow-up of AMI patients (>1 year). Furthermore, causes of death are sparsely documented. A recent study found a temporal switch from predominantly cardiac to non-cardiac causes of death after PCI over two decades [14]. Another observational study suggested a high risk of cardiac death immediately

* Correspondence: sigrun.h@online.no
[1]Department of Cardiology, Oslo University Hospital Ulleval, Postboks 4950 Nydalen, 0424 Oslo, Norway
[2]University of Oslo, Postboks 1072 Blindern, 0316 Oslo, Norway
Full list of author information is available at the end of the article

after STEMI, but the risk of death from non-cardiac causes such as cancer increased later during follow-up [15]. Still, a prolonged risk of CV events after a myocardial infarction (MI) have been documented [16], but whether gender differences in causes of death exist during long-term follow-up after AMI is unknown.

The aim of our study was to assess the risk of all-cause mortality in women compared to men during long-term follow-up after AMI, and to study whether there are gender differences in CV and cancer mortality.

Methods

Study population

All consecutive AMI patients admitted to Oslo University Hospital (OUH) Ulleval between 1 September 2005 and 31 December 2011 were included in a local AMI registry. Patients were referred to our tertiary centre, with a 24/7 service for PCI, from the region of South-Eastern Norway. The source population and method of registration has been described previously [17]. In brief, all patients admitted to OUH Ulleval alive or with on-going cardiopulmonary resuscitation and diagnosed with AMI were included in the study. The diagnosis of AMI was based on current international criteria [18]. Patients were categorised as STEMI or non-STEMI (NSTEMI) based on their index electrocardiogram (ECG).

Data collection and variables

Predefined variables were registered into a case report form by the responsible physician during hospital admission. Trained study personnel checked the report form for completeness and errors before entering the data into an electronic database. A cross check against the hospital discharge register was performed monthly and missing patients were included if they met the diagnostic criteria for AMI [18]. In a random control sample of 200 registered patients, we found >95% correspondence between registered data and the patient records, except for two variables with estimated 8% erroneous values in the registry that were not included in the regression analyses. The frequency of missing data was <7% for each variable in the registry, except for the 'smoker or ex-smoker' variable with 13% missing values.

Treatment and in-hospital mortality

The decision to perform coronary angiography and PCI was made by the treating physician. Coronary angiograms were registered as normal, with atheromatosis, or with significant stenosis defined as >50% narrowing of the lumen in one main coronary vessel or in multiple vessels (including left main stem stenosis). Relevant in-hospital medications and complications, including all-cause death, were registered.

Follow-up and cause of death

Date and cause of death was obtained by linkage of the local database with the Norwegian Cause of Death Registry containing vital status throughout 2012. Patients were censored if they were alive at the closing date 31 December 2012. Patients who had emigrated at the time of our analyses were censored at the date of last hospital contact ($n = 80$). In the competing-risks analysis of cause-specific mortality, patients were censored if alive at 31 December 2012 or if dead by other causes than the cause-specific analysis. Follow-up time was calculated from admission until censoring or death.

The Norwegian Cause of Death Registry has a 98% coverage of the Norwegian population [19]. For all deaths, a death certificate (paper form IS-1025B) with a logical sequence from the underlying to immediate cause of death must be completed by a doctor. A code from the International Classification of Disease (ICD) system is allocated to the diagnoses in the death certificate. Subsequently the underlying cause of death is identified by the IRIS computer program with the Automated Classification of Medical Entities (ACME) module, or by assessment of a professional coder. CV death was defined as death with underlying diagnoses corresponding to the ICD-10 codes I00-I99, cancer death included cause of death with code C00-C97, and death of other causes included all other underlying causes of death.

Ethics

Establishment of the local AMI registry and conduction of the study was approved by the Privacy Protection Officer at OUH. The Norwegian Data Protection Authority and the Ministry of Health and Care services provided concession for data linkage with the Norwegian Cause of Death Registry, with an exemption from the requirement of patient consent. The study was submitted to the Regional Committee for Medical Research Ethics (REK), South-East. However, the need for ethics approval from REK was waived according to national regulations (Health Personnel Act §29b). Data were anonymized before analysis.

Statistical analyses

This was a single-centre prospective cohort study. Only the patient's first admission between 1 September 2005 and 31 December 2011 was included in each cohort, so the patient was the unit of our analysis. As previous studies found an interaction between gender and type of AMI in relation to mortality [2], we analysed the STEMI and NSTEMI cohorts separately. The primary outcome was all-cause mortality during follow-up, and secondary outcomes were CV and cancer mortality during follow-up.

Differences between women and men in baseline characteristics and treatment were assessed by the Chi-square test for categorical variables and median regression for continuous variables. Odds ratio (OR) of all-cause in-hospital mortality in women compared to men was calculated by logistic regression. Kaplan-Meier survival plots were computed and gender differences in survival assessed with the log-rank test. The crude, age-adjusted and multivariate adjusted hazard ratio (HR) for all-cause mortality in women versus men were calculated by Cox proportional hazards regression. Candidate covariates for the Cox model were age, pre-hospital resuscitation, pre-hospital thrombolysis (STEMI cohort only), previous MI, previous stroke, previous revascularisation, previous peripheral arterial disease, prior hypertension, smoking, diabetes mellitus, coronary angiography, PCI, ventricular tachycardia (VT)/fibrillation (VF) >48 h, cardiogenic shock, atrioventricular block 2nd-3rd degree, atrial fibrillation, heart failure, antibiotic treatment, gastrointestinal bleeding and in-hospital stroke. Smoking was considered an important potential confounder, and with 10% (STEMI) and 15% (NSTEMI) of values missing, we used multiple imputation with 11 predictors assumed to be associated with the smoking variable. We tested for an interaction between continuous age and gender in the multivariate Cox model for all-cause mortality. We also compared the HRs for all-cause mortality in women versus men stratified by age (<70 years vs ≥70 years), with a Wald test. The proportional hazards assumption was assessed by plotting the estimated log-log survival functions for men and women against time.

The cumulative incidence function for the probability of cause-specific mortality was stratified by gender [20]. We created a stacked cumulative incidence plot to show how the total probability of one was allocated between all competing events in women and men, including the possibility of survival during follow-up. The Fine-Gray model [21] was applied to find the underlying sub-distribution hazard ratio (sHR) for competing risks of CV, cancer and other-cause mortality in women versus men during follow-up. The sHRs are not cause-specific hazards, but should be interpreted as a binary increased or decreased probability of cause-specific death when adjusted for covariates [22]. All tests were two-sided and a p-value <0.05 was considered statistically significant. Analyses were performed with STATA 13 (Statacorp LP, Texas, USA). The study confines with the STROBE (STrengthening the Reporting of OBservational studies in Epidemiology) checklist for reporting of observational studies [23].

Results
Study population
Out of 10 747 registered hospital admissions for AMI, we identified 4899 patients with STEMI (median age 63 years, 25% women) and 5159 patients with NSTEMI

(median age 70 years, 34% women) (Fig. 1). Six patients did not fulfill AMI criteria and 677 re-admissions during the period were excluded. Due to typing error in the identification key, six patients could not be linked to the Cause of Death Registry and were lost to follow-up. Baseline characteristics of the population are shown in Table 1.

Treatment and in-hospital mortality
Among STEMI patients, women were less likely to undergo coronary angiography and PCI compared to men, although the percentage receiving angiography was high (>90%) in both genders (Table 2). Women with STEMI were less likely to be treated with antiplatelet therapy, beta-blockers and statins (See Additional file 1: Appendix Table A1). A total of 104/1214 (8.6%) women died in hospital versus 185/3685 (5.0%) of men (OR 1.77 [95% CI: 1.38–2.27]). The gender difference was eliminated after adjustment (age-adjusted OR 1.08 [95% CI: 0.82–1.40]).

In the NSTEMI cohort, women were also less likely to undergo coronary angiography and PCI (Table 2) and less likely to receive treatment with antiplatelets and statins compared to men (See Additional file 1: Appendix Table A1). A total of 109/1776 (6.1%) women and 144/3383 (4.3%) of men died in hospital (OR 1.47 [95% CI: 1.14–1.90]). Again, the gender difference was eliminated after adjustment (age-adjusted OR 0.86 [95% CI: 0.65–1.13]). In-hospital complications are shown in Additional file 2: Appendix Table A2.

Long-term mortality
In the STEMI cohort, 318/1214 (26%) of women and 568/3685 (15%) of men died during a median follow-up of 1262 days (25th-75th percentile [p]: 673–1900). Fig. 2 shows Kaplan-Meier survival plots for women compared to men. The unadjusted HR for all-cause mortality was higher in women compared to men (Fig. 3). After adjustment for age and other confounders, the risk of long-term all-cause mortality was similar in both genders (adjusted HR 1.13 [95% CI: 0.98–1.32]). No gender-age interaction was found (p interaction 0.31).

In the NSTEMI cohort, 631/1776 (36%) of women and 830/3383 (25%) of men died during a median follow-up of 1043 days (25th-75th p: 537–1695, Fig. 2). The unadjusted HR for all-cause mortality was higher in women compared to men, but after adjustment for age and other confounders the risk was lower in women (Fig. 3). No significant interaction was found between continuous age and gender (p interaction 0.052). When stratifying patients into groups <70 and ≥70 years, we found no significant heterogeneity in the association with all-cause mortality (adjusted HR for women versus men <70 years 1.02 [95% CI: 0.77–1.36]; adjusted HR for patients ≥70 years 0.79 [95% CI: 0.70–0.90], p = 0.11). The log-log estimated survival curves

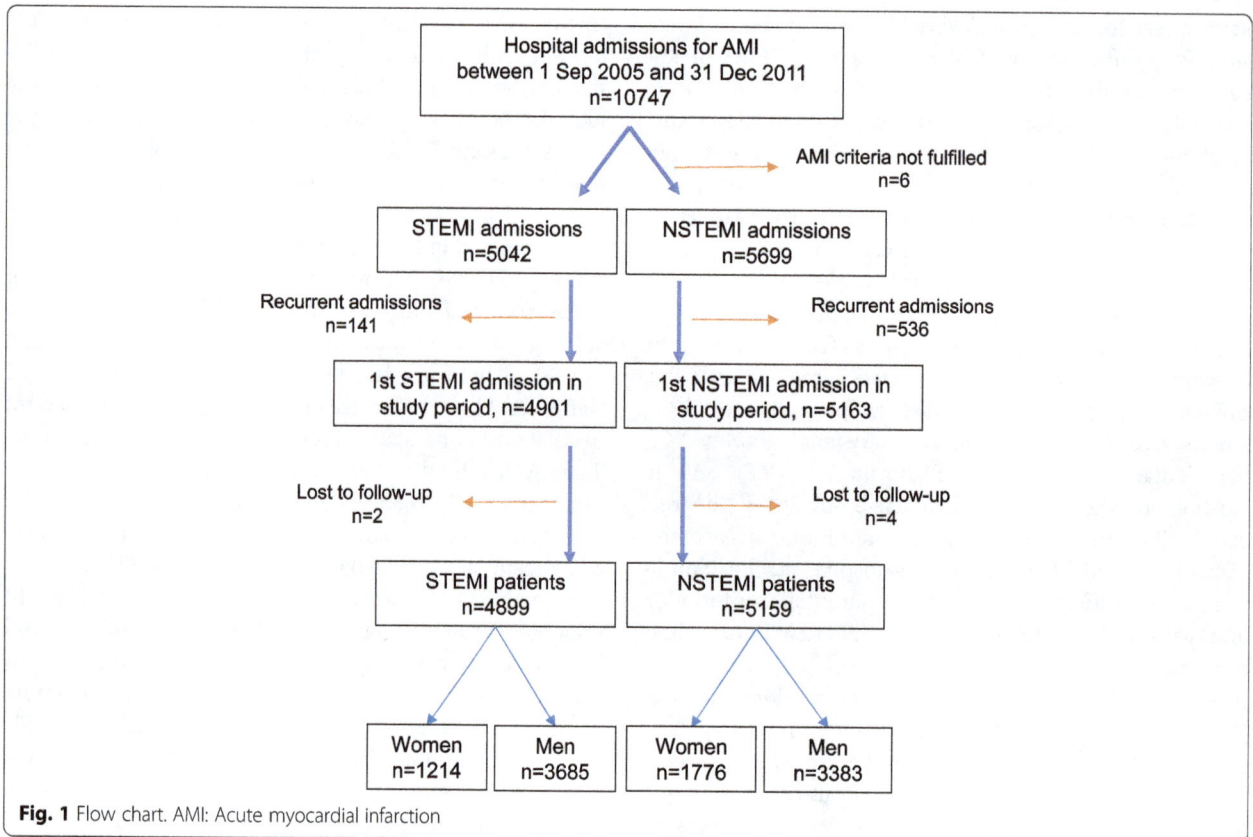

Fig. 1 Flow chart. AMI: Acute myocardial infarction

for men and women were roughly parallel for both STEMI and NSTEMI patients, thus the proportional hazards assumption was regarded valid.

Cause specific mortality

Among the 886 STEMI patients who died, CV disease was the cause of death in 67% of patients. Ten percent of women and 15% of men who died, died of cancer. Figure 4 illustrates the stacked cumulative incidence of CV, cancer and other causes of death as a function of time and shows the relationship between the competing causes of death. The calculated sHR confirms the ordering of the cumulative incidence function-plot; women with STEMI were at higher risk of CV mortality than men, but

Table 1 Baseline characteristics

	STEMI N = 4899			NSTEMI N = 5159		
	Women $n = 1214$	Men $n = 3685$	p-value	Women $n = 1776$	Men $n = 3383$	p-value
Age, years[a]	71 (60–80)	61 (53–70)	<0.0001	77 (65–85)	67 (57–77)	<0.0001
Smoker/ex-smoker, n (%)[b]	642 (62.0)	2344 (69.8)	<0.0001	731 (51.0)	1949 (66.1)	<0.0001
Diabetes mellitus, n (%)[b]	163 (13.4)	465 (12.6)	0.469	323 (18.2)	659 (19.5)	0.246
Previous hyperlipidemia, n (%)[b,c]	148 (12.2)	421 (11.5)	0.468	207 (11.7)	461 (13.7)	0.041
Previous hypertension, n (%)[b]	521 (42.9)	1163 (31.6)	<0.0001	892 (50.2)	1320 (39.0)	<0.0001
Previous MI, n (%)[b]	145 (11.9)	492 (13.4)	0.198	439 (24.7)	956 (28.3)	0.006
Previous PCI or CABG, n (%)[b]	87 (7.2)	428 (11.6)	<0.0001	267 (15.0)	838 (24.8)	<0.0001
Previous stroke, n (%)[b]	95 (7.8)	183 (5.0)	0.0002	231 (13.0)	341 (10.1)	0.002
Family history, n (%)[b,d]	160 (13.3)	606 (16.4)	0.007	158 (8.9)	438 (13.0)	<0.0001
Peripheral artery disease, n (%)[b]	60 (4.9)	143 (3.9)	0.112	121 (6.8)	258 (7.6)	0.276

MI Myocardial infarction, *PCI* Percutaneous coronary intervention, *CABG* Coronary artery bypass grafting
[a] median (25th-75th percentile)
[b] (%) = percent of patients with available information, denominator may vary
[c] Hyperlipidemia defined as treatment with lipid-lowering drugs at time of admission
[d] Coronary artery disease before age 65 years in women, 55 years in men in 1st order relatives

Table 2 Treatment

	STEMI $N = 4899$			NSTEMI $N = 5159$		
	Women $n = 1214$	Men $n = 3685$	p-value	Women $n = 1776$	Men $n = 3383$	p-value
Pre-hospital thrombolysis, n (%)[a]	105 (8.6)	429 (11.7)	0.004	-	-	-
Coronary angiography, n (%)	1115 (91.9)	3591 (97.5)	<0.0001	1200 (67.6)	2925 (86.5)	<0.0001
Normal vessels, n (%)[b]	21 (1.9)	52 (1.5)	0.307	157 (13.2)	114 (3.9)	<0.0001
Atheromatosis, n (%)[b]	23 (1.9)	48 (1.3)	0.083	126 (10.6)	136 (4.7)	<0.0001
One-vessel disease, n (%)[b]	539 (48.4)	1630 (45.5)	0.086	396 (33.2)	1145 (39.4)	0.0002
Multiple-vessel or LMS disease, n (%)[b]	530 (47.6)	1853 (51.9)	0.017	512 (43.0)	1513 (52.0)	<0.0001
Missing angiogram, n (%)[b]	2 (0.2)	8 (0.2)	NS	8 (0.7)	17 (0.6)	NS
Primary PCI, n (%)[c]	808 (66.5)	2653 (72.0)	0.0003	-	-	-
All PCI, n (%)	936 (77.0)	3160 (85.7)	<0.0001	524 (29.5)	1598 (47.2)	<0.0001
CABG, n (%)	37 (3.0)	187 (5.1)	0.003	109 (6.1)	423 (12.5)	<0.0001
Door to balloon-time, minutes[d]	38 (29–55)	36 (29–52)	0.043	-	-	-
Symptom to balloon-time, minutes[d]	270 (170–495)	245 (155–456)	0.001	-	-	-
Symptom to angiography, days[d]	-	-	-	2 (1–4)	2 (1–4)	<0.0001

LMS Left main stem, *PCI* percutaneous coronary intervention, *CABG* Coronary artery bypass grafting

(%) = percent of patients with available information, denominator may vary

[a] Pre-hospital or in local hospital

[b] among patients who underwent coronary angiography

[c] PCI ≤ 12 h from onset of symptoms, without prior thrombolysis

[d] median (25th–75th percentile)

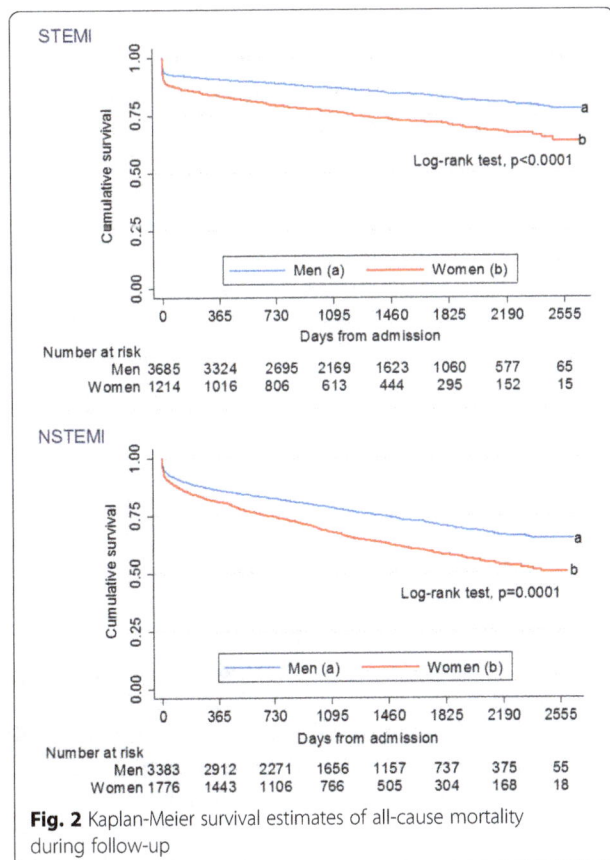

Fig. 2 Kaplan-Meier survival estimates of all-cause mortality during follow-up

the risk of cancer mortality was similar for both genders during follow-up. After adjustment for age, we found no gender differences in risk of CV nor cancer mortality during follow-up (Table 3).

Among the 1461 NSTEMI patients who died, CV disease was the cause of death in 58% of women and 54% of men, while cancer was the cause of death in 12% of women and 17% of men. Figure 4 illustrates the relationship between the competing causes of death in NSTEMI patients. After adjustment for age, there were no significant gender differences in risk of CV mortality, but a nonsignificant reduction of cancer mortality risk in women (sHR 0.76 [95% CI: 0.56–1.03], $p = 0.072$) (Table 3).

In both STEMI and NSTEMI patients the risk of death was highest the first year after AMI (Table 4). After 1 year, the annual CV mortality rate in STEMI was <2.5% in women and <1.5% in men. In NSTEMI patients, the annual CV mortality rate after 1 year was <4.5% in women and <2.5% in men (Table 4). Furthermore, annual CV mortality was higher than annual cancer mortality in both genders throughout the follow-up period (Fig. 4 and Table 4).

Discussion

In this long-term follow-up of a large AMI cohort, the main findings were: 1) Women with STEMI had similar and women with NSTEMI better long-term survival compared to men, when controlling for age and other confounding factors. 2) There were no significant gender

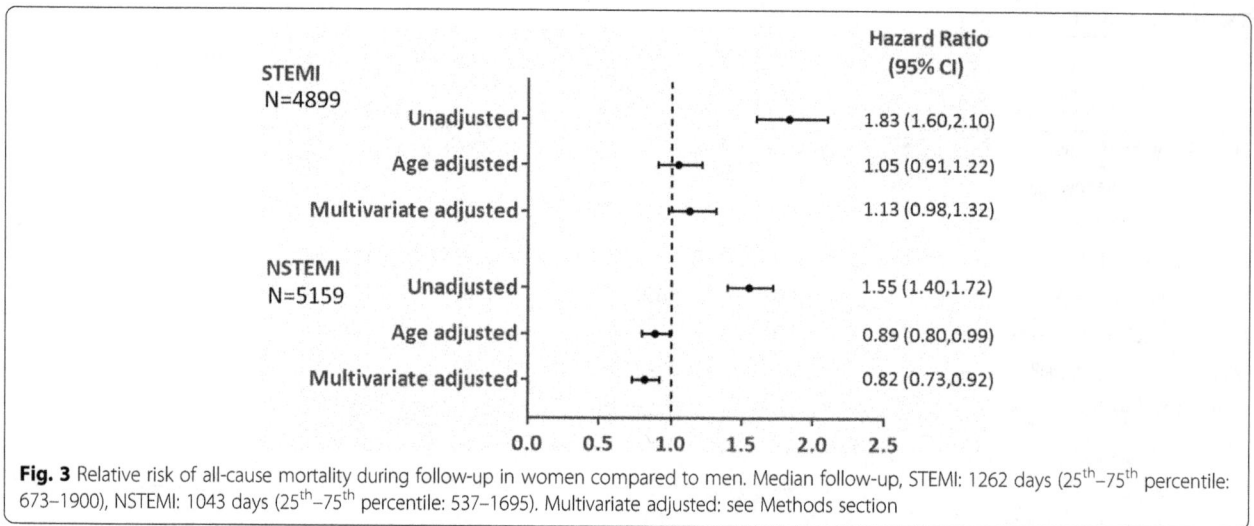

Fig. 3 Relative risk of all-cause mortality during follow-up in women compared to men. Median follow-up, STEMI: 1262 days (25th–75th percentile: 673–1900), NSTEMI: 1043 days (25th–75th percentile: 537–1695). Multivariate adjusted: see Methods section

differences in age-adjusted risk of CV nor cancer mortality.

Long-term follow-up studies after AMI (>1 year) are scarce, but needed. During seven years of follow-up, we show a similar age-adjusted risk of death among women and men with STEMI. A high proportion of both genders were treated invasively, probably contributing to the similar long-term prognosis. These results are in accordance with a recent report from Italy showing similar 1-year mortality for women and men with STEMI [12]. However, other studies of STEMI patients selected for PCI have reported a worse 1-year prognosis in women compared to men, even after adjustment for age and other confounders [8, 9].

Women with NSTEMI had 18% lower risk of long-term death compared to men, after multivariate adjustment. Lower risk in women was found already after age-adjustment, suggesting that age is the most important confounding factor when comparing long-term survival in NSTEMI women versus men. Our results correspond well with data from Sweden, confirming a 1-year survival benefit in NSTEMI women treated during 1998–2002 [24], but contradict several previous studies reporting no gender differences in risk estimates of mortality among NSTEMI patients [12, 13, 25, 26]. These studies differ with regard to study population, study period and confounding factors considered, and a comparison is not straightforward. In general, our study reflects contemporary treatment with a frequent use of invasive treatment also in women, and a much longer follow-up than most other studies. Explanations for better long-term survival in NSTEMI women could be awareness of gender differences in presentation and treatment of AMI resulting in equal opportunities for women and men [27], less extensive coronary artery disease [28] or lower

general risk burden compared to their male counterparts [29]. Among NSTEMI women in our study, normal vessels or non-significant coronary artery disease were more prevalent than in men and gender differences in treatment during hospitalization were present. Gender differences potentially exist in complete versus non-complete revascularization, drug prescription patterns, such as duration of dual antiplatelet therapy, drug compliance, and clinical follow-up influencing prognosis. Information about these factors were not available in our study, but should be included in future studies of long-term outcomes in women and men after AMI.

To our knowledge, this is the first study to elucidate the relationship between gender and risk of cause-specific mortality in an unselected AMI population. Especially in ageing clinical cohorts, an increased risk of non-CV death could influence the long-term prognosis after AMI. We did not find any significant gender differences in long-term CV mortality after adjustment for age. After 1 year, the annual CV death rate in STEMI patients in our study was low (<1.5% in men and <2.5% in women), but still higher than the annual cancer death rate throughout the follow-up period. Our results correspond to the results from a Danish study of PCI-treated STEMI patients (mean age 63 years), finding that cardiac risk beyond 30 days post-STEMI was low (<1.5% per year) [15]. In a recent report from Sweden, AMI patients (median age 74 years) who survived 1 year had a 20% risk of non-fatal MI, stroke or CV death during the next 36 months [16]. These studies along with our results all confirm a long-term risk of CV mortality and a continued need for focusing on secondary prevention measures among AMI patients of both genders.

Our finding of a non-significant tendency towards lower age-adjusted cancer mortality in NSTEMI women

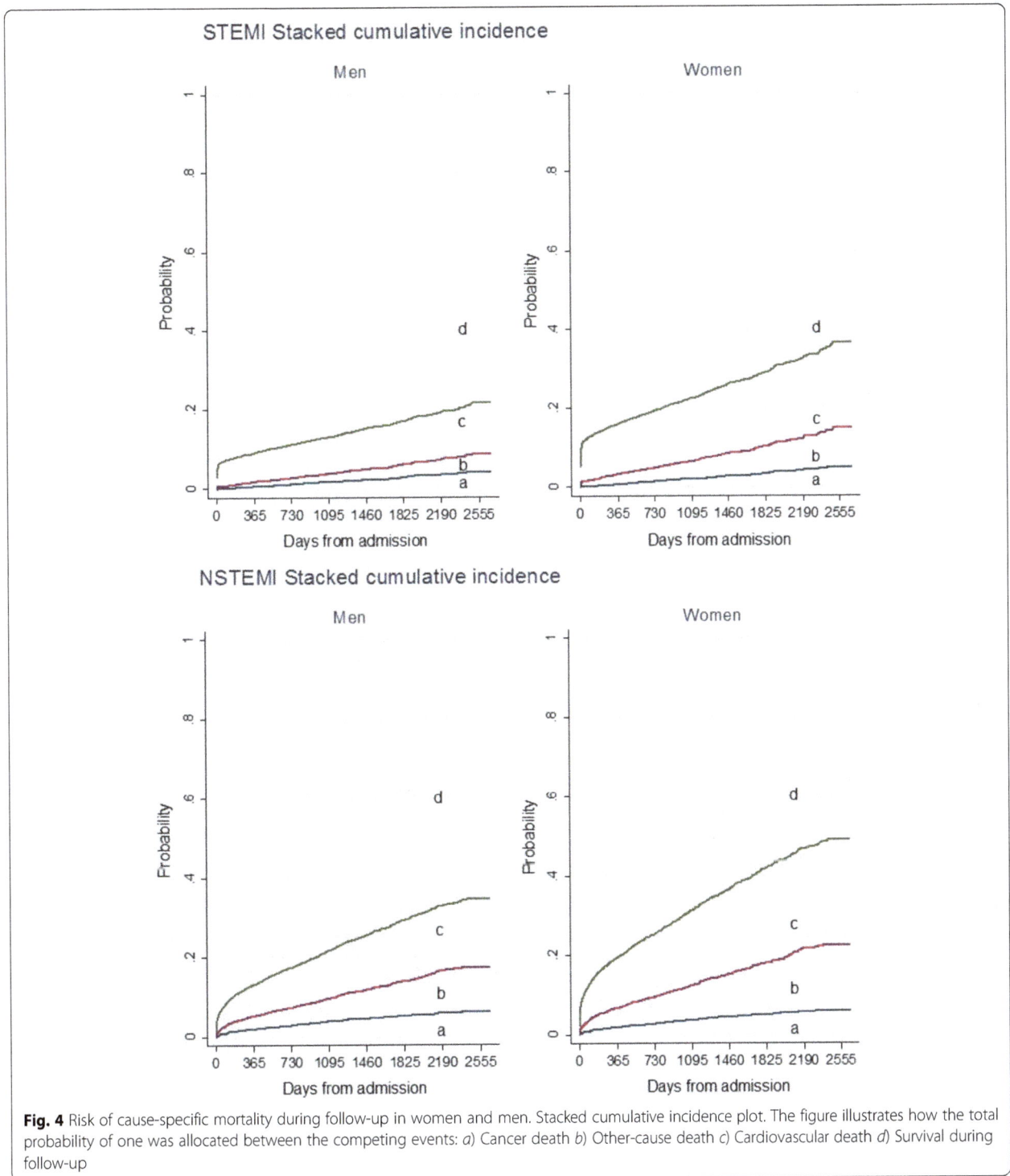

Fig. 4 Risk of cause-specific mortality during follow-up in women and men. Stacked cumulative incidence plot. The figure illustrates how the total probability of one was allocated between the competing events: *a*) Cancer death *b*) Other-cause death *c*) Cardiovascular death *d*) Survival during follow-up

compared to men needs further investigation. In Norway and Europe, men experience a higher risk of death from cancer compared to women [30, 31], and our results could reflect a higher incidence of and mortality from cancer in men diagnosed with AMI. The results of the present study must be interpreted with caution due to few cancer deaths and the relatively short follow-up period in the setting of a non-cancer cohort. Further studies are needed to register the prevalence and type of cancer in AMI patients, and should be powered to evaluate the risk of cancer death competing with cardiac death during long-term follow-up.

Table 3 Competing risks regression. Sub-distribution hazard ratios of cause-specific mortality during follow-up

	Unadjusted SHR (95% CI)	p-value	Age-adjusted SHR (95% CI)	p-value
STEMI n = 4899				
Cardiovascular death				
Women versus men	1.76 (1.49–2.08)	<0.0001	1.03 (0.87–1.22)	0.750
Cancer death				
Women versus men	1.20 (0.80–1.79)	0.378	0.79 (0.51–1.22)	0.286
Other-cause death				
Women versus men	2.21 (1.63–2.99)	<0.0001	1.26 (0.91–1.74)	0.171
NSTEMI n = 5159				
Cardiovascular death				
Women versus men	1.63 (1.42–1.87)	<0.0001	0.97 (0.84–1.12)	0.659
Cancer death				
Women versus men	0.97 (0.74–1.29)	0.852	0.76 (0.56–1.03)	0.072
Other-cause death				
Women versus men	1.52 (1.26–1.84)	<0.0001	0.90 (0.74–1.10)	0.308

SHR Sub-distribution hazard ratio, CI Confidence interval

The strengths of our study is a complete follow-up of unselected AMI patients during a 7-year period. We investigated three categories of cause of death, giving a more detailed description of mortality after AMI. We provide a descriptive analysis that indicate contemporary equal opportunities for women and men treated with AMI. Limitations were that several comorbid conditions, such as cancer, renal disease, dementia, autoimmune- and pulmonary diseases were not registered at inclusion, and may have confounded mortality risk. Heart rate and blood pressure was not registered. Follow-up did not include quality of life or physical performance, which are important measures of outcome after AMI. The causes

of death in this study were not determined by autopsy, the gold standard for identifying the cause of death. Finally, this was a single centre study from the largest university hospital in Norway, being a referral hospital for 1.5 million people in Eastern Norway. However, the results are not necessarily generalizable to other populations.

Conclusion

After adjustment for age and other confounding factors, women with STEMI had similar and women with NSTEMI had better long-term prognosis compared to

Table 4 Cumulative mortality during follow-up stratified by gender (Life table method)

	All-cause mortality % (95% CI)		Cardiovascular mortality % (95% CI)		Cancer mortality % (95% CI)	
STEMI[a]	Women	Men	Women	Men	Women	Men
1 year	16.2 (14.3–18.4)	9.2 (8.3–10.1)	12.9 (11.1–15.0)	7.6 (6.8–8.5)	0.7 (0.4–1.4)	0.6 (0.4–0.9)
2 years	20.4 (18.2–22.8)	10.9 (10.0–12.0)	15.1 (13.2–17.3)	8.6 (7.7–9.5)	2.0 (1.3–3.1)	1.1 (0.8–1.5)
3 years	23.0 (20.7–25.6)	13.0 (12.0–14.2)	16.4 (14.4–18.7)	9.6 (8.7–10.6)	2.8 (1.9–4.2)	1.7 (1.3–2.2)
4 years	26.4 (23.8–29.2)	15.3 (14.1–16.6)	18.4 (16.2–20.9)	10.5 (9.5–11.6)	3.6 (2.5–5.1)	2.4 (1.9–3.0)
5 years	28.6 (25.8–31.6)	17.1 (15.8–18.6)	19.5 (17.1–22.2)	11.3 (10.2–12.5)	3.8 (2.7–5.5)	3.0 (2.4–3.8)
NSTEMI[b]	Women	Men	Women	Men	Women	Men
1 year	18.6 (16.9–20.5)	13.6 (12.5–14.8)	12.5 (11.0–14.2)	8.4 (7.5–9.4)	2.0 (1.4–2.8)	2.0 (1.6–2.6)
2 years	25.2 (23.2–27.3)	17.3 (16.0–18.6)	16.2 (14.5–18.0)	10.6 (9.6–11.7)	3.5 (2.7–4.6)	2.8 (2.3–3.5)
3 years	31.9 (29.6–34.2)	21.3 (19.9–22.8)	20.4 (18.5–22.6)	12.4 (11.2–13.6)	4.7 (3.7–6.0)	4.0 (3.3–4.9)
4 years	36.7 (34.3–39.3)	25.2 (23.6–26.8)	23.3 (21.1–25.6)	14.3 (13.0–15.7)	5.5 (4.3–7.0)	5.0 (4.2–6.0)
5 years	42.0 (39.2–44.9)	29.3 (27.5–31.2)	26.2 (23.7–29.0)	16.4 (14.9–18.0)	5.7 (4.5–7.3)	6.3 (5.2–7.5)

CI Confidence interval
[a]Women n = 1214. Men n = 3685. Median (25th-75th percentile) follow-up: 1262 (673–1900) days
[b]Women n = 1776. Men n = 3383. Median (25th-75th percentile) follow-up: 1043 (537–1695) days

men. There were no significant gender differences in risk of CV nor cancer death during follow-up. After one year, annual risk of CV death in both genders was low, but still exceeded annual risk of death due to cancer. Possible gender differences in long-term risk of cancer death in AMI patients need further investigation.

Abbreviations
ACME: Automated Classification of Medical Entities; AMI: Acute myocardial infarction; CABG: Coronary artery bypass grafting; CI: Confidence interval; CV: Cardiovascular; ECG: Electrocardiogram; HR: Hazard ratio; ICD: International Classification of Disease; MI: Myocardial infarction; NSTEMI: Non ST-segment elevation myocardial infarction; OR: Odds ratio; OUH: Oslo University Hospital; PCI: Percutaneous coronary intervention; sHR: Sub-distribution hazard ratio; STEMI: ST-segment elevation myocardial infarction; VF: Ventricular fibrillation; VT: Ventricular tachycardia

Acknowledgements
The authors wish to thank the physicians at the Department of Cardiology, OUH Ulleval, for data collection, and the study personnel Charlotte Holst Hansen and Monica Ziener for data registration and quality control. We thank the Mid-Norway Regional Health Authority for supplying the electronic database, and the Norwegian Cause of Death registry for mortality data.

Funding
Funded by grant number 2013028 from the Scientific Board of the Southeastern Norway Regional Health Authority, Hamar, Norway.

Authors' contributions
KMK validated the data used in this study, took part in data interpretation and the statistical analyses, and drafted the manuscript. MWF was responsible for the statistical analyses of the study and participated in drafting of the manuscript. JE took part in the collection and registration of data, and in drafting of the manuscript. SH had the original idea of the study, organised the collection, registration and validation of data, participated in data interpretation and in preparation of the manuscript. All authors read and approved the final manuscript.

Competing interests
The authors declare that they have no competing interests.

Ethics approval and consent to participate
Establishment of the local AMI registry and conduction of the study was approved by the OUH Privacy Protection Officer. The establishment of a local health registry without patient consent, was based solely on information registered in the patient's medical records, and was done according to national regulations (Health Personnel Act § 26). The Norwegian Data Protection Authority (reference number 2011/18312) and the Ministry of Health and Care services (letter of 16 November 2011) provided concession for data handling and data linkage with the Norwegian Cause of Death Registry, with an exemption from the requirement of patient consent. Furthermore, the study was submitted to the Regional committee for medical and health research ethics (REK), region South-East. REK South-East found the study to be a quality of care project, thus the need for ethics approval from REK was waived according to national regulations (Health Personnel Act §29b). All data were anonymized before analysis.

Author details
[1]Department of Cardiology, Oslo University Hospital Ulleval, Postboks 4950 Nydalen, 0424 Oslo, Norway. [2]University of Oslo, Postboks 1072 Blindern, 0316 Oslo, Norway. [3]Oslo Centre for Biostatistics and Epidemiology, Research Support Services, Postboks 1110 Blindern, 0317 Oslo, Norway.

References
1. Simon T, Mary-Krause M, Cambou JP, Hanania G, Gueret P, Lablanche JM, et al. Impact of age and gender on in-hospital and late mortality after acute myocardial infarction: increased early risk in younger women: results from the French nation-wide USIC registries. Eur Heart J. 2006;27:1282–88.
2. Berger JS, Elliott L, Gallup D, Roe M, Granger CB, Armstrong PW, et al. Sex differences in mortality following acute coronary syndromes. JAMA. 2009; 302:874–82.
3. Lawesson SS, Alfredsson J, Fredrikson M, Swahn E. A gender perspective on short- and long term mortality in ST-elevation myocardial infarction–a report from the SWEDEHEART register. Int J Cardiol. 2013;168:1041–47.
4. Bonarjee VV, Rosengren A, Snapinn SM, James MK, Dickstein K. Sex-based short- and long-term survival in patients following complicated myocardial infarction. Eur Heart J. 2006;27:2177–83.
5. Vaccarino V, Parsons L, Every NR, Barron HV, Krumholz HM. Sex-based differences in early mortality after myocardial infarction. National Registry of Myocardial Infarction 2 Participants. N Engl J Med. 1999;341:217–25.
6. Champney KP, Frederick PD, Bueno H, Parashar S, Foody J, Merz CN, et al. The joint contribution of sex, age and type of myocardial infarction on hospital mortality following acute myocardial infarction. Heart. 2009;95:895–99.
7. Lawesson SS, Stenestrand U, Lagerqvist B, Wallentin L, Swahn E. Gender perspective on risk factors, coronary lesions and long-term outcome in young patients with ST-elevation myocardial infarction. Heart. 2010;96:453–59.
8. Otten AM, Maas AH, Ottervanger JP, Kloosterman A, Hof AW v't, Dambrink JH, et al. Is the difference in outcome between men and women treated by primary percutaneous coronary intervention age dependent? Gender difference in STEMI stratified on age. Eur Heart J Acute Cardiovasc Care. 2013;2:334–41.
9. de Boer SP, Roos-Hesselink JW, van Leeuwen MA, Lenzen MJ, van Geuns RJ, Regar E, et al. Excess mortality in women compared to men after PCI in STEMI: an analysis of 11,931 patients during 2000–2009. Int J Cardiol. 2014; 176:456–63.
10. Hess CN, McCoy LA, Duggirala HJ, Tavris DR, O'Callaghan K, Douglas PS, Peterson ED, Wang TY. Sex-based differences in outcomes after percutaneous coronary intervention for acute myocardial infarction: a report from TRANSLATE-ACS. J Am Heart Assoc. 2014;3:e000523. doi:10.1161/JAHA.113.000523.
11. Blomkalns AL, Chen AY, Hochman JS, Peterson ED, Trynosky K, Diercks DB, et al. Gender disparities in the diagnosis and treatment of non-ST-segment elevation acute coronary syndromes: large-scale observations from the CRUSADE (Can Rapid Risk Stratification of Unstable Angina Patients Suppress Adverse Outcomes With Early Implementation of the American College of Cardiology/American Heart Association Guidelines) National Quality Improvement Initiative. J Am Coll Cardiol. 2005;45:832–37.
12. Gnavi R, Rusciani R, Dalmasso M, Giammaria M, Anselmino M, Roggeri DP, et al. Gender, socioeconomic position, revascularization procedures and mortality in patients presenting with STEMI and NSTEMI in the era of primary PCI. Differences or inequities? Int J Cardiol. 2014;176:724–30.
13. Halvorsen S, Eritsland J, Abdelnoor M, Holst Hansen C, Risoe C, Midtbo K, et al. Gender differences in management and outcome of acute myocardial infarctions treated in 2006–2007. Cardiology. 2009;114:83–8.
14. Spoon DB, Psaltis PJ, Singh M, Holmes Jr DR, Gersh BJ, Rihal CS, et al. Trends in cause of death after percutaneous coronary intervention. Circulation. 2014;129:1286–94.
15. Pedersen F, Butrymovich V, Kelbaek H, Wachtell K, Helqvist S, Kastrup J, et al. Short- and long-term cause of death in patients treated with primary PCI for STEMI. J Am Coll Cardiol. 2014;64:2101–08.
16. Jernberg T, Hasvold P, Henriksson M, Hjelm H, Thuresson M, Janzon M. Cardiovascular risk in post-myocardial infarction patients: nationwide real world data demonstrate the importance of a long-term perspective. Eur Heart J. 2015;36:1163–70.

17. Kvakkestad KM, Abdelnoor M, Claussen PA, Eritsland J, Fossum E, Halvorsen S. Long-term survival in octogenarians and older patients with ST-elevation myocardial infarction in the era of primary angioplasty: a prospective cohort study. Eur Heart J Acute Cardiovasc Care. 2016;5:243–52.

18. Thygesen K, Alpert JS, Joint ESC/ACCF/AHA/WHF Task Force for the Redefinition of Myocardial Infarction, White HD, Jaffe AS, Apple FS, Galvani M, et al. Universal definition of myocardial infarction. Eur Heart J. 2007; 28:2525–38.

19. Pedersen AG, Ellingsen CL. Data quality in the causes of death registry. Tidsskr Nor Laegeforen. 2015;135:768–70.

20. Competing risks. In: Cleves M, GouldW, Guiterrez RG, Marchenko YV: An introduction to survival analysis using STATA. 3rd ed. Stata press. 2010; pp.365-91.

21. Fine JP, Gray RJ. A proportional hazards model for the subdistribution of a competing risk. J Am Stat Assoc. 1999;94:496–509.

22. German R. Cumulative incidence. 2012. http://data.princeton.edu/pop509/cumulativeIncidence.pdf. Accessed 9 Mar 2017.

23. STROBE Initiative. STrengthening the Reporting of OBservational studies in Epidemiology (STROBE) Checklist. ISPM University of Bern. 2007. http://strobe-statement.org/index.php?id=available-checklists. Accessed 9 Mar 2017.

24. Alfredsson J, Stenestrand U, Wallentin L, Swahn E. Gender differences in management and outcome in non-ST-elevation acute coronary syndrome. Heart. 2007;93:1357–62.

25. Vikman S, Airaksinen KE, Tierala I, Peuhkurinen K, Majamaa-Voltti K, Niemela M, et al. Gender-related differences in the management of non-ST-elevation acute coronary syndrome patients. Scand Cardiovasc J. 2007;41:287–93.

26. Alfredsson J, Lindback J, Wallentin L, Swahn E. Similar outcome with an invasive strategy in men and women with non-ST-elevation acute coronary syndromes: from the Swedish Web-System for Enhancement and Development of Evidence-Based Care in Heart Disease Evaluated According to Recommended Therapies (SWEDEHEART). Eur Heart J. 2011;32:3128–36.

27. Mollmann H, Liebetrau C, Nef HM, Hamm CW. The Swedish paradox: or is there really no gender difference in acute coronary syndromes? Eur Heart J. 2011;32:3070–72.

28. Merz CN. The Yentl syndrome is alive and well. Eur Heart J. 2011;32:1313–15.

29. Mozaffarian D, Benjamin EJ, Go AS, Arnett DK, Blaha MJ, Cushman M, et al. Heart disease and stroke statistics–2015 update: a report from the American Heart Association. Circulation. 2015;131:e29–322. doi:10.1161/CIR.0000000000000152.

30. Norwegian Institute of Public Health. Cancer mortality in Norway - fact sheet 2009. 2015 http://www.fhi.no/en/mp/chronic-diseases/cancer/cancer-mortality-in-norway—fact-s/. Accessed 9 Mar 2017.

31. Townsend N, Nichols M, Scarborough P, Rayner M. Cardiovascular disease in Europe–epidemiological update 2015. Eur Heart J. 2015;36:2696–705.

Permissions

All chapters in this book were first published in CD, by BioMed Central; hereby published with permission under the Creative Commons Attribution License or equivalent. Every chapter published in this book has been scrutinized by our experts. Their significance has been extensively debated. The topics covered herein carry significant findings which will fuel the growth of the discipline. They may even be implemented as practical applications or may be referred to as a beginning point for another development.

The contributors of this book come from diverse backgrounds, making this book a truly international effort. This book will bring forth new frontiers with its revolutionizing research information and detailed analysis of the nascent developments around the world.

We would like to thank all the contributing authors for lending their expertise to make the book truly unique. They have played a crucial role in the development of this book. Without their invaluable contributions this book wouldn't have been possible. They have made vital efforts to compile up to date information on the varied aspects of this subject to make this book a valuable addition to the collection of many professionals and students.

This book was conceptualized with the vision of imparting up-to-date information and advanced data in this field. To ensure the same, a matchless editorial board was set up. Every individual on the board went through rigorous rounds of assessment to prove their worth. After which they invested a large part of their time researching and compiling the most relevant data for our readers.

The editorial board has been involved in producing this book since its inception. They have spent rigorous hours researching and exploring the diverse topics which have resulted in the successful publishing of this book. They have passed on their knowledge of decades through this book. To expedite this challenging task, the publisher supported the team at every step. A small team of assistant editors was also appointed to further simplify the editing procedure and attain best results for the readers.

Apart from the editorial board, the designing team has also invested a significant amount of their time in understanding the subject and creating the most relevant covers. They scrutinized every image to scout for the most suitable representation of the subject and create an appropriate cover for the book.

The publishing team has been an ardent support to the editorial, designing and production team. Their endless efforts to recruit the best for this project, has resulted in the accomplishment of this book. They are a veteran in the field of academics and their pool of knowledge is as vast as their experience in printing. Their expertise and guidance has proved useful at every step. Their uncompromising quality standards have made this book an exceptional effort. Their encouragement from time to time has been an inspiration for everyone.

The publisher and the editorial board hope that this book will prove to be a valuable piece of knowledge for researchers, students, practitioners and scholars across the globe.

List of Contributors

Heidi Borgeraas, Jens Kristoffer Hertel and Jøran Hjelmesaeth
Morbid Obesity Center, Vestfold Hospital Trust, Tønsberg, Norway

Heidi Borgeraas and Jøran Hjelmesæth
Institute of Clinical Medicine, University of Oslo, Oslo, Norway

Heidi Borgeraas, Gard Frodahl Tveitevåg Svingen, Eva Kristine Ringdal Pedersen and Ottar Nygård
Department of Clinical Science, University of Bergen, Bergen, Norway

Reinhard Seifert, Hall Schartum-Hansen and Ottar Nygård
Department of Heart Disease, Haukeland University Hospital, Bergen, Norway

Ute Amann, Inge Kirchberger, Margit Heier and Christa Meisinger
MONICA/KORA Myocardial Infarction Registry, Central Hospital of Augsburg, Stenglinstr. 2, 86156 Augsburg, Germany

Ute Amann, Inge Kirchberger, Margit Heier, Annette Peters and Christa Meisinger
Institute of Epidemiology II, Helmholtz Zentrum München, German Research Center for Environmental Health (GmbH), Neuherberg, Germany

Christian Thilo and Bernhard Kuch
Department of Internal Medicine I - Cardiology, Central Hospital of Augsburg, Augsburg, Germany

Bernhard Kuch
Department of Internal Medicine/Cardiology, Hospital of Nördlingen, Nördlingen, Germany

Kymberley Thorne, John G. Williams, Ashley Akbari and Stephen E. Roberts
College of Medicine, Swansea University, Singleton Park, Swansea SA2 8PP, UK

Guo Dai, Qing Xu, Rong Luo, Jianfang Gao, Hui Chen, Yun Deng, Yongqing Li, Yuequn Wang, Wuzhou Yuan and Xiushan Wu
The Center for Heart Development, Key Laboratory of MOE for Developmental Biology and Protein Chemistry, College of Life Sciences, Hunan Normal University, Changsha, Hunan 410081, P. R. China

Xiushan Wu
The Center for Heart Development, Hunan Normal University, Changsha 410081, Hunan, P. R. China

George Mnatzaganian
School of Allied Health, Faculty of Health Sciences, Australian Catholic University, Fitzroy, Victoria 3065, Australia

George Braitberg
Department of Medicine, The University of Melbourne, Parkville, Victoria 3010, Australia
Department of Emergency Medicine, Royal Melbourne Hospital, Parkville, Victoria 3010, Australia.

Janet E. Hiller
School of Health Sciences, Faculty of Health, Arts and Design, Swinburne University of Technology, Hawthorn, Victoria 3122, Australia
Discipline of Public Health, School of Population Health, The University of Adelaide, Adelaide, South Australia 5000, Australia

Lisa Kuhn
School of Nursing and Midwifery, Faculty of Health, Deakin University, Geelong, Victoria 3220, Australia

Rose Chapman
School of Physiotherapy and Exercise Science, Faculty of Health Sciences, Curtin University, Bentley, Western Australia 6102, Australia

Qian Li, Sonia Hernández-Díaz and Frank B Hu
Department of Epidemiology, Harvard School of Public Health, Boston, MA, USA

Qian Li
Epidemiology, Worldwide Safety & Regulatory, Pfizer Inc., New York, NY, USA

Zhenqiu Lin
Center for Outcomes Research and Evaluation, Yale University School of Medicine, New Haven, CT, USA

Frederick A Masoudi
Division of Cardiology, University of Colorado Anschutz Medical Campus, Aurora, CO, USA

Jing Li, Xi L, Qing Wang and Lixin Jiang
National Clinical Research Center of Cardiovascular Diseases, State Key Laboratory of Cardiovascular Disease, Fuwai Hospital, National Center for Cardiovascular Diseases, Chinese Academy of Medical Sciences and Peking Union Medical College, 167 Beilishi Road, Beijing 100037, China

Lingling Li
Department of Population Medicine, Harvard Medical School and Harvard Pilgrim Health Care Institute, Boston, MA, USA

John A Spertus
Saint Luke's Mid America Heart Institute, Kansas City, MO, USA

Frank B Hu
Channing Division of Network Medicine, Department of Medicine, Brigham and Women's Hospital and Harvard Medical School, Boston, MA, USA
Department of Nutrition, Harvard School of Public Health, Boston, MA, USA

Hao Liang
The Ultrasonic Diagnosis and Treatment Department, Shandong Provincial Hospital affiliated to Shandong University, Jinan, Shandong, China

Yi Chen Guo, Li Ming Chen, Min Li, Wei Zhong Han and Shi Liang Jiang
Department of Cardiology, Shandong Provincial Hospital affiliated to Shandong University, No.324, Jing Wu Wei Qi Road, Jinan 250021, Shandong, People's Republic of China

Xu Zhang
Department of Endocrinology, Shandong Provincial Hospital affiliated to Shandong University, Jinan, Shandong, China

Daisuke Kitano, Tadateru Takayama, Koichi Nagashima, Masafumi Akabane, Kimie Okubo, Takafumi Hiro and Atsushi Hirayama
Division of Cardiology, Department of Medicine, Nihon University School of Medicine, 30-1 Oyaguchi-kamicho, Itabashi-ku, Tokyo 173-8610, Japan

Constantinos Ergatoudes, Erik Thunström, Annika Rosengren, Lena Björck and Michael Fu
Department of Molecular and Clinical Medicine, Institute of Medicine, Skövde, Sweden

Lena Björck and Kristin Falk
Institute of Health and Care Sciences, Sahlgrenska Academy, University of Gothenburg, Skövde, Sweden

Kristina Bengtsson Boström
R & D Centre Skaraborg Primary Care, Skövde, Sweden

Michael Fu
Department of Medicine, Section of Cardiology, Sahlgrenska University Hospital/Östra, 41651 Göteborg, Sweden

Hong Du
Cardiology Ward, the Yantai Yuhuangding Hospital, No. 20, Yuhuangding Eastern Road, Yantai 264000Shandong Province, China

Chang-yan Dong
Chinese and Western Medicine Ward, the Yantai Yuhuangding Hospital, No. 20, Yuhuangding Eastern Road, Yantai 264000, Shandong Province, China

Qiao-yan Lin
Cardiology in Intensive Care Unit, the Yantai Yuhuangding Hospital, No. 20, Yuhuangding Road, Yantai 264000Shandong Province, China

Ulrika S Pahlm, Einar Heiberg, Henrik Engblom and Håkan Arheden
Department of Clinical Physiology, Clinical Sciences, Lund University Hospital, SE-22185 Lund, Sweden

Joey F A Ubachs
Department of Cardiology, Catharina Hospital Eindhoven, Eindhoven, The Netherlands

Einar Heiberg
Centre for Mathematical Sciences, Lund University, Lund, Sweden
Department of Biomedical Engineering, Faculty of Engineering, Lund University, Lund, Sweden

David Erlinge and Matthias Götberg
Department of Cardiology, Clinical Sciences, Lund University, Lund, Sweden

Yan Dai, Jingang Yang, Zhan Gao, Haiyan Xu, Yi Sun, Yuan Wu, Xiaojin Gao, Wei Li, Yang Wang, Runlin Gao and Yuejin Yang
Department of Cardiology, Fuwai Hospital, National Center for Cardiovascular Diseases, Chinese Academy of Medical Science and Peking Union Medical College, 167 Beilishi Road, Beijing 100037, People's Republic of China

Aet Saar, Toomas Marandi, Tiia Ainla, Mai Blöndal and Jaan Eha
Department of Cardiology, University of Tartu, Tartu, Estonia
Centre of Cardiology, North Estonia Medical Centre, Tallinn, Estonia

Krista Fischer
Estonian Genome Centre, University of Tartu, Tartu, Estonia

Jaan Eha
Heart Clinic, Tartu University Hospital, Tartu, Estonia

Louise Hougesen Bjerking, Jan Skov Jensen and Rikke Sørensen
Department of Cardiology, University Hospital Gentofte, Kildegårdsvej 28, 2900 Hellerup, Denmark

Kim Wadt Hansen
Department of Cardiology, University Hospital Bispebjerg, Copenhagen, Denmark

Mette Madsen
Department of Public Health, University of Copenhagen, Copenhagen, Denmark

Jan Skov Jensen
Department of Clinical Medicine, University of Copenhagen, Copenhagen, Denmark

Pål Hasvold
Astra Zeneca Nordic Baltic, Södertälje, Sweden

Jan Kyst Madsen
Emergency Department, Holbaek Hospital, University of Copenhagen, Holbaek, Denmark

Sigrun Halvorsen
Department of Cardiology, Oslo University Hospital Ulleval and University of Oslo, Postboks 4956, Nydalen 0424, Oslo, Norway

Jarle Jortveit
Department of Cardiology, Sørlandet Hospital, Arendal, Norway

Marcus Thuresson
Statisticon, Uppsala, Sweden

Erik Øie
Department of Internal Medicine, Diakonhjemmet Hospital and Center for Heart Failure Research, University of Oslo, Oslo, Norway

Rui Zhang, Chao Lan, Hui Pei, Guoyu Duan, Li Huang and Li Li
Department of emergency, The First Affiliated Hospital of Zhengzhou University, No.1 Jianshe Road, Zhengzhou, Henan 450052, China

Wanwarang Wongcharoen, Satjatham Sutthiwutthichai, Siriluck Gunaparn and Arintaya Phrommintikul
Department of Internal Medicine, Faculty of Medicine, Chiang Mai University, Chiang Mai, Thailand

Daoyuan Si , Guohui Liu, Yaliang Tong, Cheng Zhang and Yuquan He
Department of Cardiology, China-Japan Union Hospital of Jilin University, Jilin Provincial Engineering Laboratory for Endothelial Function and Genetic Diagnosis of Cardiovascular Disease, Jilin Provincial Cardiovascular Research Institute, Xiantai Street NO.126, Changchun, Jilin, China

Saga Johansson
AstraZeneca Gothenburg, Pepparedsleden 1, S-431 83 Mölndal, Sweden

Annika Rosengren
Department of Molecular and Clinical Medicine, Sahlgrenska Academy, University of Gothenburg, Gothenburg, Sweden

Annika Rosengren
Sahlgrenska University Hospital, Gothenburg, Sweden

Kate Young
Research Evaluation Unit, Oxford PharmaGenesis, 503 Washington Ave, Newtown, PA 18940, USA

Em Jennings
AstraZeneca R&D, 132 Hills Rd, Cambridge CB2 1PG, UK

Miriam Giovanna Colombo, Inge Kirchberger, Ute Amann, Margit Heier and Christa Meisinger
MONICA/KORA Myocardial Infarction Registry, Central Hospital of Augsburg, Augsburg, Germany

Miriam Giovanna Colombo, Inge Kirchberger, Ute Amann, Margit Heier, Annette Peters and Christa Meisinger
Institute of Epidemiology II, Helmholtz Zentrum München, German Research Center for Environmental Health (GmbH), Neuherberg, Germany

Christian Thilo and Bernhard Kuch
Department of Internal Medicine I – Cardiology, Central Hospital of Augsburg, Augsburg, Germany

Bernhard Kuch
Department of Internal Medicine/Cardiology, Hospital of Nördlingen, Nördlingen, Germany

Roland von Känel and Mary Princip
Department of Consultation-Liaison Psychiatry and Psychosomatic Medicine, University Hospital Zurich, Culmannstrasse 8, CH-8091 Zurich, Switzerland

Jean-Paul Schmid
Department of Cardiology, Clinic Barmelweid, Barmelweid, Switzerland

Jürgen Barth
Complementary and Integrative Medicine, University of Zurich, Zurich, Switzerland

Hansjörg Znoj
Department of Clinical Psychology and Psychotherapy, University of Bern, Bern, Switzerland

Ulrich Schnyder
Medical Faculty, University of Zurich, Zurich, Switzerland

Rebecca E. Meister-Langraf
Department of Psychiatry, Clienia Schlössli AG, Oetwil am See, Switzerland

Birgit Steppich, Philip Groha, Martin Hadamitzky, Adnan Kastrati and Ilka Ott
Deutsches Herzzentrum der Technischen Universität München, Lazarettstr. 36, 80636 Munich, Germany

Tareq Ibrahim, Heribert Schunkert and Karl-Ludwig Laugwitz
Medizinische Klinik Klinikum rechts der Isar der Technischen Universität München, Ismaningerstr. 22, 81675 Munich, Germany

Yan Gao, Jiang-tao Li, Yu-lang Huang and He-xun Huang
Department of Cardiovascular Medicine, Shenzhen Shekou People's Hospital, Shenzhen 518067, Guangdong, China

Nanette H. Bishopric
Departments of Medicine, Molecular and Cellular Pharmacology and Pediatrics, University of Miami Miller School of Medicine, Miami, FL, USA

Hong-wei Chen
Department of Interventional Diagnosis and Treatment, Shenzhen Longhua Central Hospital, Shenzhen 518067, Guangdong, China

Miriam Giovanna Colombo, Inge Kirchberger, Ute Amann, Margit Heier and Christa Meisinger
MONICA/KORA Myocardial Infarction Registry, Central Hospital of Augsburg, Augsburg, Germany

Miriam Giovanna Colombo, Inge Kirchberger, Ute Amann and Margit Heier
Institute of Epidemiology, Helmholtz Zentrum München, German Research Center for Environmental Health (GmbH), Neuherberg, Germany

Inge Kirchberger, Ute Amann and Christa Meisinger
Chair of Epidemiology, Ludwig-Maximilians-Universität München, UNIKA-T, Augsburg, Germany

Christian Thilo and Bernhard Kuch
Department of Internal Medicine I – Cardiology, Central Hospital of Augsburg, Augsburg, Germany

Bernhard Kuch
Department of Internal Medicine/Cardiology, Hospital of Nördlingen, Nördlingen, Germany

Franziska Nairz, Christa Meisinger, Inge Kirchberger, Margit Heier and Ute Amann
Central Hospital of Augsburg, MONICA/KORA Myocardial Infarction Registry, Augsburg, Germany

Franziska Nairz, Christa Meisinger, Inge Kirchberger, Margit Heier, Annette Peters and Ute Amann
Helmholtz Zentrum München, German Research Center for Environmental Health (GmbH), Institute of Epidemiology II, Neuherberg, Germany

Franziska Nairz
Institute for Medical Informatics, Biometry and Epidemiology (IBE), LMU Munich, Munich, Germany

Christa Meisinger, Inge Kirchberger and Ute Amann
Ludwig-Maximilians-Universität München, UNIKA-T, Augsburg, Germany

Christian Thilo and Bernhard Kuch
Central Hospital of Augsburg, Department of Internal Medicine I – Cardiology, Augsburg, Germany

Bernhard Kuch
Hospital of Nördlingen, Department of Internal Medicine/Cardiology, Nördlingen, Germany

Ute Amann
KORA-Herzinfarktregister im Klinikum Augsburg/ Helmholtz Zentrum München, Stenglinstr. 2, 86156 Augsburg, Germany

Kristin Marie Kvakkestad, Jan Eritsland and Sigrun Halvorsen
Department of Cardiology, Oslo University Hospital Ulleval, Postboks 4950 Nydalen, 0424 Oslo, Norway

Kristin Marie Kvakkestad and and Sigrun Halvorsen
University of Oslo, Postboks 1072 Blindern, 0316 Oslo, Norway

Morten Wang Fagerland
Oslo Centre for Biostatistics and Epidemiology, Research Support Services, Postboks 1110 Blindern, 0317 Oslo, Norway

Index

www.ingramcontent.com/pod-product-compliance
Lightning Source LLC
Chambersburg PA
CBHW082040190326
41458CB00010B/3415

Nuclear Power: An Introduction

Edited by
Trenton Hensley

Larsen & Keller
www.larsen-keller.com

Nuclear Power: An Introduction
Edited by Trenton Hensley
ISBN: 978-1-63549-198-2 (Hardback)

目 Larsen & Keller

Published by Larsen and Keller Education,
5 Penn Plaza,
19th Floor,
New York, NY 10001, USA

Cataloging-in-Publication Data

Nuclear power : an introduction / edited by Trenton Hensley.
    p. cm.
Includes bibliographical references and index.
ISBN 978-1-63549-198-2
1. Nuclear energy. 2. Nuclear power plants. 3. Nuclear
engineering. I. Hensley, Trenton.
TK9145 .N83 2017
621.48--dc23

The publisher's policy is to use permanent paper from mills that operate a sustainable forestry policy. Furthermore, the publisher ensures that the text paper and cover boards used have met acceptable environmental accreditation standards.

Printed and bound in the United States of America.

For more information regarding Larsen and Keller Education and its products, please visit the publisher's website www.larsen-keller.com